What Other Women Are Saying About
Your Pregnancy Week by Week

"Most books only give you a month by month breakdown of what's going on with baby and mum. I like how this one gives you week by week information. I look forward to reading it each week." —RACHEL M.

"*Your Pregnancy Week by Week* has been a good friend. Reading each week and knowing what changes my baby was going through was important to me." —ANITA A.

"I have other pregnancy books but when I started reading *Your Pregnancy Week by Week*, I put the others down. This book is excellent. I highly recommend it to all new mothers." —CRYSTAL L.

"The week by week style is wonderful. It lets you know what to expect as it happens." —HEATHER H.

"I liked how it went week by week because that is how my doctor thinks, too." —REBECCA C.

"The detailed week by week information about my and my baby's changing body was excellent. It gave me something to read weekly, not just monthly." —DEANA S.

"*Your Pregnancy Week by Week* was my second Bible. I used it so much I have almost memorized it! I recommend it to everyone!" —CHRISSY M.

"*Your Pregnancy Week by Week* was very comforting, it put my mind at ease." —JENNIFER W.

"This book is full of helpful ideas that both new and experienced mothers-to-be can put to immediate use." —ZENAIDA M.

"This book is the 'A, B, C book to pregnancy'" —DORIS H.

"Reading this book is like talking to your mum about how it was being pregnant." —AMANDA S.

"All the information on a weekly basis is wonderful. I highly recommend this book to every woman expecting." —THERESA C.

"This book should be read by every mother-to-be. It gives you information week by week instead of month by month and it helped me so much." —KRISTI C.

About the Authors

Glade B. Curtis, MD, MPH, FACOG, is board-certified by the American Board of Obstetrics and Gynecology and a Fellow of the American College of Obstetricians and Gynecologists. He is in practice in Salt Lake City, Utah, is a Medical Consultant to the State of Utah Department of Health and a Medical Director of The Health Clinics of Utah.

Dr Curtis is a graduate of the University of Utah with a Bachelor of Science and a Master's Degree in Public Health (MPH). He attended the University of Rochester School of Medicine and Dentistry in New York. He interned and was a resident and chief resident in Obstetrics and Gynecology at the University of Rochester Strong Memorial Hospital, Rochester, New York.

Judith Schuler, MS, has worked with Dr Curtis for more than 22 years, as his co-author and editor. They have collaborated together on 12 books dealing with pregnancy, women's health and children's health. Ms Schuler earned a Master of Science degree in Family Studies from the University of Arizona in Tucson.

Before becoming an editor for HPBooks, where she and Dr Curtis first began working together, Ms Schuler taught at the university level in California and Arizona. She has one grown son. She divides her time between Tucson, Arizona and Laramie, Wyoming.

Consultant Editor **Dr Julian N. Robinson,** FRCOG, studied at Guys Hospital Medical School at the University Hospital in London. He has also been a research fellow in the Nuffield Department of Obstetrics and Gynaecology, Oxford University, and a Senior House Officer and Registrar in Obstetrics at both Churchill and John Radcliffe Hospitals in Oxford.

your
pregnancy™
week by week

For their assistance in preparing this British edition of *Your Pregnancy Week by Week*, special acknowledgement is owed to Judith Hannam, Sue Miller and Lily O'Connor, RGN, RM, Dip. Res. Meth., BSc (hons), a midwife at the Women's Centre, John Radcliffe Hospital, Oxford.

5TH EDITION

your
pregnancy™
week by week

Dr Glade B. Curtis, OB/GYN

Judith Schuler, MS

**Dr Julian N. Robinson, FRCOG,
Consultant Editor**

Da Capo
LIFE
LONG

A Member of the Perseus Books Group

Copyright © 2004 by Glade B. Curtis and Judith Schuler

Your Pregnancy is a trademark of Da Capo Press

Illustrations by David Fischer
Designed by Lisa Kreinbrink
Set in 11.5 point Minion by the Perseus Books Group

Cataloging-in-Publication data for this book is available from the British Library.

Originally published in the United States by Da Capo Press in 2004.
ISBN 0-7382-0976-7

Published by Da Capo Press
A Member of the Perseus Books Group
http://www.dacapopress.com

1 2 3 4 5 6 7 8 9—08 07 06 05 04

Introduction

There is an amazing array of medical information available to expectant parents these days: books, magazines, journals and online sites abound. Of course, the readability and reliability of what's out there varies greatly. Indeed, it's rare to find clinically-current information presented in prose that is digestible. *Your Pregnancy Week by Week* is such a rarity. It is an excellent single source for a comprehensive education regarding pregnancy. Importantly, it is completely up-to-date, including the latest information in rapidly evolving fields such as prenatal diagnosis and fetal surveillance. It is also refreshingly accessible and reader-friendly. The chronological style of the book lends itself both to be read through as a preparatory text or to be dipped into as a reference book for knowledge particular to a specific stage of pregnancy. For each week of pregnancy the development of the baby, maternal nutritional requirements, and the effect of maternal behavior on the baby are explained with depth and clarity.

This book was written originally for an American audience, and it has become one of the most popular guides to pregnancy in the United States. As an obstetrician who has practiced on both sides of the Atlantic, I am glad that this valuable resource is now becoming available in the United Kingdom. The information included is pertinent to all pregnant women, and I wholeheartedly recommend it to anyone searching for a relevant, clear, and modern guide to pregnancy.

—*Dr Julian N. Robinson,*
Consultant Editor

Contents

Preparing for Pregnancy *1*

Weeks 1 & 2—*Pregnancy Begins* *28*

Pregnancy Weight Gain Chart *42*

Week 3 . . . . *43*

Week 4 . . . . *54*

Week 5 . . . . *64*

Week 6 . . . . *76*

Week 7 . . . . *88*

Week 8 . . . . *98*

Week 9 . . . . *107*

Week 10 . . . . *114*

Week 11 . . . . *124*

Week 12 . . . . *133*

Week 13 . . . . *142*

Week 14 . . . . *153*

Week 15 . . . . *161*

Week 16 . . . . *168*

Week 17 . . . . *178*

Week 18 . . . . *184*

Week 19 . . . . *194*

Week 20 . . . . *204*

Week 21 . . . . *212*

Week 22 . . . . *221*

Week 23 . . . . *233*

Week 24 . . . . *242*

Week 25 . . . . *251*

Week 26 . . . . *260*

Week 27 . . . . *269*

Week 28 . . . . *281*

Week 29 . . . . *290*

Week 30 . . . . *300*

Week 31 . . . . *310*

Week 32 . . . . *322*

Week 33 . . . . *332*

Week 34 . . . . *340*

Week 35 . . . . *347*

Week 36 . . . . *354*

Week 37 . . . . *363*

Week 38 . . . . *375*

Week 39 . . . . *386*

Week 40 . . . . *402*

Week 41—*When You're Overdue* *418*

What Happens after Your Pregnancy? *424*

Resources *430*

Glossary *439*

Index *455*

Preparing for Pregnancy

Nothing compares with the miracle and magic of pregnancy. It's your chance to be involved in life's creative process. Planning ahead for this experience can improve your chances of doing well yourself and of having a healthy baby.

Your lifestyle affects your baby's health. By planning ahead, you can ensure you and your baby are exposed to good things and avoid harmful things during your pregnancy.

By the time most women realize they are pregnant, they are 1 to 2 months into their pregnancy. By the time they see their doctor/midwife, they are 2 or 3 months along. The first 12 weeks of pregnancy are extremely important because this is when the baby forms its major organ systems. Many important things can happen before you realize you are pregnant or before you see your doctor. Getting in shape for pregnancy means physical and mental preparation.

Pregnancy is a condition, not an illness; a pregnant woman is not sick. However, you will experience major changes during the course of your pregnancy. Having good general health before pregnancy can help you deal with the physical and emotional stresses of pregnancy, labour and delivery. It can help you prepare to take care of a newborn baby.

Your General Health

In recent years, an explosion of technology has resulted in new medications, medical advances and new medical treatments. Through these advances, we have learned that your health at the beginning of pregnancy and during pregnancy can have a major effect on you and your developing baby.

In the past, the emphasis was on being healthy during pregnancy. Today, most doctors suggest looking at pregnancy as lasting 12 months instead of just 9 months. This includes at least a 3-month period of preparation. Preparing your body with good general health can help you prepare for a healthy pregnancy and a healthy baby.

Preparing for Pregnancy

The following are important actions to take before you get pregnant. If you have any questions or concerns, discuss them with your doctor.

- Achieve your ideal weight at least 3 months before you conceive. Your baby's health is tied to *your* body weight when you get pregnant. Overweight pregnant women run the risk of high blood pressure and gestational diabetes; they also have a higher rate of Caesarean delivery. Underweight women may have a harder time conceiving; babies born to underweight women are more often premature and have a lower birthweight.
- Start a regular exercise programme, and stick with it. Exercising moderately before you get pregnant and continuing throughout your pregnancy can help you a great deal.
- Discuss any medications you take on a regular basis with your doctor.
- Be sure any chronic medical conditions you have are under control.

- Stop smoking. Avoid passive smoke.
- Stop drinking alcohol.
- Have your immunity to rubella and chicken pox checked. If you need vaccinations, find out how long you have to wait after you have them before you can start trying to get pregnant.
- Schedule any necessary medical tests, such as X-rays, before you stop your contraception method.
- Keep a record of your fertility cycle by using charts. Or check your fertility cycle with an ovulation-predictor kit.
- Be careful about taking dietary supplements and botanicals. Some herbs, such as St John's wort, saw palmetto and echinacea, may interfere with conception.
- Start taking folic acid—400mcg/day is recommended. Folic acid can help prevent birth defects of the brain and spinal cord, called *neural-tube defects*. It has also been shown that low levels may increase your risk of miscarriage. You need to start taking folic acid *before* you get pregnant because folic acid protects you the most during the first 28 days of pregnancy. Because you may not know when you get pregnant, begin taking it when you stop contraception and while you're trying to conceive.
- Ask your doctor to check your iron levels. You don't want to have an iron deficiency before pregnancy—this situation could make you feel even more fatigued than is normal during pregnancy.
- Check your cholesterol level; decrease high cholesterol levels with a high-fibre nutrition plan that is also low in saturated fat. High cholesterol levels may contribute to high blood pressure during pregnancy.
- Stay healthy; try to avoid infections. Wash hands frequently, have someone else change the cat litter, eat foods that are well prepared and avoid situations where you might be exposed to infection.
- Avoid hazardous chemicals at work and at home.
- Try to lessen any unnecessary stress in your life.

- Have a dental checkup; periodontal disease should be under control. Periodontal disease during pregnancy increases the risk of having a low-birthweight baby.
- Find out your HIV status.
- Know your blood type and the blood type of your baby's father.
- Together with your partner, write down your family medical histories.
- Consider how pregnancy fits into your future plans (education, career, travel).
- If appropriate, check your health insurance to see what maternity coverage it provides.

Some of the above actions may be harder to begin *during* a pregnancy. Deal with these issues before pregnancy, know you are healthy and you won't have to worry about the risks they may pose while you're pregnant. It makes sense to continue birth control until you've achieved the above.

Seeking Medical Advice

Seeing a doctor before you get pregnant is good preparation for pregnancy. Arrange for a checkup and to discuss your pregnancy plans. Then you'll know that when you do get pregnant, you are in the best possible health.

You may have a medical condition that requires attention before pregnancy. If you don't take care of it before trying to conceive, it may affect your ability to get pregnant. You may need to change medications you are taking, or you may need to make lifestyle changes.

ᔓ *Tests for You*
A general physical examination before you get pregnant helps ensure you won't have to deal with new medical problems during pregnancy. A cervical smear and a breast exam should be included in this physical. Lab tests to consider before pregnancy include tests for rubella,

blood type and Rh-factor. If you are 35 or older, a mammogram is also a good idea.

If you have been exposed to HIV or hepatitis, ask your doctor to conduct tests for these. If you have a family history of other medical problems, such as diabetes, ask whether you should have any tests to rule them out. If you have other chronic medical problems, such as anaemia or recurrent miscarriages, your doctor may suggest other specific tests.

✧ *X-rays and Other Imaging Tests*

If you are trying to conceive, ask for a pregnancy test before having any diagnostic test involving radiation, including dental work. Tests that involve radiation include *X-rays, CT scans* and *MRIs*. Use reliable contraception before these tests to make sure you are not pregnant. If you schedule these tests right after the end of your period, you can be sure you are not pregnant. If you must receive a series of these tests, continue to use contraception.

✧ *Possible Pre-pregnancy Tests*

Your doctor may conduct many tests before you become pregnant, depending on your current medical problems and your family history. Some tests you may have include:

- a physical exam
- a cervical smear
- breast exam (and mammogram if you are at least 35)
- rubella titers
- blood type and Rh-factor
- HIV (if you have been exposed to risk factors)
- hepatitis (if you have been exposed to risk factors)
- cystic fibrosis screening

Another test that is done before you become pregnant is *pre-implantation genetic diagnosis (PGD)*; it is often done if you have in vitro fertilization. With in vitro fertilization, an embryo is created outside the womb (in vitro) by mixing an egg and sperm, then it is implanted in the woman.

With PGD, a few cells are removed for genetic testing *before* the embryo is implanted to identify genes that may be responsible for some severe hereditary diseases. The goal is to select healthy embryos for implantation to avoid serious genetic disease. The technique has been used to diagnose cystic fibrosis, Down's syndrome, Duchenne muscular dystrophy, haemophilia, Tay–Sachs disease and Turner syndrome. A normal (unaffected) embryo is implanted in the uterus and allowed to develop to term (birth).

Medical History

A pre-pregnancy visit with your doctor is the best time to discuss your medical history and any problems you may have had in previous pregnancies. Ask what you can do to eliminate or to decrease chances of the same problems recurring in your next pregnancy. Past problems include ectopic pregnancy, miscarriage, previous C-sections (Caesarean deliveries) or other pregnancy complications.

This is also a good time to talk about exposure to, and problems with, sexually transmitted diseases or other infections. If you have had major surgery or any female surgery in the past, discuss it now. If you are being treated for other medical problems, discuss them with your doctor. Make plans to take medications that are safe to use during a pregnancy *before* you try to get pregnant.

Discontinuing Contraception

It's important to continue using some form of contraception until you are ready to get pregnant. If you are in the middle of treatment for a medical problem or if you are undergoing tests, finish the course of treatment or tests before trying to conceive. (If you're not using some form of birth control, you're basically trying to get pregnant.) After discontinuing your regular contraceptive, use some other birth-control method until your periods become normal. You can choose from condoms, spermicides, the sponge or a diaphragm.

✧ Birth-Control Pills or Patches

Most doctors recommend you have two or three normal periods after you stop using birth-control pills or the patch before you get pregnant. If you get pregnant immediately after stopping these contraceptives, it may be difficult to determine when you conceived. This can make it harder to determine your due date. This may not seem important now, but it will be very important to you during pregnancy and at the end of your pregnancy.

✒ *IUDs*

If you have an IUD (intrauterine device), you must have it removed before you try to conceive. However, pregnancy can occur while an IUD is in place. If you have any sign of infection with an IUD, take care of it before trying to get pregnant. The best time to remove an IUD is during a menstrual period.

✒ *Norplant*

If you use Norplant, you should have at least two or three normal menstrual cycles after it is removed before trying to get pregnant. It may take a few months for your periods to return to normal after Norplant is removed. If you get pregnant immediately after removing Norplant, it may be difficult to determine when you got pregnant and what your due date is.

✒ *Depo Provera*

Depo provera, a hormone injection used for birth control, should be discontinued for at least 3 to 6 months before trying to conceive. Wait until you have had at least two or three normal periods.

Current Medical Problems

Before you become pregnant, examine your lifestyle, diet, physical activity and any chronic medical problems you have, such as high blood pressure or diabetes. You may require extra care before and during pregnancy. Tell your doctor about any medications you currently take. Discuss any tests you may be planning to have, such as X-rays, and cover all medical problems you are being treated for. It's easier to answer questions about these problems, their treatment and their complications before you get pregnant rather than after you are pregnant.

✒ *Anaemia*

Anaemia means you do not have enough haemoglobin to carry oxygen to your body's cells. Symptoms include weakness, fatigue, shortness of breath and pale skin. *It is possible to develop anaemia during pregnancy, even if you are not anaemic before you get pregnant.* While you are pregnant, the baby makes great demands on your body for iron and iron stores. If you have low iron levels at the beginning of pregnancy, pregnancy can tip the balance and make you anaemic. Ask for a FBC (full blood count) as a part of your pre-pregnancy physical.

If you have a family history of anaemia (such as sickle-cell anaemia or thalassaemia), discuss these with your doctor *before* you get pregnant. (See Week 22 for more information on different types of anaemia.) If you take hydroxyurea to treat your sickle-cell disease, discuss whether you should continue using it while trying to conceive. We do not know whether this medication is safe during pregnancy.

ᠵ *Asthma*

Asthma affects about 1 per cent of all pregnant women. Half of those women with asthma see no change in their condition during pregnancy. For about 25 per cent, asthma improves, and for the other 25 per cent, the condition worsens.

Most asthma medications are safe to take during pregnancy, but talk to your doctor about taking any medication. Most people with asthma know what triggers attacks. While you're trying to get pregnant and during pregnancy, be especially careful to avoid things that trigger attacks. Try to get asthma under good control before trying to become pregnant. (Read more about how asthma affects pregnancy in Week 28.)

ᠵ *Bladder or Kidney Problems*

Bladder infections, commonly called *urinary-tract infections* or *UTIs*, may occur more often during pregnancy. If a urinary-tract infection is not treated, it can cause an infection of the kidneys, called *pyelonephritis*.

Urinary-tract infections and pyelonephritis are associated with premature delivery. If you have a history of pyelonephritis or repeated urinary-tract infections, you should be evaluated before you begin pregnancy.

Kidney stones may also create problems during pregnancy. Because they cause pain, it may be difficult to differentiate between kidney stones and other problems that can occur during pregnancy. Kidney stones can also cause an increased chance of urinary-tract infections and pyelonephritis.

If you have had kidney or bladder surgery, any major kidney problems or if you know your kidney function is less than normal, tell your doctor. It may be necessary to evaluate your kidney function with tests before you become pregnant.

If you have had an occasional bladder infection, don't be alarmed. Your doctor will decide whether further testing is necessary before you become pregnant. (See Week 18 for more information.)

ᴞ *Cancer*

If you have had any type of cancer in the past, tell your doctor when planning your pregnancy or as soon as you discover you are pregnant. He or she may need to make decisions about individualized care for you during this pregnancy. (See Week 30 for more information about cancer and pregnancy.)

ᴞ *Diabetes*

Diabetes is a medical problem that can have serious effects during pregnancy. Historically, women with diabetes have had problems with pregnancy, but with good control, a diabetic woman today is usually able to have a healthy pregnancy. If diabetes is *not* under control when you get pregnant, your risk of having a child with a birth defect increases 5 *times!*

If you have diabetes, it may be harder for you to become pregnant. It can also increase the chance of miscarriage, stillbirth and birth defects. These risks can be decreased by good control of blood sugar during pregnancy.

If your diabetes is not controlled, the combination of pregnancy and diabetes can be dangerous for you and your baby. Many of the problems and damage caused by diabetes occur during the first trimester (the first 13 weeks of pregnancy); poor control, however, can affect the entire pregnancy.

Pregnancy may affect diabetes by increasing your body's need for insulin. Insulin makes it possible for the body to use sugar. Most doctors recommend you have diabetes under control for at least 2 to 3 months before pregnancy begins. Controlling your diabetes may require checking your blood sugar several times a day.

If you have a family history of diabetes or suspect you might have diabetes, have it checked before getting pregnant. This will help you lower the risk of miscarriage and other problems. If you haven't had diabetes before and develop it during pregnancy, it is called *gestational diabetes*. (See Week 23.)

ᨠ *Epilepsy and Seizures*

Epilepsy includes several different problems; however, seizures are the most severe. There are two kinds of epileptic seizures—*grand mal* and *petit mal*. A mother-to-be with epilepsy has a 1 in 30 chance of having a baby with a seizure disorder. Babies also have a higher chance of birth defects, perhaps related to medications taken to control epilepsy during pregnancy.

If you take medication for epilepsy, it is important to consult your doctor before you become pregnant. Discuss the amounts and the types of medication you take. Some medications are safe during pregnancy. Most doctors will have you switch to phenobarbitone during the time you are trying to conceive and while you are pregnant.

Seizures can be dangerous to the mother and foetus. It is important for you to take your medication regularly and as prescribed by your doctor. Do not decrease or discontinue any medication on your own!

ᨠ *Heart Disease*

During pregnancy, the workload on your heart increases by about 50 per cent. If you have any kind of heart condition, tell your doctor about it before you get pregnant. Some heart problems, such as *mitral-valve prolapse*, may be serious during pregnancy and may require antibiotics at the time of delivery. Other heart problems, such as congenital heart problems, may seriously affect your health. Your doctor may advise against pregnancy in these cases. Consult your doctor about any heart condition so it can be dealt with before you become pregnant.

✣ *Hypertension*

Hypertension, or high blood pressure, can cause problems for a pregnant woman and her unborn baby. For the woman, these problems may include headaches, kidney damage or stroke. For a developing baby, high blood pressure in a mother-to-be can cause decreased blood flow to the placenta, resulting in a smaller baby or intrauterine-growth restriction (IUGR).

If you have high blood pressure before pregnancy, you must closely monitor your blood pressure during pregnancy. Your doctor may refer you to a specialist who will help you control your blood pressure.

Some high-blood-pressure medications are safe to take during pregnancy; others are not. *Do not stop or decrease any medication on your own!* This can be dangerous. If you're planning a pregnancy, ask your doctor about the medication you take for high blood pressure and its safety during conception and pregnancy.

✣ *Lupus*

Systemic lupus erythematosus (SLE) is an autoimmune disease. This means you produce antibodies to your own organs, which may destroy or damage those organs and their function. Lupus can affect many parts of the body, including joints, kidneys, lungs and the heart.

This problem can be difficult to diagnose. Lupus occurs in about 1 in 700 women between 15 and 64 years of age. In black women, it occurs once in 254 women. Lupus is found more often in women than in men, especially between the ages of 20 and 40.

There is no cure for lupus at present. Treatment is individual and usually involves taking steroids. It is best not to become pregnant while you are experiencing a flare-up. There is an increased risk of miscarriage and stillbirths in women with lupus, which requires extra care during pregnancy.

Babies born to women with lupus may have a rash, heart block and heart defects. These babies may be born prematurely or experience intrauterine-growth restriction. Talk to your doctor before you become pregnant if you have lupus. (See Week 27 for more information on lupus in pregnancy.)

✋ *Migraine Headaches*

About 15 to 20 per cent of all pregnant women suffer from migraine headaches. Many women notice an improvement in their headaches while they are pregnant. If you must take medication for headaches during pregnancy, check with your doctor ahead of time so you'll know whether the one you take is safe to use.

✋ *Thyroid Problems*

Thyroid problems can appear as either too much or too little thyroid hormone. Too much thyroid hormone, *hyperthyroidism*, results in a faster metabolism; it is usually caused by Graves' disease. The problem is often treated by surgery or medication to reduce the amount of thyroid hormone in your system. If left untreated during pregnancy, there is a higher risk of premature delivery and low birthweight. If treatment is necessary during pregnancy, there are safe medications you can take.

Too little thyroid hormone, *hypothyroidism*, is usually caused by autoimmune problems; the thyroid gland is damaged by your own antibodies. Doctors treat this problem with thyroid hormones. If left untreated, you may suffer from infertility or have a miscarriage.

If you have either thyroid problem, you should be tested before pregnancy to determine the correct amount of medication for you. Pregnancy can change medication requirements, so you will also need to be checked during pregnancy.

↜ *Other Medical Problems*

Many other specific chronic illnesses can affect a pregnancy. If you have any chronic problem or take any medication on a regular basis, talk it over with your doctor.

Current Medications

It's important for you and your doctor to consider the possibility of pregnancy each time you are given a prescription or advised to take a medication. When you are pregnant, everything changes with regard to medications.

Medications that are safe when you are not pregnant may have harmful effects when you are pregnant. Whether a medication is safe during pregnancy is not always known. Ask your doctor before changing any medication. (Some effects of medications and chemicals are discussed in Week 4.)

Most organ development in the baby occurs in the

Be Careful with Medications

During pregnancy, play it safe. Some general guidelines for medication use while you are trying to get pregnant include the following.

- Do not stop birth control unless you want to be pregnant.
- Take prescriptions exactly as they are prescribed.
- Tell your doctor if you think you might be pregnant or if you are not using birth control when a medication is prescribed.
- Do not self-treat or use medications you were given in the past for other problems.
- Never use someone else's medications.
- If you are unsure about a medication, consult your doctor *before* you use it.

first 13 weeks of pregnancy. This is an important time to avoid exposing your baby to unnecessary medications. You'll feel better and do better during pregnancy if you have medication use under control before you try to get pregnant.

Some medications are intended for short-term use, such as antibiotics for infections. Others are for chronic or long-lasting problems, such as high blood pressure or diabetes. Some medications are OK to take while you are pregnant and might even help make your pregnancy successful. Other medications may not be safe to take during pregnancy.

Vaccinations

The same rule applies to vaccinations as to X-ray tests—when you have a vaccination, use reliable contraception. Some vaccines are safe during pregnancy; some are not. A good rule of thumb is to complete vaccinations at least 3 months before trying to get pregnant.

Vaccinations are usually most harmful to a pregnancy in the first trimester. If you need a vaccination for rubella or MMR (measles, mumps, rubella) or chicken pox before you get pregnant, it is now recommended you wait at least 4 weeks after receiving it before you try to conceive.

An exception to this rule is the flu vaccine. The flu vaccine *may* be taken by a pregnant woman who will be past the 3rd month of pregnancy during the flu season. If you are advised to take the flu vaccine because of your job or for some other reason, go ahead. It's considered safe during pregnancy and while you are trying to conceive.

Fertility Monitors May Help in Achieving Pregnancy

Today we are fortunate to have many valuable tests available to predict when ovulation occurs to help a woman conceive. These tests can be done at home, and most are easy to use.

The *PERSONA*® fertility monitor helps you track where you are in your cycle by testing the hormone levels in your urine. The starter pack costs about £65.

Another ovulation test is the *First Response Fertility Monitor* which determines where you are in your cycle by monitoring your temperature. It costs about £100.

Genetic Counselling

If you're planning your first pregnancy, you are probably not considering genetic counselling. However, there may be circumstances in which genetic counselling could help you and your partner make informed decisions about childbearing. There are more than 13,000 inherited gene disorders that we know about. Each year in the UK, about 5,500 babies are born with some type of birth defect. Certain ethnic groups have a higher incidence of specific genetic defects. In addition, certain medications, chemicals and pesticides can put a couple at risk.

Genetic counselling is an information session between you and your partner and a genetic counsellor or group of counsellors. Any information you share with or receive from a genetic counsellor is confidential. It may involve one visit or several visits. If you require genetic counselling, your doctor can refer you.

Through genetic counselling, you and your partner hope to understand the possibilities or probabilities of what might affect your ability to get pregnant or your future offspring. The information you receive is not precise. Counsellors may speak in terms of 'chances' or 'odds' of a problem.

A genetic counsellor will not make a decision for you. He or she will provide information on tests you might take and what the results of those tests may indicate. When speaking with a genetic counsellor, don't hide information you feel is embarrassing or hard to talk about. It is important to give him or her as much information as possible.

Ask your doctor if you should seek genetic counselling. Most couples who need genetic counselling do not find out they needed it until after they have a child born with a birth defect. You might consider genetic counselling if any of the following apply to you.

- You will be at least 35 years old at the time of delivery.
- You have delivered a child with a birth defect.
- You or your partner has a birth defect.

- You or your partner has a family history of Down's syndrome, mental retardation, cystic fibrosis, spina bifida, muscular dystrophy, bleeding disorders, skeletal or bone problems, dwarfism, epilepsy, congenital heart defects or blindness.
- You or your partner has a family history of inherited deafness (antenatal testing can identify congenital deafness caused by the Connexin–26 gene, allowing parents and medical personnel the opportunity to manage the problem immediately).
- You and your partner are related (consanguinity).
- You have had recurrent miscarriages (usually three or more).
- You *and* your partner are descended from Ashkenazi Jews (risk of Tay–Sachs disease or Canavan's disease).
- You or your partner are of African descent (risk of sickle-cell anaemia).
- Your partner is at least 40 years old. (Medical information shows a father in his forties may have an increased chance of fathering a child with a birth defect. See page 18 for more information.)

Some of the information you need may be difficult to gather, especially if you or your partner was adopted. You may know little or nothing of your family's medical history. Discuss this with your doctor before you become pregnant. If you learn about the chances of problems before getting pregnant, you won't be forced to make difficult choices after becoming pregnant. The primary goal in genetic counselling is the same as other goals in pregnancy—early diagnosis and prevention of problems.

Pregnancy after 35

More women are choosing to marry after they have established their career, and more couples are choosing to start their families at a later age. Today, doctors are seeing more older first-time mothers, and more of these mothers are having safe, healthy pregnancies than women their age did in the past.

We have found that an older woman considering pregnancy has two major concerns. She wants to know how the pregnancy will affect her and how her age will affect her pregnancy. There is a slight increase in the possibility of complications for the mother and baby when the mother is older. You may also want to read our book, *Your Pregnancy after 35*, which focuses primarily on pregnancy in older women.

A pregnant woman older than 35 may be more likely to face increased risks of the following:

• a baby born with Down's syndrome
• high blood pressure
• pelvic pressure or pelvic pain
• pre-eclampsia
• Caesarean delivery
• multiple births
• placental abruption
• bleeding and other complications
• premature labour

An older pregnant woman must also deal with problems a younger woman might not face. A broad simplification of this is that it is easier to be pregnant when you are 20 than it is when you are 40. Chances are, by age 40 you have a job or other children making demands on your time. You may find it harder to rest, exercise and eat right.

Maternal problems associated with increasing age include most of the chronic illnesses that tend to appear as age increases. High blood pressure is one of the more common pregnancy complications in women over 35 (see Week 31). There is also a higher incidence of pre-eclampsia (see Week 31). Older women who give birth have a slightly higher risk of abnormalities and problems, including premature labour, pelvic pressure and pelvic pain.

The chance of diabetes, as well as complications of diabetes, increases with age. Researchers cite figures showing that twice as many women over age 35 have complications with diabetes. In the past, hypertension (high blood pressure) and diabetes were major complications in any pregnancy. With today's advances, we can manage these complications of pregnancy quite well.

❧ *Down's Syndrome*

Through medical research, we know older women are at higher risk of giving birth to a child with Down's syndrome, although many of these pregnancies end in miscarriage or stillbirth. Various tests are offered to an older woman during pregnancy to determine whether a baby will have Down's syndrome. It is the most common chromosomal defect detected by amniocentesis. (See Week 16 for more information on amniocentesis.)

The risk of delivering a baby with Down's syndrome increases as you get older. Look at the following statistics:

- at age 25 the risk is 1 in 1300 births
- at 30 it is 1 in 965 births
- at 35 it is 1 in 365 births
- at 40 it is 1 in 109 births
- at 45 it is 1 in 32 births
- at 49 it is 1 in 12 births

But there is also a positive way to look at these statistics. If you're 45, you have a 97 per cent chance of *not* having a baby with Down's syndrome. If you're 49, you have a 92 per cent chance of delivering a child without Down's syndrome. If you are concerned about the risk of Down's syndrome because of your age or family history, discuss it with your doctor.

❧ *Father's Age*

Research shows a father's age may also be important to a pregnancy. Chromosomal abnormalities that cause birth defects occur more often in older women and in men over 40. Men over 55 have twice the normal risk of fathering a child with Down's syndrome. The chance of chromosomal problems increases with the increase in the age of the father. Some researchers recommend that men father their children before age 40. However, there is still some controversy about this.

ᔔ *Your General Health*

Important questions to consider before getting pregnant when you are older include those about your general health. Are you fit for pregnancy? If you are older, you can maximize your chances of having a successful pregnancy by being as healthy as possible *before* you become pregnant.

Most researchers recommend a baseline mammogram be done at age 35. Have this test before you become pregnant. Paying attention to general recommendations for your diet and your health care are also important in preparing for pregnancy.

Your Nutrition before Pregnancy

Most people feel better and work better when they eat a well-balanced diet. Planning and following a good diet before pregnancy ensures that your developing foetus receives good nutrition during the first few weeks or months of pregnancy.

Usually a woman takes good care of herself once she knows she is pregnant. By planning ahead, you will guarantee that your baby has a healthy environment for the entire 9 months of pregnancy, not for just the 6 or 7 months after you discover you truly are pregnant. When you make your nutrition plan, you are preparing the environment in which your baby will be conceived and will develop and grow.

ᔔ *Weight Management*

Before trying to get pregnant, pay attention to your weight; you don't want to be too overweight or too underweight. Either condition can make pregnancy more difficult for you.

Do *not* diet during pregnancy or while you are trying to conceive. Don't take diet pills, unless you're using reliable contraception. Consult your doctor if you are considering a special diet for weight reduction or weight gain before you try to get pregnant. Dieting may cause temporary deficiencies in vitamins and minerals that both you and your developing baby need.

✂ Be Careful with Vitamins, Minerals and Herbs

Don't self-medicate with large amounts or unusual combinations of vitamins, minerals or herbs. You *can* overdo it. Certain vitamins, such as vitamin A, can cause birth defects if used in excessive amounts.

As a general rule, stop all extra supplementation at least 3 months before pregnancy. Eat a well-balanced diet and take folic acid or one prenatal vitamin a day.

✂ Folic Acid

Folic acid is a B vitamin (B_9) that can contribute to a healthy pregnancy. If a mother-to-be takes 0.4 mg (400 micrograms) of folic acid each day, starting 3 or 4 months *before* pregnancy begins, it may protect her developing baby against various birth defects of the spine and brain, called *neural-tube defects*.

One of these defects, *spina bifida*, affects up to 1,200 pregnancies in the UK every year. It develops in the first few weeks of pregnancy. Studies have shown that about 75 per cent of all cases can be prevented if a mother-to-be takes folic acid. As you plan your pregnancy, ask your doctor about supplementation.

In 1998, the US government ordered that some grain products, such as flour, breakfast cereals and pasta, be fortified with folic acid. In the UK, the Committee on Medical Aspects of Food and Nutrition (COMA) recommended in January 2000 that folic acid be added to flour. As yet nothing more has happened. It is found in many other foods, too. A varied diet can help you reach your goal. Many common foods contain folic acid, including:

asparagus • avocados • bananas • black beans • broccoli • citrus fruits and juices • egg yolks • fortified breads and cereals • green beans • leafy green vegetables • lentils • liver • peas • plantains • spinach • strawberries • tuna • wheat germ • yoghurt

✍ Begin Good Eating Habits

Often, a woman carries her pre-pregnancy eating habits into her pregnancy. Many women eat on the run and pay little attention to what they eat most of the day. Before pregnancy, you may be able to get away with this. However, because of the increased demands on you and the requirements of your developing baby, this won't work when you do become pregnant.

The key to good nutrition is balance. Eat a balanced diet. Going to extremes with vitamins or fad diets can be harmful to you and your growing baby. It could even make you feel run-down during pregnancy.

✍ Specific Considerations

Specific factors to consider before getting pregnant include whether you follow a vegetarian diet, the amount of exercise you do, whether you skip meals, your diet plan (are you trying to lose or gain weight?) and any special dietary needs you might have.

If you eat a special diet because of medical problems, consult your doctor about it. Much information is available through your doctor or your local hospital about good diets and healthy nutrition.

Many diets go to extremes

> ### *Can You Help Avoid Morning Sickness in Pregnancy?*
>
> A recent study showed that women who ate high amounts of saturated fat—the kind found in cheese and red meat—in the year *before* they got pregnant had a higher risk of suffering severe morning sickness during pregnancy. If you're planning a pregnancy, you may want to cut down on these foods.

that you may be able to tolerate, but these extremes can be harmful to a developing baby. It is important to discuss dieting with your doctor ahead of time. You don't want to find out when you are 8 weeks pregnant that you are malnourished because of dieting.

Exercise before Pregnancy

Exercise is good for you—before you become pregnant and during pregnancy. Benefits may include weight control, a feeling of well-being and increased stamina or endurance, which will become important later in pregnancy.

Begin exercising regularly before you become pregnant. Making adjustments in your lifestyle to include regular exercise will benefit you now and make it easier to stay in shape throughout pregnancy.

Exercise can be carried to extremes, however, which can cause problems. While you are trying to get pregnant, avoid intense training. Don't try to increase your exercise programme. This is not a good time to play competitive sports that involve pushing yourself to the maximum.

It's important to find exercise you enjoy and will continue on a regular basis, in any kind of weather. Concentrate on improving strength in your lower back and abdominal muscles to help during your pregnancy.

If you have concerns about exercise before or during pregnancy, discuss them with your doctor. Exercise you tolerate well and can do easily before pregnancy may be more difficult for you during pregnancy.

Many hospitals and health clubs or spas have exercise programmes specifically for pregnant women. See Week 3 for more information about exercise, including guidelines, suggestions and possible problems.

The best approach to exercise is a balanced one. Regular exercise that is enjoyable helps you feel better and enjoy your pregnancy more. It will also provide your developing baby with a healthier environment.

Substance Use before Pregnancy

In the past, little was understood about drug or alcohol abuse, and not a lot could be done to help a person with these problems. Today healthcare providers are able to give suggestions and provide care for those who use or abuse drugs, alcohol or other substances. Don't be embarrassed to confide in your doctor about substance use. Your doctor's concern is for you and your baby.

Tip for Pre-pregnancy

Even though you know you aren't pregnant, treat your body as if you were during your preparation period. When you do get pregnant, you'll be on the right track for eating, exercising and avoiding harmful substances.

We have learned much about drug and alcohol use and the effect on pregnancy in recent years. We now believe the safest approach to drug or alcohol use during pregnancy is *no use at all.*

It makes sense to solve these problems before pregnancy. By the time you realize you're pregnant, you may already be 8 or 10 weeks along. Your baby goes through some of its most important developmental stages in the first 13 weeks of pregnancy. You might use drugs and not realize you are pregnant. Few women would take these substances if they knew they were pregnant. Stop using any substance you don't need at least 3 months before trying to conceive!

Research into these problems continues, showing that use of drugs or alcohol during pregnancy may affect a child's IQ, attention span and learning ability. To date, no safe level of these substances has been determined.

Drug use before pregnancy is serious business. Fortunately, there is help for those who use drugs. Get help before you become pregnant. Preparing for pregnancy may be a good reason for you and your partner to change your lifestyle.

ᴄᴏ *Common Substances of Abuse*

Tobacco. We have known for a long time that smoking affects foetal development. Mothers who smoke during pregnancy are more likely to have low-birthweight babies or babies with intrauterine-growth restriction. Ask for help to stop smoking before you become pregnant. Your doctor should be receptive to this request. (See Weeks 1 & 2 for tips on quitting.)

Alcohol. In the past, some believed a small amount of alcohol during pregnancy was OK. Today, we believe *no amount* of alcohol is safe to drink during pregnancy. Alcohol crosses the placenta and directly affects your baby. Heavy drinking during pregnancy can cause foetal alcohol syndrome (FAS) or foetal alcohol exposure (FAE), discussed in Weeks 1 & 2.

Cocaine. Cocaine has been shown to affect the baby throughout pregnancy, not just during the first trimester. If you use cocaine during the first 12 weeks of pregnancy, you run a higher risk of miscarriage. Cocaine can also cause severe deformities in a foetus. The type of defect it causes depends on the point at which cocaine is used in the pregnancy.

Dad Tip If your partner is making lifestyle changes to prepare for pregnancy, such as giving up smoking or not drinking alcohol, support her in her efforts. Quit these habits, too, if you share them.

Infants born to mothers who use cocaine during pregnancy have been found to have long-term mental deficiencies. Sudden infant death syndrome (SIDS) is also more common in these babies. Many babies born to women who use cocaine are stillborn.

Cocaine affects the mother-to-be, too. It is a stimulant and increases the user's heart rate and blood pressure. Women who use the drug during pregnancy have a higher rate of placental abruption, which is the premature separation of the placenta from the uterus.

In some parts of the United States, more than 10 per cent of all pregnant women use cocaine at some time during their pregnancy. Figures for the UK are unavailable, but it is likely that in some areas cocaine use is significant. Stop using cocaine before you stop using birth control. Damage to the embryo (later the foetus) can occur as early as 3 days after conception!

Marijuana. Marijuana (hashish) is dangerous during pregnancy because it crosses the placenta and enters the baby's system. It can have long-lasting effects on babies exposed before birth. Research has shown that a mother's marijuana use during pregnancy can affect cognitive function, decision-making ability and future-planning ability in her child. Use can also affect a child's verbal reasoning and memory.

If your partner smokes marijuana, encourage him to stop. One study showed that the risk of SIDS was twice the average for children if their father smoked marijuana. The risk is present if the male smokes before conception. Researchers believe the THC in marijuana may adversely affect sperm and the growing foetus.

Work and Pregnancy

You may need to consider your job when you plan a pregnancy. Many women do not know they are pregnant until the early stages of the

Are You in the Armed Forces?

Are you currently serving in the Armed Forces or planning to enter one of the services soon? If so, as you prepare for your pregnancy, there are some things to keep in mind.

Studies have shown that women who get pregnant while they are on active duty may face many challenges, including some risks to their developing foetuses. The pressure to meet military body-weight standards can have an effect on a mother-to-be's health. Many women also have low iron stores and lower-than-normal folic-acid levels due to poor dietary habits. As we discuss on page 20, folic acid is extremely important early in pregnancy, and you must have adequate iron stores throughout pregnancy. In addition, some aspects of a job may pose hazards, such as standing for prolonged periods, heavy lifting and exposure to toxic chemicals. All of these factors can impact on your pregnancy.

If you're planning on getting pregnant during your service commitment, work hard to reach your ideal weight a few months before you conceive, then maintain that weight. Be sure your folic-acid intake is adequate and your iron stores are at an acceptable level by following a well-balanced food plan and eating foods high in these substances. You may also want to take prenatal vitamins. If you are concerned about hazards related to your work, discuss it with a superior. Find out if you're pregnant before receiving any vaccinations or inoculations.

It's important to take care of yourself and your baby. Start by making plans now to have a healthy pregnancy. Also see the discussion of *Pregnancy in the Armed Forces* in Week 14.

pregnancy are already behind them. It's wise to plan ahead. Learn about things you are exposed to at work.

Some jobs might be considered harmful during pregnancy. Some substances you might be exposed to at work, such as chemicals, inhalants, radiation or solvents, could be a problem while you're pregnant. Much of this chapter has discussed your lifestyle and how you take care of yourself. It is important to consider things you are exposed to at work as part of your lifestyle. Continue reliable contraception until you know the environment at work is safe.

Other important work-related considerations are the types of benefits or insurance coverage you have and your company's maternity-leave programme. It makes sense to check into this before getting pregnant. With the expense of having a baby, it could cost you several thousand pounds if you don't plan ahead.

Women who stand for long periods have smaller babies. If you have had a premature delivery in the past or if you have had an incompetent cervix, a job that requires you to stand a great deal may not be the wisest choice for you during pregnancy. Talk to your doctor about your work situation.

Sexually Transmitted Diseases

Infections or diseases passed from one person to another by sexual contact are called *sexually transmitted diseases* (STDs). These infections can affect your ability to get pregnant and can harm your developing baby. The type of contraception you use may have an effect on the likelihood of your contracting an STD. Condoms and spermicides can lower the risk of getting an STD. You are more likely to get a sexually transmitted disease if you have more than one sexual partner.

Some STD infections can cause *pelvic inflammatory disease* (PID). PID is serious because it can spread from the vagina and cervix through the uterus and involve the Fallopian tubes and ovaries. The result can be scarring and blockage of the tubes, making it difficult or

impossible for you to become pregnant or making you more susceptible to an ectopic pregnancy (see Week 5).

✕ *Protecting Yourself from STDs*

Part of planning and preparing for pregnancy includes protecting
yourself against STDs. Take the following actions.

- Use a condom (regardless of what other type of contraception
  you might be using).
- Limit the number of sexual partners you have.
- Have sexual contact only with those you are sure do not have
  multiple sexual partners.

Ask for treatment if you think you have a sexually transmitted disease. Get tested if you have any chance of having an STD, even if you
haven't had any symptoms.

Weeks 1 & 2

Pregnancy Begins

*T*his is an exciting time for you—having a baby growing inside you is an incredible experience! This book will help you understand and enjoy your pregnancy. You will learn what is going on in your body and how your baby is growing and changing.

You are not alone in your pregnancy. Thousands of women successfully complete a pregnancy every year. In fact, the average number of babies born every day in the UK is 1,800. More than half a million— 660,000—are born every year.

One focus of this book is to help you see how your actions and activities affect your health and well-being and that of your growing baby. If you're aware of how a particular test at a particular time, such as an X-ray, will affect the developing foetus, you may decide on another course of action. If you understand how taking a certain drug can harm your baby or cause long-lasting effects, you may decide not to use it. If you know a poor diet can cause heartburn or nausea in you or delayed growth in your baby, you may choose to eat nutritiously. If you are aware of how much your actions affect your pregnancy, you may be able to choose wisely, free yourself from worry and enjoy your pregnancy a great deal more.

Material in this book is divided into weeks of pregnancy. Illustrations help you see clearly how you and your baby are changing and growing each week. General topics each week cover areas of special concern as well as how big your baby is, how big you are and how your actions affect your baby.

The information in this book is *not* meant to take the place of any discussion with your doctor/midwife. Be sure you discuss any and all concerns with him or her. Use this material as a starting place in your dialogue. It may help you put your concerns or interests into words.

Signs and Symptoms of Pregnancy

Many changes in your body can indicate pregnancy. If you have one or more of the following symptoms and you believe you could be pregnant, contact your doctor:

- missed menstrual period
- nausea, with or without vomiting
- food aversions or food cravings
- fatigue
- frequent urination
- breast changes and breast tenderness
- new sensitivity or feelings in your pelvic area
- metallic taste in your mouth

What will you notice first? It's different for every woman. When your expected menstrual period does not begin, it may be the first sign of pregnancy.

When Is Your Baby Due?

The beginning of a pregnancy is actually calculated from the beginning of your last menstrual period. That means, for your doctor's computational purposes, you are pregnant 2 weeks before you actually conceive! This can be confusing, so let's examine it more closely.

Definitions of Time

Gestational age (menstrual age)—Begins from the first day of your last period, which is actually about 2 weeks *before* you conceive. This is the age most doctors use to discuss your pregnancy. Average length of pregnancy is 40 weeks.

Ovulatory age (fertilization age)—Begins the day you conceive. Average length of pregnancy is 38 weeks.

Trimester—Each trimester lasts about 13 weeks. There are three trimesters in a pregnancy.

Lunar months—A pregnancy lasts an average of 10 lunar months (28 days each).

↷ Calculating Your Due Date

Most women don't know the exact date of conception, but they are usually aware of the beginning of their last period. This is the point from which a pregnancy is dated. A due date is important in pregnancy because it helps your doctor determine when to perform certain tests or procedures. It also helps estimate the baby's growth and may indicate whether you are overdue. For most women, the fertile time of the month (ovulation) is around the middle of their monthly cycle or about 2 weeks before the beginning of their next period.

Pregnancy lasts about 280 days, or 40 weeks, from the beginning of the last menstrual period. You can calculate your due date by counting 280 days from the first day of bleeding of your last period. Or count back 3 months from the date of your last period and add 7 days. This also gives you the approximate date of delivery. For example, if your last period began on February 20, your due date is November 27.

Calculating a pregnancy this way gives the gestational age (menstrual age). This is how most doctors and midwives keep track of time during pregnancy. It is different from ovulatory age (fertilization age), which is 2 weeks shorter and dates from the actual date of conception.

Some medical experts are now suggesting that instead of a 'due date,' women be given a 'due week'—a 7-day window of time during which delivery may occur. This time period would fall between 39½ and 40½ weeks. Because so few women (only 5 per cent) deliver on their actual due date, this 7-day period could conceivably help ease a mum-to-be's anxiety about when her baby will be born.

Many people count the time during pregnancy using weeks. It's really the easiest way. But it can be confusing to remember to begin counting from when your period starts and that you don't become pregnant until about 2 weeks later. For example, if your doctor says you're 10 weeks pregnant (from your last period), conception occurred 8 weeks ago.

You may hear references to your stage of pregnancy by trimester. *Trimesters* divide pregnancy into three periods, each about 13 weeks long. This helps group together developmental stages. For example, your baby's body structure is largely formed and his or her organ systems develop during the first trimester. Most miscarriages occur during the first trimester. During the third trimester, most maternal problems with pregnancy-induced hypertension or pre-eclampsia occur.

You may even hear about lunar months, referring to a complete cycle of the moon, which is 28 days. Because pregnancy is 280 days from the beginning of your period to your due date, pregnancy lasts 10 lunar months.

⌁ 40-Week Timetable

In this book, pregnancy is based on a 40-week timetable. Using this method, you actually become pregnant during the third week. Details of your pregnancy are discussed week by week beginning with Week 3. Your due date is the end of the 40th week.

Each weekly discussion includes the actual age of your growing baby. For example, in Week 8, you'll see the following:

Week 8 *(gestational age)*
Age of Foetus—6 Weeks *(fertilization age)*

In this way, you'll know how old your developing baby is at any point in your pregnancy.

It's important to understand a due date is only an estimate, not an exact date. As we've already said, only 1 out of 20 women delivers on her due date. It's a mistake to count on a particular day (your due date or an earlier date). You may see that day come and go and still not have your baby. Think of your due date as a goal—a time to look forward to and to prepare for. It's helpful to know you're making progress.

No matter how you count the time of your pregnancy, it's going to last as long as it's going to last. But a miracle is happening—a living human being is growing and developing inside you! Enjoy this wonderful time in your life.

✣ *Your Menstrual Cycle*

Menstruation is the normal periodic discharge of blood, mucus and cellular debris from the cavity of the uterus. The usual interval for menstruation is 28 days, but this can vary widely and still be considered normal. The duration and amount of menstrual flow can vary; the usual duration is 4 to 6 days.

Two important cycles actually occur at the same time—the ovarian cycle and the endometrial cycle. The *ovarian cycle* provides an egg for fertilization. The *endometrial cycle* provides a suitable site for implantation of the fertilized egg inside your uterus. Because endometrial changes are regulated by hormones made in the ovary, the two cycles are intimately related.

The ovarian cycle produces an egg (ovum) for fertilization. There are about 2 million eggs in a newborn girl at birth. This decreases to about 400,000 in girls just before puberty. The maximum number of eggs is actually present *before* birth. When a female foetus is about 5 months old (4 months before birth), she has about 6.8 million eggs!

Some women (about 25 per cent) experience lower abdominal pain or discomfort on or about the day of ovulation, called *mittelschmerz*. It

Tip for Weeks 1 & 2
Over-the-counter pregnancy tests are reliable and can be positive (indicate pregnancy) as early as 10 days after conception.

is believed to be caused by irritation from fluid or blood from the follicle when it ruptures. The presence or absence of this symptom is not considered proof that ovulation did or did not occur.

Your Health Affects Your Pregnancy

Your health is one of the most important factors in your pregnancy. Good nutrition, proper exercise, sufficient rest and attention to how you care for yourself all affect your pregnancy. Throughout this book, we provide information about medications you may take, medical tests you may need, over-the-counter substances you might use and many other topics that may concern you. This information is necessary for you to be aware of how your actions affect your health and the health of your developing baby.

The health care you receive can also affect your pregnancy and how well you tolerate being pregnant. Good health care is important to the development and well-being of your baby.

ᠵ *Choices in Childbirth*

As soon as your pregnancy has been confirmed, visit your doctor/midwife. He or she will be able to advise you on the types of care available in your area. In more populous parts of the country, you will be able to choose the hospital in which you give birth, though this may not be the case in more rural areas. Almost everybody, however, should have various options about the kind of antenatal care they receive. If your doctor cannot give you all the information you need, contact your local team of community midwives or local maternity unit (there is no substitute for going and finding out what it can offer you) or talk to other women you know who are pregnant or have recently had babies. If, at any point, you feel you have made the wrong choice, you are entitled to change your mind at any time during your pregnancy.

Once you have chosen a hospital, find out as much as you can by asking questions such as:

- Can my partner stay with me all the time? Will they ever be asked to leave?
- Will I have the same midwife throughout labour?
- Can I bring my own midwife to attend to me?
- Will I be able to move around freely?
- Does the hospital have a birthing pool?
- What kinds of pain relief are available?
- What are the hospital policies on episiotomies, Caesareans and induction?
- Will my baby be with me at night?
- Will I be able to feed my baby whenever I want?
- Will my partner be able to stay with me the first night after the birth?

When choosing the type of antenatal care you want, it is useful to ask yourself questions such as whether being cared for by the same person or team throughout pregnancy and labour are important to you, whether you would like your medical carers to be female, whether you are prepared, or able, to travel to antenatal care, and who you would like to have for your antenatal care? A midwife, your GP, or alternate visits between the midwife and doctor?

Whatever type of care you choose, it should start as soon as possible, as taking measurements and doing tests early in pregnancy give a baseline against which changes are measured as the pregnancy progresses.

Finding the Right Antenatal Care for You. Antenatal clinics may be held at your local surgery, where you will see either your family doctor or one of the community midwives. Alternatively, a midwife may be able to visit you at home. This is referred to as *GP/community midwife care*. You will need to visit a hospital, however, for some antenatal investigations, e.g. anomaly scan of approximately 19–21 weeks.

Another option is *team midwifery*. This is a group of about six midwives who work either in a hospital or in the community visiting expectant mothers at home. By the time your baby is due, you'll have met most of the team looking after you, so there will be a familiar face at the birth.

A third option is consultant care, where you attend the *hospital antenatal clinic* for some of your antenatal care. The rest of your care is shared with the doctor or midwife. This specialist care is usually offered to women who have had problems with a previous pregnancy, or have an illness such as diabetes that needs close monitoring.

If continuity of care is very important to you, you may want to consider employing an *independent midwife*. This option guarantees you one-to-one attention. It is expensive, though it is usually possible to pay by instalments.

How Your Actions Affect Your Baby's Development

It's never too early to start thinking about how your activities and actions can affect your growing baby. Many substances you normally use may have adverse effects on the baby you carry. These substances include drugs, tobacco, alcohol and caffeine. Below are discussions of cigarette smoking and alcohol use. Either of these activities can harm a developing baby. Other substances are discussed throughout the book.

ᴗ Cigarette Smoking

Smoking cigarettes has harmful effects on a pregnancy. A pregnant woman who smokes 20 cigarettes a day (one pack) inhales tobacco smoke more than 11,000 times during an average pregnancy! And when you smoke, your baby does, too. What we mean by that is cigarette smoke crosses the placenta to your baby. A recent study showed that when this occurs, a baby is exposed to *much higher concentrations of nicotine* than its mother. This higher concentration could lead to nicotine withdrawal in baby after his or her birth.

Tobacco smoke contains many harmful substances, such as nicotine, carbon monoxide, hydrogen cyanide, tars, resins and some cancer-causing agents (carcinogens). These substances may be responsible singly or together for damaging your developing baby.

Nicoderm Patch, Nicorette Gum and Zyban

Many studies have shown the harmful effects of cigarette smoking during pregnancy. You may be wondering if you can use an aid to help you stop smoking, such as the patch, gum or the stop-smoking pill. The specific effects on foetal development of these three devices are unknown.

Nicotrol, available as an inhaler, a nasal spray, gum or patch, is a popular aid used for smoking cessation. Nicotrol is sold under the brand names *Nicoderm* and *Nicorette;* it is also sold generically. All Nicotrol preparations contain nicotine and are *not* recommended for use during pregnancy.

Zyban (bupropion hydrochloride) is an oral medication that is a non-nicotine aid to help with smoking cessation. This medication is also marketed as the antidepressant Wellbutrin or Wellbutrin SR. Zyban is not recommended for use by pregnant women.

If you are pregnant, researchers advise avoiding gum, the patch and the pill. Discuss the situation with your doctor if you have questions.

Scientific evidence has shown smoking during pregnancy increases the risk of foetal death or foetal damage. Smoking interferes with a woman's absorption of vitamins B and C and folic acid. Lack of folic acid can result in neural-tube defects and increases the risk of pregnancy-related complications in a mother-to-be.

For more than 30 years, we have known infants born to mothers who smoke weigh less by about 200 g (7 oz). That is why cigarette packages carry a warning to women about smoking during pregnancy. Decreased birthweight is directly related to the number of cigarettes the expectant mother smoked. These effects don't appear in her other babies if the mother doesn't smoke with other pregnancies. There is a direct relationship between smoking and impaired foetal growth.

A growing baby is greatly affected by its mother's smoking. Smoking causes narrowing of the capillaries in the placenta; the capillaries carry blood, oxygen and other nutrients to the baby. This narrowing can lead to a reduction in the nourishment baby receives from you, which can lead to low birthweight and smaller-in-stature (shorter) babies.

Children born to mothers who smoked during pregnancy have been observed to have lower IQ scores and increased incidence of reading disorders than children of non-smokers. The incidence of minimal-brain-dysfunction syndrome (hyperactivity) has also been reported to be higher among children of mothers who smoked during pregnancy.

Cigarette smoking during pregnancy increases the risk of miscarriage and foetal death or death of a baby soon after birth. The risk is also directly related to the number of cigarettes the pregnant woman smokes. The risk may increase as much as 35 per cent in a woman who smokes more than one pack of cigarettes a day.

Smoking also increases the incidence of serious complications in a mother-to-be. An example of this is placental abruption, discussed in detail in Week 33. The risk of developing placental abruption increases by almost 25 per cent in moderate smokers and more than 65 per cent in heavy smokers.

Placenta previa (discussed in Week 35) also occurs more frequently among smokers. The rate of occurrence increases by 25 per cent in moderate smokers and 90 per cent in heavy smokers.

Tips for Stopping Smoking

- Make a list of things you can do instead of smoking, especially activities that involve using your hands, such as puzzles or needlework.
- List things you'd like to buy for yourself or your baby. Set aside the money you normally spend on cigarettes to buy these items.
- Identify all your 'triggers'—what brings on an urge to smoke. Make plans to avoid them or to handle them differently.
- Instead of smoking after meals, brush your teeth, wash dishes or go for a walk.
- If you always smoke while driving, clean your car inside and out, and use an air freshener. Sing along with the radio or a cassette tape. Listen to an audiobook. Take a bus or the train for a while.
- Drink lots of water.

If you continue to have trouble stopping, a recent study determined that using a 'quitter's hotline' for help is twice as effective as going it alone. You can talk directly to someone who has been through the same experience. If you're interested, contact QUIT's trained counsellors on 0800 002200 or www.quit.org.uk, or call the NHS Smoking Helpline on 0800 1690169 or online at www.givingupsmoking.co.uk.

What can you do? The answer sounds simple but isn't—quit smoking. In more realistic terms, a woman who smokes during pregnancy will benefit from reducing or stopping cigarette use before or during pregnancy—and so will her developing baby. Some studies indicate that a non-smoker and her unborn baby exposed to secondary smoke (cigarette smoke in the environment) are exposed to nicotine and other harmful substances. Perhaps pregnancy can serve as good motivation for everyone in the family to stop smoking!

✣ *Alcohol Use*

Alcohol use by a pregnant woman carries risk. Moderate drinking has been linked to an increased chance of miscarriage. Excessive alcohol consumption during pregnancy often results in foetal abnormalities. Chronic use of alcohol in pregnancy can lead to abnormal foetal development called *foetal alcohol syndrome (FAS)*.

FAS is characterized by growth restriction before and after birth, and defects in limbs, the heart and facial characteristics of children are also seen. Facial characteristics are recognizable—the nose is upturned and short, the upper jawbone is flat and the eyes look 'different.' An FAS child may also have behavioural problems.

FAS children often have impaired speech, and their fine and gross motor functions are impaired. The infant mortality rate is 15 to 20 per cent.

Most studies indicate women would have to drink four to five drinks a day for FAS to occur. But mild abnormalities have been associated with two drinks a day (30 ml/1 fl oz of alcohol). These milder birth defects are the result of *foetal alcohol exposure* (FAE), a condition that can result from very little alcohol. This has led many researchers to conclude there is *no safe level of alcohol consumption* during pregnancy.

Taking drugs with alcohol increases the chances of damage to a baby. Analgesics, antidepressants and anticonvulsants cause the most concern. Some researchers have suggested the father's heavy alcohol consumption before conception may also result in foetal alcohol syndrome. Alcohol intake by the father has been cited as one possible

cause of intrauterine-growth restriction.

As a precaution, be very careful
about over-the-counter cough
and cold remedies you may use.
Many contain alcohol—some as
much as 25 per cent!

Some women want to know
if they can drink socially. There
is a great deal of disagreement
about it because there is no
known safe level of alcohol con-

Alcohol in Cooking

Most pregnant women know they
should avoid alcohol during pregnancy but what about recipes
that call for alcohol? A good rule
of thumb is it's probably OK to
eat a food that contains alcohol if
it has been baked or simmered
for at least 1 hour. Cooking for
that length of time evaporates
most of the alcohol content.

sumption during pregnancy. Why take chances? For the health and
well-being of your developing baby, abstain from alcohol during pregnancy. Responsibility for preventing these problems rests squarely on
your shoulders!

Your Nutrition

If your weight is normal before pregnancy, you need to increase your
calorific intake during pregnancy. During the first trimester (first 13
weeks), you should eat a total of about 2200 calories a day. During the
second and third trimesters, you probably need an additional 300 calories each day.

Extra calories provide the energy
your body needs for you and your
growing baby. Your baby uses the energy to create and to store protein,
fat and carbohydrates. It needs energy for foetal body processes to
function. The extra calories also sup-

Dad Tip Give your
partner a lot of hugs. Many women
enjoy more hugging and cuddling
during this very special time.

port changes your body is going through. Your uterus increases in size,
and your blood volume increases by about 50 per cent.

Although this book is designed to take you through your pregnancy by examining one week at a time, you may seek specific information. Because the book cannot include *everything* you need *before* you know you're looking for it, check the index, beginning on page 455, for a particular topic. For example, if you're searching for information early in your pregnancy on ways to snack healthily, check the index for various page references. We may not cover the subject until a later week.

You can meet most of your nutritional needs by eating a well-balanced, varied diet. The *quality* of your calories is important, too. If a food grows in the ground or on a tree (meaning it's fresh), it's probably better for you than if it comes out of a box or can.

Be cautious about adding the extra 300 calories to your nutrition plan—it doesn't mean doubling your portions. A medium apple and a carton of low-fat yoghurt add up to 300 calories!

You Should Also Know

↭ *Hepatitis in Pregnancy*

Hepatitis is a viral infection of the liver. It is one of the most serious infections that can occur during pregnancy. Hepatitis B is responsible for nearly half the cases of hepatitis in the UK. It is transmitted by sexual contact or reuse of hypodermic needles.

Those at risk for contracting hepatitis B include people with a history of intravenous drug use, a history of sexually transmitted diseases or exposure to people or blood products that contain hepatitis B. The B type can be transmitted to the developing foetus of a pregnant woman.

Hepatitis symptoms include the following:

• nausea
• flu-like symptoms
• jaundice (yellow skin)
• dark urine
• pain in or around the liver or upper-right abdomen

Hepatitis B is diagnosed by blood tests, which are now offered to all women at the beginning of their pregnancy. If you test positive, your baby may receive *immune globulin* (antibodies to fight hepatitis) after delivery. It is now recommended that all newborns from mothers tested positive for hepatitis B receive a hepatitis vaccine shortly after birth.

If you want to chart your pregnancy weight gain, we've provided a chart on the following page just for that purpose. The weeks listed are weeks when you may have an antenatal appointment. If your appointment doesn't fall on that exact week, cross out the week number that we have listed and mark down which week you made your visit to the doctor or midwife.

Chart Your
Pregnancy Weight Gain

Weight Before Pregnancy Begins _____

Week	Weight at Antenatal Appointment	Weight Gain
8	_____	_____
12	_____	_____
16	_____	_____
20	_____	_____
24	_____	_____
28	_____	_____
30	_____	_____
32	_____	_____
34	_____	_____
36	_____	_____
37	_____	_____
38	_____	_____
39	_____	_____
40	_____	_____

Total pregnancy weight gain _____

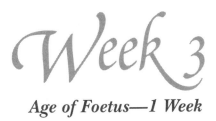

Week 3

Age of Foetus—1 Week

How Big Is Your Baby?

The embryo growing inside you is very small. At this point, it is only a group of cells, but it is multiplying and growing rapidly. The embryo is the size of the head of a pin and would be visible to the naked eye if it weren't inside you. The group of cells doesn't look like a foetus or baby; it looks like the illustration on page 45. During this first week, the embryo is about 0.150 mm (0.006 in) long.

How Big Are You?

In this third week of pregnancy, you won't notice any changes. It's too soon! Few women know they have conceived. Remember, you haven't even missed a period yet.

How Your Baby Is Growing and Developing

A great deal is happening, even though your pregnancy is in its earliest stage. Ovaries lie free in your pelvis (or peritoneal cavity). They are close to the uterus and Fallopian tube. At the time of ovulation, the end of the tube (called the *fimbria*) lies close to the ovary. Some researchers believe this tube opening covers the area on the ovary where the egg (ovum) is released at the time of ovulation. The release site on the ovary is called the *stigma*.

During intercourse, an average of 2 to 5 ml (0.06 to 0.15 fl oz) of semen is deposited in the vagina. Each millilitre contains an average of 70 million sperm; each ejaculation contains 140 to 350 million sperm. Only about 200 sperm actually reach the egg in the tube. *Fertilization* is the joining together of one sperm and an egg.

ᕽ *Fertilization of the Egg*

Fertilization is believed to occur in the middle part of the tube, called the *ampulla*, not inside the uterus. Sperm travel through the uterine cavity and out into the tube to meet the egg.

When the sperm and egg join, the sperm must pass through the outer layer of the ovum, the *corona radiata*. The sperm then digests its way through another layer of the ovum, the *zona pellucida*. Although several sperm may penetrate the outer layers of the ovum, usually only one sperm enters the ovum and fertilizes it.

Boy or Girl?

Your baby's sex is determined at the time of fertilization by the type of sperm (male or female) that fertilizes the egg. A Y-chromosome-bearing sperm produces a boy, and an X-chromosome-bearing sperm produces a girl.

After the sperm penetrates the ovum, the sperm head attaches to its surface. The membranes of the sperm and ovum unite, enclosing them in the same membrane or sac. The ovum reacts to this contact with the sperm by making changes in the outer layers so no other sperm can enter.

Once the sperm gets inside the ovum, it loses its tail. The head of the sperm enlarges and is called the *male pronucleus*; the ovum is called the *female pronucleus*. The chromosomes of the male and female pronuclei intermingle. When this happens, extremely small bits of information and characteristics from each partner unite. This

Blastomere

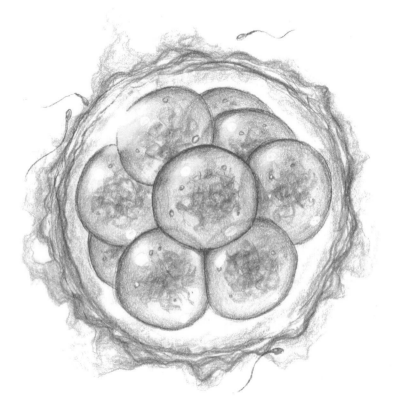

Nine-cell embryo 3 days after fertilization. The embryo is made up of many blastomeres; together they form a blastocyst.

chromosomal information gives each of us our particular characteristics. The usual number of chromosomes in each human is 46. Each parent supplies 23 chromosomes. Your baby is a combination of chromosomal information from you and your partner.

ᴥ *Embryonic Development Begins*

The developing ball of cells is called a *zygote*. The zygote passes through the uterine tube on its way to the uterus as the division of cells continues. These cells are called a *blastomere*. As the blastomere continues to divide, a solid ball of cells is formed, called a *morula*. The gradual accumulation of fluid within the morula results in the formation of a *blastocyst*, which is tiny.

During the next week, the blastocyst travels through the uterine tube to the cavity of the uterus (3 to 7 days after fertilization in the tube). The blastocyst lies free in the uterine cavity as it continues to grow and to develop. About a week after fertilization, it attaches to the uterine cavity (implantation), and cells burrow into the lining of the uterus.

Changes in You

Some women can tell when they ovulate. They may feel mild cramping or pain, or they may have an increased vaginal discharge. Occasionally at the time of implantation of the fertilized egg into the uterine cavity, a woman may notice a small amount of bleeding.

It's too early for you to notice many changes. Your breasts haven't started to enlarge and you aren't starting to 'show.' That lies ahead! (See the discussion in Weeks 1 & 2 for signs and symptoms of pregnancy.)

How Your Actions
Affect Your Baby's Development

Exercise is an important part of life for many women. The more we learn about health, the more the advantages of regular exercise become evident. Regular exercise may decrease your risk of developing several medical problems, including cardiovascular disease, osteoporosis (softening of bones), depression, premenstrual syndrome (PMS) and obesity.

There are many types of exercise to choose from before, during and after pregnancy. Each offers its own advantages. Aerobic exercise is very popular with women who want to keep in shape. Muscle-building exercises are also a popular way to tone and to increase strength. Many women combine the two. Good exercise choices for pregnant women include brisk walking, stationary bicycling, swimming and aerobic exercise designed especially for pregnant women.

ꝏ Aerobic Exercise

For cardiovascular fitness, aerobic exercise is the best. You must exercise at least 3 times a week at a sustained heart rate of 110 to 120 beats a minute, maintained for at least 15 continuous minutes. The rate of 110 to 120 beats a minute is an approximate target for people of different ages.

If you exercised aerobically before pregnancy, you can probably continue aerobic exercise at a somewhat lower rate. If you have any problems, such as bleeding or premature labour, you and your doctor will have to choose another programme.

It is unwise to start a strenuous aerobic exercise programme or to increase training during

Target Heart Rates		
Age (years)	Target heart rate (beats/minute)	Max. heart rate (beats/minute)
20	150	200
25	117–146	195
30	114–146	190
35	111–138	185
40	108–135	180
45	105–131	175
50	102–131	170

(US Department of Health and Human Services)

pregnancy. If you haven't been involved in regular, strenuous exercise before pregnancy, walking and swimming are probably about as involved as you should get with exercise.

Before you begin any exercise programme, discuss it with your midwife or doctor. Together you can develop a programme consistent with your current level of conditioning and your exercise habits.

ᴥ *Muscle Strength*

Some women exercise for muscle strength. To strengthen a muscle, there has to be resistance against it. There are three different kinds of muscle contractions—isotonic, isometric and isokinetic. *Isotonic exercise* involves shortening the muscle as tension is developed, such as when you lift a weight. *Isometric exercise* causes the muscle to develop tension but doesn't change its length, such as when you push against a stationary wall. *Isokinetic exercise* occurs when the muscle moves at a constant speed, such as when you swim.

Cardiac and skeletal muscles cannot usually be strengthened at the same time. Strengthening skeletal muscles requires lifting heavy weights, but you can't lift these heavy weights long enough to strengthen the cardiac muscle.

Weight-bearing exercise is the most effective way of promoting increased bone density to help avoid osteoporosis. Other advantages of exercise include flexibility, coordination, improvement in mood and alertness. Stretching and warming up muscles before and after exercise help you improve flexibility and avoid injury.

ᴥ *Should You Exercise during Pregnancy?*

As a pregnant woman, you are probably concerned about the risks of exercise. Can you or should you exercise when you're pregnant?

Pregnant women need cardiovascular fitness. Women who are physically fit are better able to perform the hard work of labour and delivery. Exercise during pregnancy is not without some risk, however. Risks to the developing baby can include any of the following:

- increased body temperature
- decreased blood flow to the uterus
- possible injury to the mother's abdominal area

You can exercise during pregnancy if you do it wisely. Avoid raising your body temperature above 38.9°C (102°F). Aerobic exercise can raise your body temperature higher than this, so be careful. A rise in body temperature can be increased by dehydration. Avoid prolonged aerobic exercise, particularly during hot weather.

While exercising aerobically, blood can be diverted to the exercising muscle or skin and away from other organs, such as the uterus, liver or kidneys. A lower workload during pregnancy is advised to avoid potential problems. Now is *not* the time to try to set new records or to train for a forthcoming marathon! During pregnancy, keep your heart rate below 140 beats a minute.

ꝛ *General Exercise Guidelines*
Before beginning any exercise programme, consult your doctor about any medical problems or pregnancy problems.

- Begin any exercise programme before you become pregnant.
- Begin exercising gradually. Start with 15-minute workout sessions, with 5-minute rest periods in between.
- Check your heart rate every 15 minutes. Don't let it exceed 140 beats a minute (bpm). An easy way to calculate your pulse is to count the number of heartbeats by feeling the pulse in your neck or wrist for 15 seconds. Multiply by 4. If your pulse exceeds 140 bpm, rest until your pulse drops below 90.
- Allow enough time to warm up and to cool down.
- Wear comfortable clothing during exercise, including clothing that is warm enough or cool enough, and good, comfortable athletic shoes that offer maximum support.
- Do not allow yourself to become overheated.
- Exercise on a regular basis.
- Avoid risky sports, such as horse riding or water skiing.
- Increase the number of calories you consume.
- When you're pregnant, be careful about getting up and lying down.
- After the 4th month of pregnancy (16 weeks), don't lie on your back while exercising. This can decrease blood flow to the uterus and placenta.
- When you finish exercising, lie on your left side for 15 to 20 minutes.

Dad Tip Bring home flowers for no special occasion.

℘ Possible Problems

Stop exercising and consult your doctor if you experience bleeding or loss of fluid from the vagina while exercising, shortness of breath, dizziness, severe abdominal pain or any other pain or discomfort. Consult your doctor, and exercise only under his or her supervision, if you experience (or know you have) an irregular heartbeat, high blood pressure, diabetes, thyroid disease, anaemia or any other chronic medical problem.

Tip for Week 3 Talk with your doctor before starting an exercise programme during pregnancy. If you have been exercising, cut back your level of exercise to no more than 80 per cent of your pre-pregnancy level.

Talk to your doctor about exercise if you have a history of three or more miscarriages, an incompetent cervix, intrauterine-growth restriction, premature labour or any abnormal bleeding during pregnancy.

How Your Actions Affect Your Baby's Development

℘ Aspirin Use

Almost any medication taken during pregnancy can have some effect on your baby. The reason there are warnings about aspirin is because aspirin use can increase bleeding. It causes changes in the platelet function; platelets are important in blood clotting. This is particularly important to know if you are bleeding during pregnancy or if you are at the end of your pregnancy and close to delivery. Small doses of aspirin may be acceptable during pregnancy; see the box opposite. **Note:** Do *not* take any amount of aspirin without discussing it with your doctor first!

Read labels on any medication you take to see if it contains aspirin. Avoid using aspirin or any products that contain aspirin unless you first discuss it with your doctor.

If you need a pain reliever or a medication to reduce fever, and you cannot reach your doctor for advice, paracetamol is one over-the-counter medication you can use for a short while with little fear of complications or problems for you or your baby. For further information about over-the-counter medication use during pregnancy, see Week 7.

Your Nutrition

Folic acid, also referred to as *folate, folacin* or *vitamin B₉,* is important to you during pregnancy. Studies indicate taking folic acid during pregnancy may help prevent or decrease the incidence of neural-tube defects, which are defective closures of the neural tube during early pregnancy. Some of these defects include *spina bifida*, when the base of the spine remains open, exposing the spinal cord and nerves; *anencephaly*, congenital (present at birth) absence of the brain and spinal cord; and *encephalocele*, a protrusion of the brain through an opening in the skull.

> ### *Taking Low-dose Aspirin during Pregnancy*
>
> Even though you have heard warnings about taking aspirin during pregnancy, research has shown there may be situations in which aspirin use is beneficial. Researchers now believe that taking a *very low dose* of aspirin in the evening may be good insurance against some pregnancy complications, such as premature labour and high blood pressure. Discuss it with your doctor. Low-dose aspirin, which contain 81½ mg of aspirin, may be prescribed. A woman who takes low doses of aspirin is advised to begin taking it *before* week 16 because the protective effect is not as evident if she begins taking it later.

A folic-acid deficiency can also result in anaemia in the mother-to-be. Additional folic acid may be necessary with multiple foetuses or when the mother suffers from Crohn's disease or alcoholism.

A prenatal vitamin contains 0.8 mg to 1 mg of folic acid. This is usually sufficient for a woman with a normal pregnancy. Researchers believe spina bifida may be prevented if the mother-to-be takes 0.4 mg of folic acid a day, beginning before pregnancy and continuing through the first 13 weeks. This is suggested for all pregnant women. A pregnant woman's body excretes four or five times the normal amount of folic acid. Because folic acid is not stored in the body for very long, it must be replaced every day.

Some grain products, including flour, breakfast cereals and pasta, are fortified with folic acid. Eating 45 g (1½ oz) of fortified breakfast cereal, with milk, and drinking a glass of orange juice supplies about half of your folic-acid requirement for one day. Folic acid is found naturally in many other foods, too, such as fruits, vegetables, brewer's yeast, soya beans, whole-grain products and dark, leafy vegetables. A well-balanced diet can help you reach your folic-acid-intake goal. Also see the list of foods that are good folic-acid sources in Preparing for Pregnancy.

You Should Also Know

ᝑ Bleeding during Pregnancy

Bleeding during pregnancy causes concern. In the first trimester, bleeding can make you worry about the well-being of your baby and the possibility of a miscarriage. (We discuss miscarriage in Week 8.)

Bleeding during pregnancy is *not* unusual. Some researchers estimate that 1 in 5 pregnant women bleeds during the first trimester. Although it makes you worry about possible problems, not all women who bleed have a miscarriage.

Bleeding at the time of implantation is mentioned on page 46. This can occur as the blastocyst burrows into the uterine lining. At this point, you won't know you are pregnant because you haven't missed a period. If this happens, you may just think your period is starting.

As your uterus grows, the placenta forms and vascular connections are made. Bleeding may occur at this time. Strenuous exercise or intercourse may also cause some bleeding. If this occurs, stop your activities and check with your doctor, who will advise you what to do.

If bleeding causes your doctor concern, he or she may order an ultrasound exam. Sometimes ultrasound can show a reason for bleeding, but during this early part of pregnancy, there may be no discernible reason for it.

Most doctors suggest resting, decreasing activity and avoiding intercourse when bleeding occurs. Surgery or medication are not helpful and are unlikely to make a difference. Call your doctor if you experience any bleeding. He or she will advise you what to do.

Benefits of Pregnancy

- Allergy and asthma sufferers may feel better during pregnancy because the natural steroids produced during pregnancy help reduce their symptoms.
- Pregnancy may help protect against breast cancer and ovarian cancer. The younger a woman is when she starts having babies, and the more pregnancies she has, the greater the benefit.
- Migraine headaches often disappear during the second and third trimesters of pregnancy.
- Menstrual cramps are a thing of the past during pregnancy. An added benefit—they may not return after your baby is born!
- Endometriosis (when endometrial tissue attaches to parts of the ovaries and other sites outside the uterus) causes pelvic pain, heavy bleeding and other problems during menstruation for some women. Pregnancy can stop growth of endometriosis.

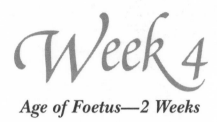

Week 4

Age of Foetus—2 Weeks

If you've just found out you're pregnant, you might want to begin by reading the previous chapters.

How Big Is Your Baby?

Your developing baby is still tiny. Its size varies from about 0.36 mm to about 1 mm (0.014 in to 0.04 in) in length. One millimetre is half the size of a letter 'o' on this page.

How Big Are You?

At this point, your pregnancy doesn't show at all. You haven't gained weight, and your figure hasn't changed. The illustration on page 55 gives you an idea of how small your baby is, so you can see why you won't notice any changes yet.

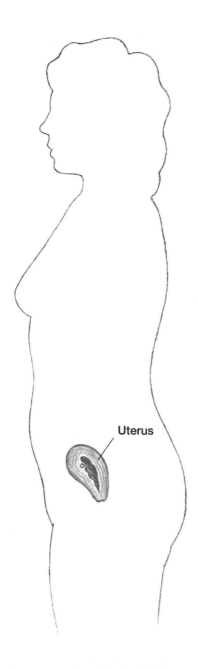

Uterus

Pregnancy at around 4 weeks (foetal age—2 weeks).

How Your Baby Is Growing and Developing

Foetal development is still in the very early stages, but many great changes are taking place! The implanted blastocyst is embedded more deeply into the lining of your uterus, and the amniotic cavity, which will be filled with amniotic fluid, is starting to form. The placenta is forming; it plays an important role in hormone production and transport of oxygen and nutrients. Vascular networks that contain maternal blood are becoming established.

∽ Germ Layers

Different layers of cells are developing. They are called *germ layers* and develop into specialized parts of your baby's body, such as various organs. There are three germ layers—the *ectoderm, endoderm* and *mesoderm.*

The ectoderm will become the nervous system (including the brain), the skin and the hair. The endoderm develops into the lining of the gastrointestinal tract, the liver, pancreas and thyroid. From the mesoderm comes the skeleton, connective tissues, blood system, urogenital system and most of the muscles.

Changes in You

You are probably expecting a period around the end of this week. When it doesn't occur, pregnancy may be one of the first things you think of!

∽ The Corpus Luteum

When you ovulate, the egg leaves the ovary. The area on the ovary where the egg comes from is called the *corpus luteum.* If you become pregnant, it is called the *corpus luteum of pregnancy.* The corpus luteum forms immediately after ovulation at the site of the ruptured follicle where the egg is released. It looks like a small sac of fluid on the ovary. It undergoes rapid blood-vessel development in preparation for producing hormones, such as progesterone, to support a pregnancy before the placenta takes over.

The importance of the corpus luteum is the subject of much debate. It is believed to be essential in the early weeks of pregnancy because it produces progesterone. The placenta takes over this function between 8 and 12 weeks of pregnancy. The corpus luteum lasts until about the 6th month of pregnancy, when it shrinks, although normal corpus lutea have been found with full-term pregnancies. Successful pregnancies have also occurred when the corpus luteum was removed because of a ruptured cyst as early as the 20th day after a menstrual period or about the time of implantation.

How Your Actions Affect Your Baby's Development

During pregnancy, nearly every parent worries whether their baby will be perfect. Most parents worry unnecessarily. Major birth defects are apparent in only about 3 per cent of all newborns at birth. Of those 3 per cent, are causes of these abnormalities known? Could they have been prevented?

ᑐ *Abnormal Foetal Development*
Teratology is the study of abnormal foetal development. An exact cause or reason for a birth defect is found in less than half of all cases. Obstetricians, midwives and GPs providing care to pregnant women are often asked about substances (teratogens) that may be harmful. A *teratogen* is a substance that can produce birth defects, including major and minor structural deformities and abnormalities in the way organs function. Researchers have been unable to prove the danger of some agents we believe are harmful. They *have* proved the harm of other agents.

Some agents cause major defects if exposure occurs at a specific, critical time in foetal development. But they may not be harmful at other times. Once the foetus has completed major development, usually by the 13th week, the effect of a certain substance may be only growth restriction or smaller organ size rather than large structural defects. One example is rubella. It can cause many anatomical defects, such as heart malformations, if the foetus is infected during the first trimester of pregnancy. A rubella infection occurring later is less serious.

ᴄ⳽ *Individual Response to Exposure*
Individual responses to particular agents and to different doses of agents vary greatly. Alcohol is a good example. Large amounts appear to have no effect on some foetuses, while other foetuses may be harmed by low amounts.

Animal studies provide much of our information about possible harmful agents. This information can be helpful but cannot always be applied directly to humans. Other information comes from situations in which women were exposed who did not know they were pregnant or that a particular substance could be harmful. Information gathered from these instances is difficult to apply directly to a particular pregnancy.

> *Tip for Week 4*
> Passive smoking may harm a non-smoking woman and her developing baby. Ask those who smoke to refrain from smoking around you during your pregnancy.

A list of known teratogens and the effects they may have on an embryo or foetus appears on pages 59–60. If you have taken any of these substances, discuss them as soon as possible with your doctor for your peace of mind. If testing or follow-up is necessary, he or she will advise you.

ᴄ⳽ *Drug Use*
Information about the effects of a specific drug on a human pregnancy comes from cases of exposure before the pregnancy is discovered. These 'case reports' help researchers understand possible harmful effects but leave gaps in our knowledge. For this reason, it can be difficult or impossible to make exact statements about particular drugs and their effects. The charts on pages 59 and 60 list possible effects of various substances.

If you use drugs, be honest with your doctor. Ask questions about drugs and drug use. Tell your doctor about anything you take or have taken that may affect your baby. The victim of drug use is your baby. A

Effects of Various Substances on Foetal Development

Many substances can affect your baby's early development. Below is a list of substances and their effects on a developing foetus. This list is of common prescription drugs and chemicals. A second list, which contains other substances, can be found on page 60.

Common Prescription Drugs and Other Chemicals

Drug or Chemical	Possible Effects on Your Baby
Androgens (male hormones)	ambiguous genital development (depends on dose given and when given)
Angiotensin-converting enzyme (ACE) inhibitors (enalapril, captopril)	foetal and neonatal death
Anticoagulants	bone and hand abnormalities, intrauterine-growth restriction (IUGR), central-nervous-system and eye abnormalities
Antithyroid drugs (propylthiouracil, iodide)	hypothyroidism, foetal goiter
Carbamazepine	birth defects, spina bifida
Chemotherapeutic drugs (methotrexate)	increased risk of miscarriage, fetal death and birth defects
Coumadin derivatives (warfarin)	haemorrhage (bleeding), birth defects, an increase in miscarriage and stillbirth
Diethylstilbestrol (DES)	abnormalities of female reproductive organs (in females and males), infertility
Folic-acid antagonists (methotrexate)	increased risk of miscarriage, foetal death and birth defects
Isotretinoin (Roaccutane)	increased miscarriage rate, nervous-system defects, facial defects, cleft palate
Lead	increased miscarriage and stillbirth rates
Lithium	congenital heart disease
Organic mercury	cerebral atrophy, mental retardation, spasticity, seizures, blindness
Phenytoin (Epanutin, Pentran)	IUGR, microcephaly
Streptomycin	hearing loss, cranial-nerve damage
Tetracycline	hypoplasia of tooth enamel, discoloration of permanent teeth
Thalidomide	severe limb defects
Trimethadione	cleft lip, cleft palate, IUGR, miscarriage
Valproic acid	neural-tube defects
Vitamin A and derivatives (etritinate, retinoids)	foetal death and birth defects
X-ray therapy	microcephaly, mental retardation, leukaemia

(Modified from ACOG Technical Bulletin 84, Teratology, February, 1985, American College of Obstetricians and Gynecologists)

Drugs and Other Substances to Avoid

Drug	Possible Effects on Your Baby
Alcohol	foetal abnormalities, foetal alcohol syndrome (FAS), foetal alcohol exposure (FAE), IUGR
Amphetamines	placental abruption, IUGR, foetal death
Barbiturates	possible birth defects, withdrawal symptoms, poor eating habits, seizures
Benzodiazepines (including Valium and Librium)	increased chance of congenital malformations
Caffeine	decreased birthweight, smaller head size, breathing problems, sleeplessness, irritability, jitters, poor calcium metabolism, IUGR, mental retardation, microcephaly, various major malformations
Cocaine/crack	miscarriage, stillbirth, congenital defects, severe deformities in a foetus, long-term mental deficiencies, sudden infant death syndrome (SIDS)
Ecstasy	long-term learning problems, memory problems
Glues and solvents	shortened stature, low birthweight, small head, joint and limb problems, abnormal facial features, heart defects
Ketamine	behavioural problems, learning problems
Marijuana and hashish	attention-deficit disorder (ADD), attention-deficit hyperactivity disorder (ADHD), memory problems, impaired decision-making ability
Methamphetamines	IUGR, difficulty bonding, tremors, extreme fussiness
Nicotine	miscarriage, stillbirth, neural-tube defects, low birthweight, lower IQ, reading disorders, minimal-brain dysfunction syndrome (hyperactivity)
Opioids such as morphine, heroin	congenital abnormalities, premature birth, IUGR, withdrawal symptoms in baby

drug problem may have serious consequences that your doctor/midwife can best deal with if he or she knows about your drug use in advance.

If your partner uses marijuana, it's a good idea for him to stop, too. Researchers have found that children born to men who smoke marijuana have twice the risk of experiencing SIDS (sudden infant death syndrome) after birth. This occurred whether the father smoked before pregnancy, during pregnancy or after the baby's birth.

Your Nutrition

You must be prepared to gain weight during your pregnancy. It's necessary for your health and the health of your growing baby. Getting on the scales and seeing your weight rise may be very hard for you. Acknowledge now that it's OK to gain weight. You don't have to let yourself go—you can control your weight by eating carefully and nutritiously. But you *need* to gain enough weight to meet the needs of your pregnancy.

Many years ago, women were not allowed to gain much weight—sometimes only 5.4 to 6.8 kg (12 to 15 lb) for their entire pregnancy! Today, we know that restricting weight gain to this extent is not healthy for the baby or the mother-to-be. However, the American Association for Cancer Research has demonstrated an important reason to watch your weight during pregnancy. They found that normal-weight women who gained more than 17.2 kg (38 lb) during a singleton pregnancy were at higher risk for developing breast cancer after menopause. Not shedding that extra weight after pregnancy also contributed to higher risk.

Gain weight slowly. Don't let yourself go, just because you're pregnant. You may be eating for two, but you don't have to eat twice as much! The amount of weight you gain during the first trimester is important. The amount you gain in the *first 13 weeks* has been found to correlate more closely with your baby's birth weight than the amount of weight you put on later in pregnancy. If you gain a lot of weight during the first trimester, your baby may be large. Conversely, if you don't gain very much weight in early pregnancy, you may have a lower-birthweight baby.

You probably won't be able to eat all you want during pregnancy, unless you are one of the lucky women who doesn't have a problem with calories. Even then, you must pay strict attention to the foods you choose, and eat healthily. Eat nutritious foods. Avoid those with empty calories (lots of sugar and fat). Choose fresh fruits and vegetables. Avoid caffeine when possible. We discuss many of these subjects in later weeks.

You Should Also Know

৵ *Environmental Pollutants and Pregnancy*

Some environmental pollutants may be harmful to a developing baby. Avoiding exposure to these pollutants is important for a mother-to-be. The box on the opposite page provides information on specific pollutants.

What Can You Do? There is a lack of clear information on the safety of many chemicals in our environment. The safest course of action is to avoid exposure when possible, whether by oral ingestion or through the air you breathe. It may not be possible to eliminate all contact with every possible chemical. If you know you will be around various chemicals, wash your hands well before eating. Not smoking cigarettes also helps.

> *Ɗad Ꞇip* **Make it a habit to pull out your favourite pregnancy book, such as *Your Pregnancy Week by Week*, and read together about what is happening each week in your pregnancy.**

One reassuring fact is that most of the chemicals tested have produced illness in the mother-to-be before damage to her growing baby occurred. An environment that is healthy for you will be healthy for your developing baby.

৵ *Health of the Baby's Father*

Can the father's health and drug or alcohol use affect the health of the developing baby?

In recent years, more attention has been given to the father's contribution in pregnancy. We now believe if a father is over 40, it may increase the risk of Down's syndrome, although there is not a great deal of evidence to support this theory. A father's drug habit at the time of conception may influence the outcome of a pregnancy. Evidence is scanty, but there does appear to be an effect. Why take the chance?

৵ *Do You Take Paxil?*

If you take the antidepressant Paxil, discuss its use with your doctor. The charity MIND is campaigning for its licence to be withdrawn, and

Some Pollutants to Avoid during Pregnancy

Lead

The toxicity of lead has been known for centuries. In the past, most lead exposure came from the atmosphere. Today, exposure may come from many sources, including some petrol (now regulated), water pipes, solders, storage batteries, construction materials, paints, dyes and wood preservatives.

Lead is easily transported across the placenta to the baby. Toxicity can occur as early as the 12th week of pregnancy, which could result in lead poisoning in the baby. Avoid exposure to lead. If you might be exposed in your workplace, discuss it with your doctor.

Mercury

Mercury has a long history as a potential poison to a pregnant woman. Reports of fish contaminated with mercury have been linked to cerebral palsy and microcephaly.

PCBs

Our environment has been significantly contaminated with polychlorinated biphenyls (PCBs). PCBs are mixtures of several chemical compounds.

Most fish, birds and humans now have measurable amounts of PCBs in their tissues. Some experts have suggested that pregnant women limit their intake of fish (to avoid exposure to mercury and PCBs), particularly if a woman is exposed to PCBs where she works. See the discussion of fish in Week 26.

Pesticides

Pesticides cover a large number of agents used to control unwanted plants and animals. Human exposure is common because pesticides are used extensively. Those of most concern contain several agents—DDT, chlordane, heptachlor, lindane and others.

research has shown that taking the medication during your third trimester could expose your baby to potential problems, including respiratory distress, jaundice and low blood sugar. Although these problems are usually temporary, why take the risk? Other treatment options may be available, so ask your doctor about them. You may need to start other treatment options early in pregnancy.

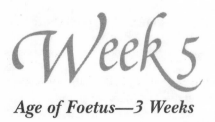

Week 5

Age of Foetus—3 Weeks

If you've just found out you're pregnant, you might
want to begin by reading the previous chapters.

How Big Is Your Baby?

Your developing baby hasn't grown a great deal. It's about 1.25 mm
(0.05 in) long.

How Big Are You?

At this point, there are still no big changes in you. Even if you are
aware you're pregnant, it will be awhile before others notice your
changing figure.

How Your Baby Is Growing and Developing

As early as this week, a plate that will later become the heart has developed. The central nervous system (brain and spinal cord), and muscle

and bone formation are beginning to take shape. During this time, your baby's skeleton is also starting to form.

Changes in You

Many changes are occurring now. You may be aware of some of them; others will be evident only after some kind of test.

✐ *Pregnancy Tests*

Home pregnancy tests have become more sensitive, which makes early diagnosis of pregnancy more common. Tests detect the presence of *human chorionic gonadotropin* (HCG), a hormone of early pregnancy. A pregnancy test can be positive before you have even missed a period!

Many tests can provide positive results (you are pregnant) 10 days after you become pregnant. You might want to wait until you have missed a period before investing money and emotional energy in pregnancy tests, whether done at a hospital, in a clinic or at home. The best time to take a home pregnancy test is the first day *after your missed period* or any time thereafter. If you take the test too early, you may get a false-negative result, meaning you are really pregnant when the test says you're not! False-negative results occur for 50 per cent of the women who take the test *too early.*

Dad Tip Clean or vacuum the house without being asked.

Most home tests range in price from £8 to £15. They vary in how effective they are in helping you 'diagnose' your pregnancy. Hospitals, GP practices and clinics offer free pregnancy testing, which can save you some money.

✐ *Nausea and Vomiting*

An early symptom of pregnancy for some women is nausea, with or without vomiting; it is often called *morning sickness.* The condition affects nearly 70 per cent of all pregnant women. Whether it occurs in the

morning or later in the day, it usually starts early and improves throughout the day as you become active. Morning sickness can begin around
the 6th week of pregnancy. Take heart—morning sickness usually improves and disappears around the end of the first trimester (week 13).
Hang in there, and keep in mind that this condition is temporary.

Many women have nausea. It doesn't usually cause enough trouble
to require medical attention. However, a condition called *hyperemesis
gravidarum* (severe nausea and vomiting) causes a great deal of vomiting, which results in loss of nutrients and fluid. The pregnant woman is
often treated in the hospital with intravenous fluids and medications.
Hypnosis has also been used successfully in treating the problem.

If you experience severe nausea and vomiting, if you cannot eat or
drink anything or if you feel so ill that you cannot carry on your daily
activities, call your doctor or local community midwives. Your first antenatal appointment may not be scheduled for a while, but there's no
reason you should suffer. There may be some simple suggestions your
doctor or midwife can offer that will help. Reassurances that this situation is normal and your baby is OK can be comforting.

There is no completely successful treatment for the normal nausea
and vomiting of pregnancy. A pill to help relieve the symptoms of
morning sickness marketed in the UK under the name Debendox is
available once again in the United
States. Sold under the trade name
Bendectin, it was removed in the
early 1980s because some claimed
it caused birth defects. However,
studies have not supported these
claims and have actually proved it
is safe to use during pregnancy. As
yet, however, it is unavailable in the UK.

Tip for Week 5

**Precaution: Be careful about using
over-the-counter cough and cold
remedies. Many contain alcohol—
some as much as 25 per cent.**

Acupressure, acupuncture and massage may also prove helpful in
dealing with nausea and vomiting. Acupressure wristbands, worn for
motion and seasickness, help some women feel better.

You may have heard about acupressure wrist bands that can help some women with nausea. Another device that goes beyond acupressure is available in the US and via the Internet. This band has been on the market since 1997 and has been used to relieve motion sickness and the nausea and vomiting many people experience with chemotherapy. A new study shows it also works to help relieve morning sickness.

Patented and sold under the name *ReliefBand*, it is about the size of a large watch and worn like a wristwatch on the inside of your wrist. Using gentle electrical signals, it stimulates the nerves in the wrist; this stimulation is believed to interfere with messages between the brain and stomach that cause nausea. It has various stimulation levels that allow you to adjust signals for maximum control for your individual comfort. It can be used when nausea begins, or you can wear it before you feel ill. This device does not interfere with eating or drinking. It is water resistant and shock resistant, so you can wear it just about any time!

This is an extremely important period in the development of your baby. Don't expose your unborn baby to herbs, over-the-counter treatments or any other 'remedies' for nausea that are not known to be safe during pregnancy. Discuss different ways to deal with nausea with your doctor or midwife.

Some Actions You Can Take. Eat small meals more frequently to help you feel better. Experts agree that you should eat what appeals to you—foods that are appealing may be the ones you can keep down more easily right now. If that means jam doughnuts and orange squash, go for it! Some women find that protein foods settle more easily in their stomachs; these foods include cheese, eggs, peanut butter and non-fatty meats. Also see the discussion in the Nutrition section.

Be sure you keep up your fluid intake, even if you can't keep food down. Dehydration is a lot more serious than not eating for a while. If you vomit a great deal, you may want to choose fluids that contain electrolytes to help replace those you lose when you vomit. Ask your doctor or midwife what fluids he or she recommends.

Be Prepared for Morning Sickness!

It may be a good idea to carry your own 'morning sickness' emergency travelling bag. You may find it comes in handy, especially if you suffer from nausea and vomiting throughout the day. In a sturdy bag, pack along some opaque plastic bags (plastic grocery sacks are a good choice) without holes, wet wipes, tissue or napkins to wipe your face and mouth, a small bottle of water to rinse your mouth and teeth, a toothbrush and toothpaste to brush away stomach acids and a small bottle of breath spray or breath mints. With your emergency bag along, you'll feel confident you can handle this temporary side effect of pregnancy, no matter where you are.

If You're Absent from Work. If morning sickness causes you to be absent from your job, you do *not* need a doctor's note verifying the problem unless you are absent for more than 7 days.

Other Changes You May Notice

In early pregnancy, you may need to urinate frequently. It can continue during most of your pregnancy and become particularly annoying near delivery, as your uterus enlarges and puts pressure on your bladder.

You may notice changes in your breasts. Tingling or soreness in the breasts or nipples is common. You may also see a darkening of the areola or an elevation of the glands around the nipple. See Week 13 for more information on how your breasts are affected by pregnancy.

Another early symptom of pregnancy is fatigue or tiring easily. This common symptom may continue throughout pregnancy. Be sure to take your prenatal vitamins and any other medications prescribed by your doctor, and get enough rest. If you experience fatigue, avoid sugar and caffeine; either can make the problem worse.

How Your Actions
Affect Your Baby's Development

◌ *When Should You Visit the Doctor/Midwife?*

One of the first questions you may ask yourself when you suspect you're pregnant is, 'When should I see my doctor/midwife?'

Good antenatal care is necessary for the health of the baby and mother-to-be. Make an appointment to see your doctor as soon as you are reasonably sure you're pregnant. This could be as early as a few days after a missed period.

◌ *Getting Pregnant while Using Birth Control*

If you have been using some type of birth control, tell your doctor. No method is 100 per cent effective. Occasionally a method fails, even oral contraceptives. If you are sure you're pregnant, stop taking the pill and set up an appointment as soon as possible. Don't become overly alarmed if this happens to you; talk to your doctor about it.

Pregnancy can also occur with an intrauterine device (IUD) in place. If this happens, see your doctor immediately. Discuss whether the IUD should be removed or left in place. In most cases, an attempt is made to remove the IUD. If left in place, the risk of miscarriage increases slightly.

Spermicides used alone, or with a condom, sponge or diaphragm, may be in use when pregnancy occurs. They have not been shown to be harmful to a developing baby.

Your Nutrition

As discussed previously, you may have to deal with nausea and vomiting during pregnancy. Not every woman suffers from it, but many women do. The same hormone—HCG (human chorionic gonadotropin)—that makes a home pregnancy test change colour causes morning sickness. If you suffer this discomfort, you may be happy to know that HCG levels taper off near the end of the first trimester, so your nausea and vomiting should improve then. If you experience morning sickness, try some of the following suggestions.

- Eat small meals frequently to keep your stomach from being over-full.
- Drink lots of fluid.
- Find out what foods, smells or situations make you nauseated. Avoid them when possible.
- Avoid coffee because it stimulates stomach acid.
- A high-protein snack before bed may help stabilize blood sugar.
- Sometimes a high-carbohydrate snack before bed helps.
- Ask your partner to make you some dry toast in the morning before you get up; eat it in bed. Or keep crackers or dry cereal near the bed to nibble on before you get up in the morning. They help absorb stomach acid.
- Keep your bedroom cool at night, and air it out often. Cool, fresh air may help you feel better.
- Get out of bed slowly.
- If you take an iron supplement, take it an hour before meals or 2 hours after a meal.
- Nibble on raw ginger, or pour boiling water over it and sip the 'tea.'
- Salty foods help some women with nausea.
- Lemonade and watermelon may help alleviate symptoms.

ॐ *Weight Gain during Pregnancy*

The amount of weight women gain during pregnancy varies greatly. It may actually range from weight loss to a total gain of 22.5 kg (50 lb) or more.

We know complications increase at the extremes of these weight changes. Because of this, it's difficult to set one figure as an 'ideal' weight gain during pregnancy. How much weight you gain is affected by your weight before you became pregnant. Many experts quote a weight-gain figure of 285 g (10 oz) a week until 20 weeks, then 450 g (1 lb) a week from 20 to 40 weeks.

Other researchers have suggested weight-gain amounts acceptable for underweight, normal weight and overweight women. See the box to the right.

If you have any questions about your weight gain during pregnancy, discuss them with your doctor/midwife. He or she will advise you on how much weight you should gain during your pregnancy.

Average Pregnancy Weight Gain	
Body Type	Acceptable Gain
Underweight	13 to 18 kg (28 to 40 lb)
Normal weight	11 to 16 kg (25 to 35 lb)
Overweight	7 to 11 kg (15 to 25 lb)

Dieting while you're pregnant is not a wise idea, but that doesn't mean you shouldn't watch your calorific intake. You should! It's important for your baby to get proper nutrition from the foods you eat. Choose foods for the nutrition they provide for you and your growing baby.

You Should Also Know

✋ *What Sex Will Your Baby Be?*
You can guess the sex of your child as well as your doctor—often better! As we've mentioned, the sex of your baby is determined when the egg is fertilized by the baby's father's sperm.

Many couples ask for ways to 'get a boy' or 'get a girl' before they try to get pregnant. In a few cases, and only for medical reasons, sperm separation is used. Male and female sperm are separated, and artificial insemination deposits the selected sperm in the woman. It's not a foolproof method, and it is expensive. This procedure may be done when there is a sex-specific problem, such as a family history of haemophilia or Duchenne muscular dystrophy.

✋ *Ectopic Pregnancy*
As described in Weeks 1 & 2, fertilization occurs in the Fallopian tube. The fertilized egg travels through the tube to the uterus, where it implants on the cavity wall. An *ectopic pregnancy* occurs when the

egg implants outside the uterine cavity, usually in the tube itself. Ninety-five per cent of all ectopic pregnancies occur in the tube (hence the term *tubal pregnancy*). Other possible sites of implantation are the ovary, cervix or other places in the abdomen. The illustration on the opposite page shows some possible locations of an ectopic pregnancy.

In the UK, ectopics happen in about 0.25 to 1 per cent of all pregnancies. It is, however, becoming more common. Researchers believe STDs (sexually transmitted diseases) are the cause, especially chlamydia and gonorrhoea. If you have had an STD in the past, tell your doctor at your first antenatal visit. And be sure to tell him or her if you have had a previous ectopic pregnancy.

Ectopic pregnancy occurs in 1 of every 100 pregnancies. Chances of an ectopic pregnancy occurring increase with damage to the Fallopian tubes from pelvic inflammatory disease (PID), from other infections, such as a ruptured appendix, from infertility, endometriosis, sexually transmitted diseases and prior tubal or abdominal surgery. Other factors that contribute to an increased risk of ectopic pregnancy include smoking, exposure to DES (diethylstilbestrol) during your mother's pregnancy and increase in a mother-to-be's age. If you have had a previous ectopic pregnancy, there is a 12 per cent chance of recurrence. Use of an intrauterine device (IUD) also increases the chance of ectopic pregnancy.

✄ *Symptoms of an Ectopic Pregnancy*
Symptoms of ectopic pregnancy, which occur in the first 12 weeks of pregnancy, include:

- cramps
- tenderness in the lower abdomen
- bleeding or brown spotting
- shoulder pain, caused by blood from the ruptured tube irritating the peritoneum in the area between the chest and stomach
- weakness, dizziness or fainting, caused by blood loss
- nausea

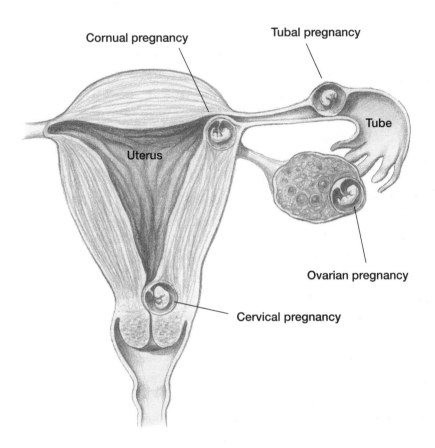

Possible locations of an ectopic (tubal) pregnancy.

It may be difficult for your doctor to diagnose an ectopic pregnancy because many of these symptoms can be present in a normal pregnancy.

Diagnosing Ectopic Pregnancy. To test for an ectopic pregnancy, human chorionic gonadotropin (HCG) is measured. The test is called a *quantitative HCG*. The level of HCG increases rapidly in a normal pregnancy and doubles in value about every 2 days. If HCG levels do not increase as they should, an abnormal pregnancy is suspected. In the case of an ectopic pregnancy, the woman may have a high HCG level with no sign by ultrasound of a pregnancy inside the uterus.

Ultrasound testing is helpful in diagnosing an ectopic pregnancy. (We discuss ultrasound in detail in Week 11.) A tubal pregnancy may be visible in the tube during ultrasound examination. Doctors may see blood in the abdomen from rupture and bleeding or a mass in the area of the Fallopian tube or the ovary.

Our ability to diagnose an ectopic pregnancy has improved with use of laparoscopy. Tiny incisions are made in the area of the bellybutton and in the lower-abdominal area. Doctors view the inside of the abdomen and the pelvic organs with a small instrument called a *laparoscope*. They can see an ectopic pregnancy if one is present.

An attempt is made to diagnose a tubal pregnancy before it ruptures and damages the tube, which could make it necessary to remove the entire tube. Early diagnosis also attempts to avoid the risk of internal bleeding from a ruptured, bleeding tube.

Most ectopic pregnancies are detected around 6 to 8 weeks of pregnancy. The key in early diagnosis involves communication between you and your doctor about any symptoms and their severity.

Treatment for Ectopic Pregnancy. With an ectopic pregnancy, the doctor's goal is to remove the pregnancy while preserving fertility. Surgical treatment requires general anaesthesia, laparoscopy or laparotomy (a larger incision and no scope) and recovery from surgery. In many instances, it is necessary to remove the Fallopian tube, which affects future fertility.

A non-surgical treatment of an unruptured ectopic pregnancy involves the use of a cancer drug, methotrexate. Methotrexate is given intraveneously in the hospital or at an outpatient clinic. Methotrexate is cytotoxic; it terminates the pregnancy. HCG levels should decrease after this treatment, which indicates the pregnancy has been terminated. Symptoms should improve.

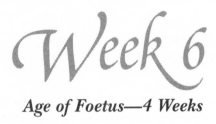

Week 6

Age of Foetus—4 Weeks

If you've just found out you're pregnant, you might want to begin by reading the previous chapters.

How Big Is Your Baby?

The crown-to-rump length of your growing baby is 2 to 4 mm (0.08 to 0.16 in). *Crown-to-rump* is the sitting height or distance from the top of the baby's head to its rump or buttocks. This measurement is used more often than crown-to-heel length because the baby's legs are most often bent, making that determination difficult.

Occasionally, with the proper equipment, a heartbeat can be seen on ultrasound by the 6th week. Ultrasound is discussed in detail in Week 11.

How Big Are You?

You may have gained some weight by now. If you have been nauseated and not eating well, you may have lost weight. You have been pregnant for 1 month, which is enough time to notice some changes in your body. If this is your first pregnancy, your abdomen may not have changed much. Or you may notice your clothes are getting a little tighter around the waist. You may be gaining weight in your legs or other places, such as your breasts.

How Your Baby Is Growing and Developing

This is the beginning of the *embryonic period* (from conception to week 10 of pregnancy; or from conception to week 8 of foetal development). It is a period of extremely important development in your baby! At this time, the embryo is most susceptible to factors that can interfere with its development. Most malformations originate during this critical period.

As the illustration on page 78 shows, the result of this growth is a body form showing the head and tail area. Around this time, the neural groove closes and early brain chambers form. The eyes are also forming, and limb buds appear. The heart tubes fuse, and heart contractions begin. This can be seen on ultrasound.

Changes in You

✺ *Heartburn*

Heartburn discomfort *(pyrosis)* is one of the most common complaints of pregnancy. It may begin early, although generally it becomes more severe later in pregnancy. It is usually caused by the backing up *(reflux)* of gastric and duodenal contents into the oesophagus. This occurs more frequently during pregnancy for two reasons—food moves more slowly through the intestines and the stomach is compressed as the uterus enlarges and moves up into the abdomen.

Symptoms are not severe for most women. Eat small, frequent meals, and avoid some positions, such as bending over or lying flat. One sure way to get heartburn is to eat a large meal, then lie down! (This is true for anyone, not just pregnant women.)

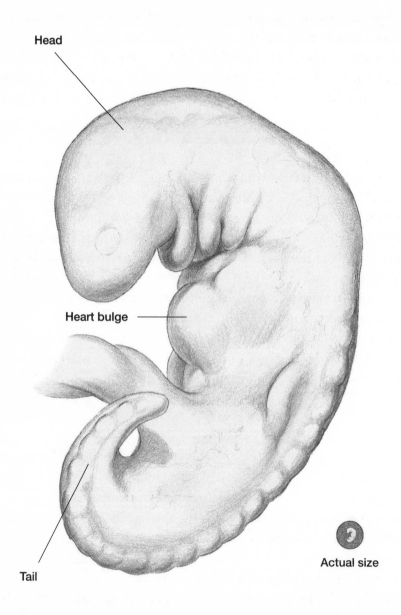

Head

Heart bulge

Tail

Actual size

Embryo at 6 weeks of pregnancy (foetal age—4 weeks). It is growing rapidly.

Some antacids provide considerable relief, including aluminum hydroxide, magnesium trisilicate and magnesium hydroxide. Follow your doctor's advice or the instructions on the packet relating to pregnancy. Don't overdo taking antacids! Avoid sodium bicarbonate because it contains excessive amounts of sodium that may cause you to retain water.

ᢌ *Constipation*
Your bowel habits will probably change during pregnancy. Most women notice some constipation, often accompanied by irregular bowel movements. Haemorrhoids may occur more often (see Week 14).

You can help avoid constipation problems during pregnancy. Increase your fluid intake. Exercise also helps. Many doctors suggest a mild laxative, such as milk of magnesia or prune juice, if you have problems. Certain foods, such as bran and prunes, can increase the bulk in your diet, which may help relieve constipation.

Do not use laxatives, other than those mentioned, without your doctor's OK. If constipation is a continuing problem, discuss treatment at an antenatal visit. Try not to strain when you have a bowel movement, if you are constipated. Straining can lead to haemorrhoids.

How Your Actions Affect Your Baby's Development

During pregnancy, a sexually transmitted disease can harm your growing baby. Take care of any STD as soon as possible!

ᢌ *Genital Herpes Simplex Infection*
Often a herpes infection during pregnancy is a reinfection, not a primary infection. Infection in the mother is associated with higher risks of premature delivery and low-birthweight infants. If a pregnant woman has an outbreak, which is not the first episode, her baby's risk of being infected during delivery is very low. However,

when membranes rupture, an active infection can travel upwards towards the uterus. If there are active herpes lesions in or near the birth canal near or at the time of labour, a caesarean section may be done to protect the baby. Most women can have a normal delivery if theirs is not a primary infection and if they do not have signs of active infection with the virus during this time.

✌ Yeast Infections (Monilial Vulvovaginitis)

Yeast (monilial) infections are more common in pregnant women than in non-pregnant women. They have no major negative effect on pregnancy, but they may cause you discomfort and anxiety.

Yeast infections are sometimes harder to control when you're pregnant. They may require frequent retreatment or longer treatment (10 to 14 days instead of 3 to 7 days). Creams used for treatment are usually safe during pregnancy. Your partner does not need to be treated.

A newborn infant can get thrush after passing through a birth canal infected with monilial vulvovaginitis. Treatment with nystatin is effective. Avoid the use of fluconazole (Diflucan); it may not be safe to use during pregnancy.

✌ Trichomonal Vaginitis

This infection has no major effects on pregnancy. However, a problem in treatment may arise because some doctors believe metronidazole, the drug of choice, shouldn't be taken in the first trimester of pregnancy. Most doctors will prescribe metronidazole for a bad infection after the first trimester.

✌ HPV—Human Papillomavirus (Condyloma Acuminata)

Human papillomavirus (HPV) is the virus that causes venereal warts, also called *condyloma acuminata*. Some strains of HPV cause genital warts; some strains of genital warts can lead to cancer of the cervix and cancer of the genitals.

If you do have genital warts, tell your doctor at your first antenatal appointment. During pregnancy, certain treatments, such as laser ablation or acids, should be avoided. Discuss the problem with your doctor.

If you have extensive venereal warts, a Caesarean delivery may be necessary to avoid heavy bleeding. Warty skin tags often enlarge during pregnancy. In rare instances, they have blocked the vagina at the time of delivery. Infants have also been known to get *laryngeal papillomas* (small benign tumours on the vocal cords) after delivery.

↜ *Gonorrhoea*

Gonorrhoea presents risks to a woman and her partner, and to her baby when it passes through the birth canal. The baby may contract *gonorrhoeal ophthalmia*, a severe eye infection. Eye drops are used in newborns to prevent this problem. Other infections may also result. Gonorrhoeal infections in the mother are treated with penicillin or other medications that are safe to use during pregnancy.

↜ *Syphilis*

Detection of a syphilis infection is important for you, your partner and your growing baby. Fortunately this rare infection is also treatable. If you notice any open sore on your genitals during pregnancy, have your doctor check it. Syphilis can be treated effectively with penicillin and other medications that are safe to use in pregnancy.

↜ *Chlamydia*

You may have heard or read about chlamydia. It is the cause of more sexually transmitted diseases in the UK than any other organism. In 1999, there were 32,544 known new infections in women, though the actual number may be up to 90 per cent higher because in many cases the bacterium does not cause any symptoms. Infection is caused by a germ that invades certain types of healthy cells. Infection may be passed through sexual activity, including oral sex.

Between 20 and 40 per cent of all sexually active women have probably been exposed to chlamydia at some time. Infection can cause serious problems if left untreated, but these problems can be avoided with treatment.

Chlamydia is most likely to occur in young people who have more than one sexual partner. It may also occur in women who have other sexually transmitted diseases. Some doctors believe chlamydia occurs more commonly in women who take oral contraceptives. Barrier methods of contraception, such as diaphragms and condoms used with spermicides, may offer protection from infection.

One of the most significant complications of chlamydia is pelvic inflammatory disease (PID), a severe infection of the upper genital organs involving the uterus, the Fallopian tubes and even the ovaries. There may be pelvic pain, or there may be no symptoms at all. PID can result from an untreated infection that spreads throughout the pelvic area. Chlamydia is one of the main causes of PID. If a PID infection is prolonged or recurrent, the reproductive organs, Fallopian tubes and uterus may be damaged, with formation of adhesions. Surgery may be required to repair them. If tubes are damaged, scar tissue can increase the risk of ectopic (tubal) pregnancy and may make it harder to get pregnant (infertility).

Chlamydia in Pregnancy. During pregnancy, a mother-to-be can pass the infection to her baby as it comes through the birth canal and vagina. The baby has a 20 to 50 per cent chance of getting chlamydia if the mother has it. It may cause an eye infection, but that is easily treated. Complications that are more serious include pneumonia, which may require hospitalization of the baby.

Research has shown that chlamydial infection may be linked to ectopic pregnancy. One study showed 70 per cent of the women studied who had an ectopic pregnancy also had chlamydia. If a woman is trying to get pregnant, she may want to be screened for this STD, which can be treated easily.

Tip for Week 6 If you have questions between your antenatal visits, call your doctor's surgery or your midwife. It's OK to call; as a matter of fact, your carer *wants* you to call to get correct medical information. You'll probably feel more comfortable when your questions are answered.

Testing for Chlamydia. Chlamydia can be detected by a cell culture, but as we've said, more than half of those infected have no symptoms. Symptoms that may appear include burning or itching in the genital area, discharge from the vagina, painful or frequent urination, or pain in the pelvic area. Men may also experience symptoms. Rapid diagnostic tests can be done in the doctor's surgery. They can provide a result quickly, possibly even before you go home.

Chlamydia is usually treated with tetracycline, but this drug should not be given to a pregnant woman. During pregnancy, erythromycin may be the drug of choice. After treatment, your doctor may want to do another culture to make sure the infection is gone. If you're concerned about a possible chlamydial infection, discuss it at a antenatal visit. Your doctor will advise you.

ˣˀ *HIV and AIDS*

HIV (human immunodeficiency virus) is the virus that causes AIDS (acquired immune deficiency syndrome). In 1997, 265 mothers in the UK were known to be HIV positive and as a result about 50 babies were born with the virus. By the end of June 2003 a total of 3,584 children born to HIV infected mothers had been reported. Research has shown that an infected woman can pass the virus to her baby as early as the 8th week of pregnancy. It is important to tell your doctor if you are HIV positive or think you might be.

The exact number of people infected with HIV is unknown. Currently it is estimated that 41,200 people in the UK are living with HIV/AIDS, about 30 per cent of whom are undiagnosed.

Women at greatest risk include current or former intravenous drug users and women whose sexual partners have used drugs intravenously or engaged in bisexual activities. Women with sexually transmitted diseases, those who engage in prostitution or those who received blood transfusions before screening began are also at higher risk. If you are unsure about your risk, seek counselling about testing for the AIDS virus.

A woman infected with HIV may not have symptoms. There may be a period of weeks or months when tests do not reveal the presence of the virus. In most cases, antibodies can be detected 6 to 12 weeks after exposure. In some cases, this latent period can be as long as 18 months. Once the test is positive, a person may remain free of symptoms for a variable amount of time. For every patient with AIDS, we believe there are 20 to 30 infected individuals who have no symptoms.

There is no evidence of transmission through casual contact with water, food or environmental surfaces. There is no evidence the virus can be transmitted with Anti-D. (See Week 16.) A mother can pass HIV to her baby before birth or during its birth. We know that 90 per cent of all cases of HIV in children are due to transmission related to pregnancy—mother to baby during pregnancy, childbirth or breastfeeding.

Pregnancy may hide some AIDS symptoms, which makes the disease harder to discover. Because the illness can be a serious threat to an unborn child, counselling and psychological support are critical.

There is some positive news for women who suffer from AIDS. We know if a woman is in the early course of the illness, she may have an uneventful pregnancy, labour and delivery. Her baby has a risk of being infected during pregnancy, birth or breastfeeding. However, research shows that the risk of a woman infected with HIV passing the virus to her baby can now be greatly reduced and nearly eliminated. If she takes AZT during pregnancy and has a Caesarean delivery, she reduces the risk of passing the virus to about 2 per cent! Studies have not found any birth defects linked to the use of these medications. However, if an infection is left untreated, there's a 25 per cent chance her baby will be born with the virus.

Testing for AIDS. Testing comprises two tests—the ELISA test and the Western Blot test. The ELISA is a screening test. If positive, it should be confirmed by the Western Blot test. Both tests involve testing blood to measure antibodies to the virus, not the virus itself. No test should be considered positive until the Western Blot test is done. It is believed to be more than 99 per cent sensitive and specific.

HIV/AIDS and Pregnancy. If you are HIV positive, expect more blood tests during pregnancy. These tests help your doctor assess how well you are doing as a pregnant woman. Breastfeeding is not recommended for women who are HIV positive. However, pasteurised breastmilk does not contain the virus. The pasteuriser costs approximately £50.

Your Nutrition

To get the nutrition you need during your pregnancy, you must be selective in your food choices. You *cannot* eat whatever you want. Eating the right foods, in the correct amounts, takes planning. Eat foods high in vitamins and minerals, especially iron, calcium, magnesium, folic acid and zinc. You also need fibre and fluids to help alleviate any constipation problems.

Some of the foods you should eat, and the amounts of each, are listed below. You should try to eat these foods every day. Ways to get enough of each food group are discussed in the following weeks. Check out each weekly discussion for nutrition tips. Foods to help your baby grow and develop include:

Understanding Serving Portions of the Food Pyramid

Many people today overeat because they do not understand what constitutes a 'portion' or 'serving,' as determined by the Food Pyramid. You may believe it will be difficult for you to eat all the portions you need for the health of your growing baby.

To learn the *correct* serving size for each of the food groups, as listed below, ask your doctor for some guidelines. For example, a 100-g (3½-oz) serving of breakfast cereal can actually be *three* grain servings!

- bread, cereal, pasta and rice—at least 6 servings/day
- fruits—3 to 4 servings/day
- vegetables—4 servings/day
- meat and other protein sources—2 to 3 servings/day
- dairy products—3 to 4 servings/day
- fats, sweets and other 'empty' calorie foods—2 to 3 servings/day

You Should Also Know

↜ Your First Visit to the Doctor/Midwife
Your first antenatal visit may be one of your longest. There's a lot to accomplish. If you saw your doctor before you got pregnant, you may have already discussed some of your concerns.

Feel free to ask questions to get an idea of how your doctor/midwife will relate to you and your needs. This is important as your pregnancy progresses. During pregnancy, there should be an exchange of ideas. Consider what your doctor/midwife suggests and why. It's important to share your feelings and ideas. Your doctor/midwife has experience that can be valuable to you during pregnancy.

What Will Happen? What should you expect at this first visit? First, your doctor or midwife will ask for a history of your medical health. This includes general medical problems and any problems relating to your gynaecological and obstetrical history. He or she will ask about your periods and recent birth-control methods. If you've had an abortion or a miscarriage, or if you've been in the hospital for surgery or for some other reason, it's important information. If you have old medical records, bring them with you.

Your doctor needs to know about any medication you take or any medication you are allergic to. Your family's medical history may also be important, such as the occurrence of diabetes or other chronic illness.

Laboratory tests may be done at this first visit or on a subsequent visit. If you have questions, ask them. If you think you may have a 'high-risk' pregnancy, discuss it with your doctor/midwife.

$Dad Tip$ **Bring home her favourite dinner, or cook it yourself, if she's not suffering a lot of nausea and/or vomiting.**

Under new guidelines issued at the end of 2003, first-time mothers will see their family doctor or midwife 10 times rather than the traditional 14 (where mothers were asked to return every 4 weeks for the first 7 months, then every 2 weeks until the last month, then every week), and those who already have children will have only 7 such checks. If problems arise, however, you may be scheduled for more frequent visits.

Ways to Have a Great Pregnancy

Every woman wants to have a happy, healthy pregnancy. Start now to help ensure that yours will be the best it can be! Try the following.

Prioritize—Examine what you need to do to help yourself and your growing baby. Do what you need to do, decide what else you can do and let the rest go.

Involve others in your pregnancy —When you include your partner, other family members and friends in your pregnancy, it helps them understand what you are going through so they can be more understanding and supportive.

Treat others with respect and love—You may be having a hard time, especially at the beginning of your pregnancy. You may have morning sickness. You may find adjusting to the role of 'mum-to-be' difficult. People will understand if you take the time to let them know how you feel. Show respect and appreciation for their concern. Treat them with kindness and love, and they will respond in kind.

Create memories—It takes some planning, but it is definitely worth it. When you're pregnant, it seems like it will go on forever. However, speaking from experience, we can tell you it passes very quickly and is soon a memory. Take steps to document the many changes that are occurring in your life right now. Include your partner in all this. Have him jot down some of his thoughts and feelings. Take his picture, too! You'll be able to look back and share the highs and lows with him, and in the years ahead, you and your kids will be glad you did.

Relax when you can—Easing the stress in your life is very important now. Do things that help you relax and focus on what is important in your lives right now.

Enjoy this time of preparation—All too soon your pregnancy will be over, and you'll be a new mother, with all the responsibilities of being a mum and a partner! You may have other responsibilities, too, in your professional or personal life. This is a time to concentrate on your couple relationship and on the many changes you will be experiencing in the near future.

Focus on the positive—You may hear negative things from friends or family members, such as scary stories or sad tales. Ignore them. Most pregnancies work out fine!

Don't be afraid to ask for help—Your pregnancy is important to others, too. Friends and family will be pleased if you ask them to be involved.

Get information—There are many sources today, such as books, magazine articles, television programmes, radio interviews and the Internet.

Smile—You're part of a very special miracle that is happening to you and your partner!

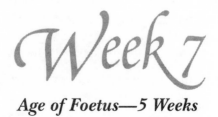

Week 7

Age of Foetus—5 Weeks

If you've just found out you're pregnant, you might
want to begin by reading the previous chapters.

How Big Is Your Baby?

Your baby goes through an incredible growth spurt this week! At the
beginning of the 7th week, the crown-to-rump length of your growing
baby is 4 to 5 mm (0.16 to 0.2 in). This is about the size of a cap gun
pellet. By the end of the week, your baby has more than doubled in
size, to about 1.1 to 1.3 cm (½ in).

How Big Are You?

Although you are probably quite anxious to show the world you're
pregnant, there still may be little noticeable change. Changes will come
soon, though.

How Your Baby Is
Growing and Developing

Leg buds are beginning to appear as short fins. As you can see on page 90, arm buds have grown longer; they have divided into a hand segment and an arm-shoulder segment. The hand and foot have a digital plate where the fingers and toes will develop.

The heart bulges from the body. By this time, it has divided into right and left heart chambers. The primary *bronchi* are present in the lungs; bronchi are air passages in the lungs. The cerebral hemispheres, which make up the brain, are also growing. Eyes and nostrils are developing.

Intestines are developing, and the appendix is present. The pancreas, which produces the hormone insulin, is also present. Part of the intestine bulges into the umbilical cord. Later in your baby's development, it will return to the abdomen.

Changes in You

Changes are occurring gradually. You still probably won't 'show,' and people won't be able to tell you're pregnant unless you tell them. You may be gaining weight throughout your body, but you should have gained only a kilogram or so (a couple of pounds) this early in your pregnancy.

If you haven't gained weight or if you have lost a little, it isn't unusual. It will go the other direction in the weeks to come. You may still be experiencing morning sickness and other symptoms of early pregnancy.

How Your Actions
Affect Your Baby's Development

～ *Using Over-the-Counter Medications and Preparations*
Many people don't consider over-the-counter (OTC) preparations as medication, and they take them at will, pregnant or not. Some

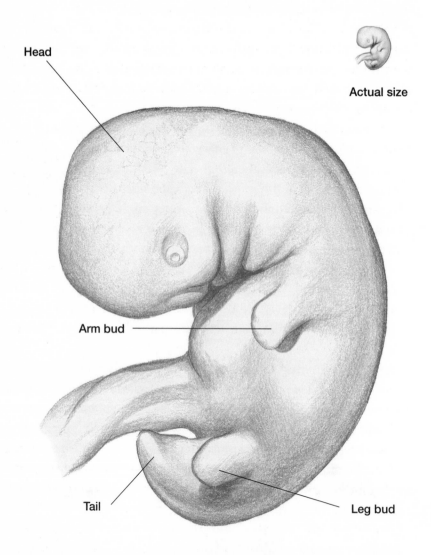

Head

Actual size

Arm bud

Tail

Leg bud

Your baby's brain is growing and developing. The heart has divided into right and left chambers.

researchers believe non-prescription, or over-the-counter, medication usage actually *increases* during pregnancy.

OTC medications and preparations may not be safe during pregnancy. Use them with as much caution as any other drug! Many over-the-counter preparations are combinations of medications. For example, pain medication can contain aspirin, caffeine and phenacetin. Cough syrups or sleep medications can contain as much as 25 per cent alcohol. This is no different than drinking wine or beer during pregnancy.

Tip for Week 7 Don't take any over-the-counter medications for longer than 48 hours without consulting your doctor. If a problem doesn't resolve, your doctor may have another treatment plan for you.

There are quite a few OTC medications to be careful with during pregnancy, including ibuprofen (Motrin, Nurofen), naproxen (Naprosyn), ketoprofen (Orudis), famotidine (Pepcid), cimetidine (Tagamet), hydrocortisone and any medication containing iodine. Because experience with use of these medications during pregnancy is limited, it's best to avoid them. Take them *only* under the supervision of your doctor.

Read packet labels and packet inserts about safety during pregnancy—nearly all medications contain this information. Some antacids contain sodium bicarbonate, which increases your intake of sodium (this can be important to avoid if you have water-retention problems). Antacids can also cause constipation and increased gas. Some antacids contain aluminum, which can cause constipation and affect the metabolism of other minerals (phosphate). Others contain magnesium; excessive use of these may cause magnesium poisoning.

Some over-the-counter medications and preparations can be used safely during pregnancy, if you use them wisely. Check the list below:

- analgesics and pain relievers—paracetamol (Panadol)
- decongestants—chlophenamine (Piriton)
- nasal spray decongestants—oxymetazoline (Dristan Long-Lasting)

- cough medicine—dextromethorphan (Robitussin; Vicks Medinite)
- stomach relief—antacids (Maalox, milk of magnesia)
- throat relief—throat lozenges
- laxatives—bulk-fibre laxatives (Celevac)

If you think your symptoms or discomfort are more severe than they should be, call your doctor/midwife. Follow his or her advice. In addition, take good care of yourself. Exercise, eat correctly and keep a positive mental attitude about your pregnancy.

Using Paracetamol

Most doctors and researchers believe paracetamol is OK to use during pregnancy. It's hard to avoid because the drug is in over 200 products! However, recent studies have found that it is easy to overdose on the medication because it *is* in so many medications. You may not be aware that paracetamol is contained in various products you may take to treat a single problem. Taking multiple products to treat a condition or illness could be dangerous. *Always read labels* if you are thinking about taking more than one product to help relieve your symptoms. For example, take only *one* medication to treat a cold or flu symptoms, and always take the correct dose!

Your Nutrition

Dairy products can be very important to you during pregnancy. They contain calcium, which is important to you and your baby. They also contain vitamin D, which aids in calcium absorption.

Calcium helps keep your bones healthy, and baby needs it to develop strong bones and teeth. Other important reasons to get enough calcium in your diet are it may help prevent high blood pressure, and it may also lower your risk of pre-eclampsia. In addition, your body stores calcium in the latter part of pregnancy to draw on if you breastfeed.

✌ *How Much Calcium Do You Need?*

How much calcium should you take in each day? Recommended for pregnant women is 1200 mg a day (1½ times the recommended amount for non-pregnant women). Your prenatal vitamin supplies about 300 mg, so be sure you eat enough of the right foods to get the other 900 mg.

Read food labels for information on the calcium content of packaged foods. Keep track of the number of milligrams (mg) of calcium in the foods you eat. Every day, write down the amount of calcium in each of the foods you consume, and keep a running total to be sure you're getting 1200 mg each day.

✌ *Some Good Sources of Calcium*

Milk, cheese, yoghurt and ice cream are good calcium sources. Other foods that contain calcium include broccoli, pak choi, kale, spinach, salmon, sardines, chickpeas, sesame seeds, almonds, cooked dried beans, tofu and trout. Some foods are now calcium fortified, such as orange juice, breads, cereals and grains. Check your supermarket shelves.

Some dairy foods you may choose, and their serving sizes, include the following:

- cottage cheese—325 g (13 oz)
- processed cheese—55 g (2 oz)
- hard cheese (Parmesan or Romano)—25 g (1 oz)
- sardines, canned (with bones)—85 g (3 oz)
- milk—240 ml (8 fl oz)
- Cheddar—45 g (1½ oz)
- yoghurt (plain or flavoured)—240 ml (8 fl oz)

If you want to keep your calorie intake low, choose low-fat dairy products. Some choices include skimmed milk, low-fat yoghurt and low-fat cheese. Calcium content is unaffected in low-fat dairy products.

✃ *Other Ways to Get Calcium*

You can increase the amount of calcium in your diet in other ways. Add powdered non-fat milk to recipes, such as soup, mashed potatoes and meat loaf. Make fruit shakes with fresh fruit and milk; add a scoop of frozen yoghurt or ice cream. Cook rice and oatmeal in skimmed or semi-skimmed milk.

✃ *Some Precautions with Calcium*

Some foods interfere with the body's absorption of calcium. Salt, tea, coffee, protein and unleavened bread decrease the amount of calcium absorbed.

If your doctor decides you need calcium supplementation, calcium carbonate combined with magnesium (to aid calcium absorption) is a good choice. Avoid any supplement derived from animal bones, oyster shells or dolomite because it may contain lead.

Note: Your body cannot absorb more than 500 mg of calcium at a time, so spread your intake out over the course of the day. At breakfast, if your meal consists of calcium-fortified orange juice, calcium-fortified bread, cereal with milk and a carton of yoghurt, you may be taking in a lot more than 500 mg, but your body won't be able to absorb it.

Dad Tip Buy a present for your partner and the baby.

✃ *Calcium Supplement*

Some doctors prescribe calcium supplementation. Calcium is important for every pregnant woman. It helps build strong bones and teeth in the baby and helps keep your bones healthy. During pregnancy, you need 1200 to 1500 mg a day. That's about 3 to 4 glasses of skimmed milk a day.

✃ *Lactose Intolerance*

If you're lactose intolerant, there are still many sources of calcium available to you. As mentioned earlier, look for calcium-fortified products. Rice milk and soya milk can provide calcium and vitamin D. If you like cheese, hard cheeses, such as Cheddar, Gouda, Parmesan and Gruyère, contain a lower lactose content.

A Caution for Listeriosis

Avoid unpasteurized milk and any foods made from unpasteurized milk. Also avoid soft cheeses such as Camembert, Brie, feta and Roquefort. These products are a common source of *listeriosis,* a form of food poisoning. Undercooked poultry, red meat, seafood, deli meats and hot dogs can contain listeriosis. Cook all meat and seafood thoroughly before eating. Be careful about cross contamination of foods. If you place raw seafood or hot dogs on a counter or other surface during preparation, thoroughly wash the surface with soap and water or a disinfectant *before* you place any other food on that surface.

The medicines Milkaid and Lactrase (lactase enzyme), which are available from Biocare Ltd at www.biocare.co.uk, contain a natural enzyme that helps the body break down lactose, the complex sugar found in products and food. When lactose is not properly digested, it can cause gas, bloating, cramps and diarrhoea. There are no warnings or precautions for this medication during pregnancy; however, check with your doctor *before* you use it.

✌ *Do You Need Extra Iron?*

Nearly all diets that supply a sufficient number of calories for appropriate weight gain contain enough minerals (except iron) to prevent mineral deficiency. During pregnancy, your iron requirement increases. Very few women have sufficient iron stores to meet pregnancy demands. During a normal pregnancy, blood volume increases by about 50 per cent. A large amount of iron is required to produce those additional blood cells.

Iron needs are most important in the latter half of pregnancy. Most women don't need to take iron supplements during the first trimester. If prescribed at this time, they can worsen symptoms of nausea and vomiting.

The iron content of prenatal vitamins can irritate your stomach. Iron supplements may also cause constipation. Even if you need them, you may not be able to take iron supplements until after the first trimester.

Prenatal Vitamins

Prenatal vitamins are usually prescribed for a pregnant woman during pregnancy. Some women begin taking prenatal vitamins while they are trying to get pregnant. Supplements contain the daily amounts of vitamins and minerals recommended for you during pregnancy.

Your prenatal vitamin is different from a regular multivitamin because of its iron and folic-acid content. These are the most important supplements for you in pregnancy. Prenatal vitamins are often best tolerated if you take them with meals or at night before bed.

Prenatal vitamins contain many essential ingredients for the development of your baby and your continued good health. That's why you should take them every day until your baby is born. A typical prenatal vitamin contains the following:

- calcium to build baby's teeth and bones, and to help strengthen your own
- copper to help prevent anaemia, and to help baby's bone formation
- folic acid to reduce the risk of neural-tube defects and to help in blood-cell production
- iodine to help control metabolism
- iron to prevent anaemia, and to help baby's blood development
- vitamin A for general health and body metabolism
- vitamin B_1 for general health and body metabolism
- vitamin B_2 for general health and body metabolism
- vitamin B_3 for general health and body metabolism
- vitamin B_6 for general health and body metabolism
- vitamin B_{12} to promote blood formation
- vitamin C to aid in your body's absorption of iron
- vitamin D to strengthen baby's bones and teeth, and to help your body use phosphorus and calcium
- vitamin E for general health and body metabolism
- zinc to help balance fluids in your body and to aid nerve and muscle function

✌ Zinc

Research has found that zinc may be helpful to a thin or underweight woman during pregnancy. We believe this mineral helps a thin woman increase her chances of giving birth to a bigger, healthier baby.

✌ Fluoride Supplementation

The value of fluoride and fluoride supplementation in a pregnant woman is unclear. Some researchers believe fluoride supplementation during pregnancy results in improved teeth in the child; not everyone agrees. Fluoride supplementation in a pregnant woman has not been proved harmful to her baby. Some prenatal vitamins contain fluoride.

You Should Also Know

✂ *Sexual Intimacy during Pregnancy*

Many couples question whether it is wise or permissible to have sexual intercourse during pregnancy. Sexual relations are usually OK for a healthy pregnant woman and her partner.

Sex doesn't just mean sexual intercourse. There are many ways for couples to be sensual together, including giving each other a massage, bathing together and talking about sex. Whatever you do, be honest with your partner about how you're feeling—and keep a sense of humour!

Can Sex during Pregnancy Hurt the Baby? Many men wonder if sexual activity can harm a growing baby. Neither intercourse nor orgasm should be a problem if you have a low-risk pregnancy.

The baby is well protected by the amniotic sac and amniotic fluid. Uterine muscles are strong, and they protect the baby. A thick mucus plug seals the cervix, which helps protect against infection.

If you have questions, bring them up at an antenatal visit. This may be especially helpful if your partner goes with you to your appointments. If he doesn't, assure him there should be no problems if your doctor/midwife gives you the go-ahead.

Frequent sexual activity should not be harmful to a healthy pregnancy. Usually a couple can continue the level of sexual activity they are used to. If you are concerned, discuss it when you visit your doctor/midwife.

Some doctors recommend abstinence from intercourse during the last 4 weeks of pregnancy, but not all doctors agree with this. Discuss it with your doctor/midwife.

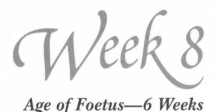

Week 8

Age of Foetus—6 Weeks

If you've just found out you're pregnant, you might
want to begin by reading the previous chapters.

How Big Is Your Baby?

By your 8th week of pregnancy, the crown-to-rump length of your baby
is 1.4 to 2 cm (½ to ¾ in). This is about the size of a kidney bean.

How Big Are You?

Your uterus is getting bigger, but it probably still isn't big enough for
you to be showing, especially if this is your first pregnancy. You will
notice a gradual change in your waistline and the fit of your clothes.

Tip for Week 8 Wash your hands
thoroughly throughout the day, especially after
handling raw meat or using the bathroom. This
simple activity can help prevent the spread of
many bacteria and viruses that cause infection.

How Your Baby Is
Growing and Developing

Your baby is continuing to grow and to change rapidly during these early weeks. Compare the illustration on page 100 with the illustration for the 7th week of pregnancy. Can you see the incredible changes?

Eyelid folds are forming on the face and nerve cells in the retina are beginning to develop. The tip of the nose is present. Ears are forming, internally and externally.

In the heart, the aortic and pulmonary valves are present and distinct. Tubes leading from the throat to the functioning part of the lungs are branched, like the branches of a tree. The body's trunk area is getting longer and straightening out.

Elbows are present, and the arms and legs extend forward. Arms have grown longer. They bend at the elbows and curve slightly over the heart. The digital rays, which become fingers, are notched. Toe rays are present on the feet.

Changes in You

ᴄᴠ *Changes in Your Uterus*

Before pregnancy, your uterus was about the size of your fist. After 6 weeks of growth, it is about the size of a grapefruit. As you progress through pregnancy and your uterus grows, you may feel cramping or even pain in your lower abdomen or your sides. Some women feel tightening or contractions of the uterus.

The uterus tightens or contracts throughout pregnancy. If you don't feel this, don't worry. However, when contractions are accompanied by bleeding from the vagina, call your doctor.

ᴄᴠ *Sciatic-Nerve Pain*

Many women experience an occasional excruciating pain in their buttocks and down the back or side of their legs as pregnancy progresses. This is called *sciatic-nerve pain*. The sciatic nerve runs behind the

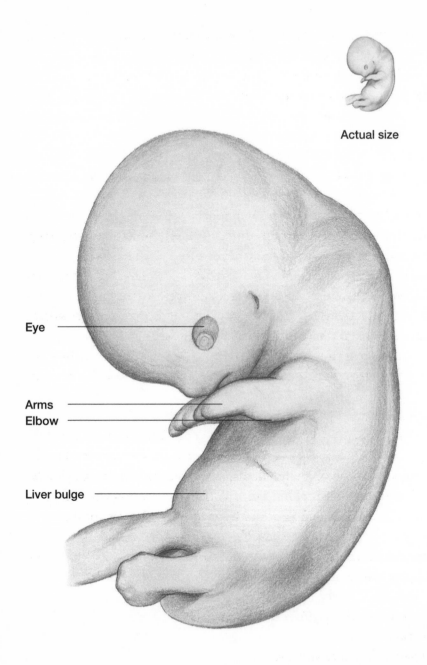

Actual size

Eye

Arms
Elbow

Liver bulge

Embryo at 8 weeks (foetal age—6 weeks). Crown-to-rump length is about 20 mm (0.8 in). Arms are longer and bend at the elbows.

uterus in the pelvis to the legs. We believe pain is caused by pressure on the nerve from the growing, expanding uterus.

The best treatment for the pain is to lie on your opposite side. This helps relieve pressure on the nerve.

How Your Actions Affect Your Baby's Development

✢ *Avoid Roaccutane*

Some women notice an improvement in their acne during pregnancy. But this doesn't happen for everyone.

Roaccutane (isotretinoin) is commonly prescribed for the treatment of acne. **Do not take Roaccutane during pregnancy!** Taken during the first trimester, Roaccutane is responsible for a higher frequency of miscarriages and malformations of the foetus.

If you are pregnant or think you might be pregnant, don't take Roaccutane. Use reliable birth control to avoid pregnancy if you use this product.

✢ *Miscarriage*

Miscarriage occurs when a pregnancy ends before the embryo or foetus can survive on its own outside the uterus, during the first 20 weeks of pregnancy. After 20 weeks, loss of a pregnancy is called a *stillbirth*. Nearly every pregnant woman thinks about miscarriage during pregnancy, but it occurs in only about 15 per cent of all pregnancies.

Some Common Signs of Miscarriage. Some signs you can be alert for that may indicate a miscarriage may be about to occur include:

- vaginal bleeding
- cramps
- pain that comes and goes
- pain that begins in the small of the back and moves to the lower abdomen
- loss of placenta (or foetal) tissue

What Causes a Miscarriage? We don't usually know, and are often unable to find out, what causes a miscarriage. The most common finding in early miscarriages is an abnormality in the development of the embryo. Studies indicate more than half of all early miscarriages have chromosomal abnormalities.

Many factors can affect the embryo and its environment, including radiation, chemicals (drugs or medications) and infections. Called *teratogens*, these adverse factors are discussed in depth in Week 4.

We believe various maternal factors are important in some miscarriages. Unusual infections, such as listeriosis, toxoplasmosis and syphilis, have been implicated in miscarriages.

Ðad Tip If you have pets, take over their care during your partner's pregnancy. Change the cat's litter box (she should *never* do this while pregnant). Walk the dog (the pull on the leash might hurt her back). Buy food and other pet supplies (to save her back from the strain of lifting big food bags). Make and keep vet appointments.

We have no concrete evidence that deficiency of any particular nutrient or even a moderate deficiency of all nutrients causes a miscarriage. Women who smoke have a higher rate of miscarriage. Alcohol is also blamed for an increase in miscarriages.

The trauma of an accident or major surgery has been related to an increase in miscarriages, although this is difficult to verify. An incompetent cervix (see Week 24) is a cause of pregnancy loss after the first trimester. Many women have blamed emotional upset or trauma for a miscarriage, but this is hard to prove.

Below is a discussion of different types and causes of miscarriage. It is included to alert you about what to watch for if you have any symptoms of a miscarriage. If you have questions, discuss them with your doctor.

Threatened Miscarriage. A threatened miscarriage may be presumed when there is a bloody discharge from the vagina during the first half of pregnancy. Bleeding may last for days or even weeks. There may not be any cramping or pain. Pain may feel like a menstrual cramp or a mild backache. Resting in bed is about all you can do, although being active does not cause miscarriage. No procedure or medication can keep a woman from miscarrying.

Threatened miscarriage is a common diagnosis because 20 per cent of all women experience bleeding during early pregnancy but not all miscarry.

Inevitable Miscarriage. An inevitable miscarriage occurs with the rupture of membranes, dilatation of the cervix and passage of blood clots and even tissue. Miscarriage is almost certain under these circumstances. The uterus usually contracts, expelling the foetus or products of conception.

Incomplete Miscarriage. With an incomplete miscarriage, the entire pregnancy may not be passed at once. Part of the pregnancy is passed while part of it remains in the uterus. Bleeding may be heavy and continues until the uterus is empty.

Missed Miscarriage. A missed miscarriage can occur with prolonged retention of an embryo that died earlier. There may be no symptoms or bleeding. The time period from when the pregnancy failed to the time the miscarriage is discovered is usually weeks.

Habitual Miscarriage. This term usually refers to three or more consecutive miscarriages.

If You Have Problems. If you have problems, notify your doctor immediately! Bleeding often appears first, followed by cramping. Ectopic pregnancy must also be considered. A quantitative HCG may be useful in identifying a normal pregnancy, but a single test report usually won't help. Your doctor needs to repeat the test over a period of several days.

Ultrasound may help if you are more than 5 gestational weeks into your pregnancy. You may continue to bleed, but seeing your baby's heartbeat and a normal-appearing pregnancy may be reassuring. If the first ultrasound is not reassuring, you may be asked to wait a week or 10 days, then repeat the ultrasound.

The longer you bleed and cramp, the more likely you are having a miscarriage. If you pass all of the pregnancy, bleeding stops and cramping goes away, you may be done with it. However, if everything is not expelled, it may be necessary to perform a *dilatation and curettage* (D&C) to empty the uterus. It is preferable to do this so you won't bleed for a long time, risking anaemia and infection.

Some women are given the hormone progesterone in an effort to help them keep a pregnancy. The use of progesterone to prevent miscarriage is controversial. Doctors do not agree on its use or its effectiveness.

Rh-Sensitivity and Miscarriage. If you're Rh-negative and you have a miscarriage, you will need to receive Anti-D. This applies *only* if you are Rh-negative. Anti-D is given to protect you from making antibodies to Rh-positive blood. (This is discussed in Week 16.)

If You Have a Miscarriage. One miscarriage can be traumatic; two in a row can be very difficult to deal with. Repeated miscarriages occur due to chance or 'bad luck' in most cases.

Most doctors don't recommend testing to find a reason for miscarriage unless you have three or more miscarriages. Chromosome analysis can be done, and other tests can be performed to investigate the possibility of infections, diabetes and lupus.

Don't blame yourself or your partner for a miscarriage. It is usually impossible to look back at everything you've done, eaten or been exposed to and find the cause of a miscarriage.

Your Nutrition

It's hard to eat nutritiously for *every* meal. You may not always get the nutrients you need, in the amounts you need. On the opposite page is a chart showing where you can get the various nutrients you should be eating every day. Your prenatal vitamin is *not* a substitute for food, so don't count on it to supply you with essential vitamins and minerals. Food is important, too!

Sources of Food Nutrients

Nutrient (Daily Requirement)	Food Sources
Calcium (1200 mg)	dairy products, dark leafy vegetables, dried beans and peas, tofu
Folic acid (0.4 mg)	liver, dried beans and peas, eggs, broccoli, whole-grain products, oranges, orange juice
Iron (30 mg)	fish, liver, meat, poultry, egg yolks, nuts, dried beans and peas, dark leafy vegetables, dried fruit
Magnesium (320 mg)	dried beans and peas, cocoa, seafoods, whole-grain products, nuts
Vitamin B_6 (2.2 mg)	whole-grain products, liver, meat
Vitamin E (10 mg)	milk, eggs, meat, fish, cereals, leafy vegetables, vegetable oils
Zinc (15 mg)	seafood, meat, nuts, milk, dried beans and peas

You Should Also Know

∽ *Blood Tests Your Doctor/Midwife May Order*

On your first or second visit, routine blood tests are performed. These include an FBC (full blood count), blood type and Rh-factor, immunity against rubella (German measles), syphilis (VDRL) and hepatitis B. Many areas offer testing for H.I.V. A sample of urine is also obtained for urinalysis and sent to the Laboratory for culture.

Other tests are done as required. Tests are not performed at each visit; they are carried out at the beginning of pregnancy as needed.

∽ *Toxoplasmosis*

If you have a cat, you may be concerned about *toxoplasmosis*. The disease is spread by eating raw, infected meat or by contact with infected cat faeces. It can cross the placenta to your baby. Usually an infection in the mother has no symptoms.

Infection during pregnancy can lead to miscarriage or an infected infant at birth. Antibiotics, such as pyrimethamine, sulfadiazine and erythromycin, can be used to treat toxoplasmosis, but the best plan is prevention. Hygienic measures prevent transmission of the disease.

Avoid exposure to cat faeces (get someone else to change the cat litter). Wash hands thoroughly after petting your cat, and keep your cat off counters and tables. Wash your hands after contact with meat and soil. Cook all meat thoroughly. Avoid cross contamination of foods while preparing and cooking them.

Medical Conditions and 'Safe' Medications to Use during Pregnancy

Condition	Drugs of Choice that Are Safe to Use
Acne	benzoyl peroxide (gel), clindamycin (gel), erythromycin (gel)
Asthma	inhalers—beta-adrenergic antagonists, corticosteroids, ipratropium
Bacterial infection	clindamycin, co-trimoxazole, erythromycin, nitrofurantoin
Bipolar disorder	chlorpromazine, haloperidol
Coughs	cough lozenges, dextromethorphan, diphenhydramine, codeine (short term)
Depression	fluoxetine, tricyclic antidepressants
Headache	paracetamol
Hypertension	hydralazine, methyldopa
Hyperthyroidism	propylthiouracil
Migraines	codeine, dimenhydrinate
Nausea and vomiting	doxylamine plus pyridoxine
Peptic ulcer disease	antacids, rantidine

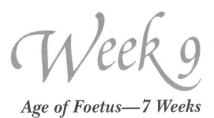

Week 9

Age of Foetus—7 Weeks

If you've just found out you're pregnant, you might
want to begin by reading the previous chapters.

How Big Is Your Baby?

The crown-to-rump length of the embryo is 2.2 to 3 cm (1 to 1¼ in).
This is close to the size of a medium green olive.

How Big Are You?

Each week your uterus grows larger with the baby growing inside it.
You may begin to see your waistline growing thicker by this time.

How Your Baby Is
Growing and Developing

If you could look inside your uterus, you'd see many changes in your
baby. The illustration on page 109 shows some of them.

Your baby's arms and legs are longer. Hands are flexed at the wrist and meet over the heart area. They continue to extend in front of the body. Fingers are longer, and the tips are slightly enlarged where touch pads are developing. The feet are approaching the midline of the body and may be long enough to meet in front of the torso.

The head is more erect, and the neck is more developed. The eyelids almost cover the eyes. Up to this time, the eyes have been uncovered. External ears are evident and well formed. Your baby now moves its body and limbs. This movement may be seen during an ultrasound exam.

The baby looks more recognizable as a human being, although it is still extremely small. It is probably impossible to distinguish a male from a female. External organs (external genitalia) of the male and female appear very similar and will not be distinguishable for another few weeks.

Changes in You

༚ *Weight Change*

Most women are interested in their weight during pregnancy; many watch their weight closely. As strange as it may seem, gaining weight is an important way to monitor the well-being of your developing baby. Even though your weight gain may be small, your body is growing.

How Is Pregnancy Weight Distributed?

5.4 kg (12 lb)	Maternal stores (fat, protein and other nutrients)
1.8 kg (4 lb)	Increased fluid volume
900 g (2 lb)	Breast enlargement
900 g (2 lb)	Uterus
3.4 kg (7½ lb)	Baby
900 g (2 lb)	Amniotic fluid
680 g (1½ lb)	Placenta (connects mother and baby; brings baby nourishment and takes away waste)

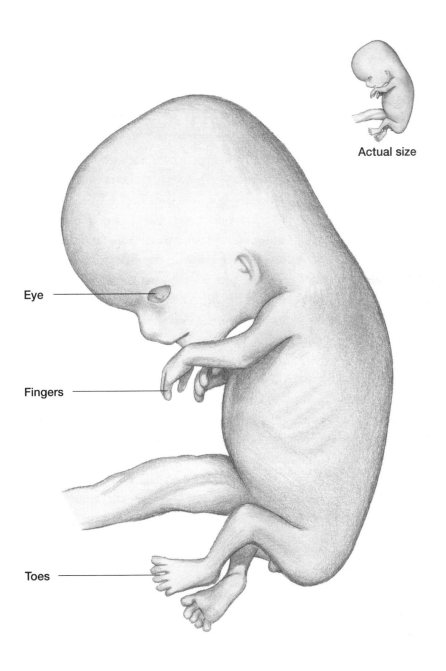

Actual size

Eye

Fingers

Toes

Embryo at 9 weeks of pregnancy (foetal age—46 to 49 days). Toes are formed and feet are more recognizable. Crown-to-rump length is about 25 mm (1 in).

✐ Increased Blood Volume

Your blood system changes dramatically during pregnancy. Your blood volume increases greatly—to about 50 per cent more than before you became pregnant. However, this amount varies from woman to woman.

Increased blood volume is important. It is designed to meet the demands of your growing uterus. This increase does not include the blood in the embryo, whose circulation is separate (foetal blood does not mix with your blood). More blood in your system protects you and your baby from harmful effects when you lie down or stand up. The increase is also a safeguard during labour and delivery, when some blood is lost.

The blood-volume increase begins during the first trimester. The largest increase occurs during the second trimester. It continues to increase but at a slower rate during the third trimester.

Blood is composed of fluid (plasma) and cells (red blood cells and white blood cells). Plasma and cells play an important role in your body's function.

Fluid and cells increase to different degrees. Usually there is an initial rise in plasma volume followed by an increase in red blood cells. The increase in red blood cells increases your body's demand for iron.

Red blood cells and plasma both increase during pregnancy; plasma increases more. This increase in plasma can cause anaemia. If you're anaemic, especially during pregnancy, you may feel tired, fatigue easily or experience a general feeling of ill health. (See Week 22 for a discussion of anaemia.)

How Your Actions
Affect Your Baby's Development

✐ Saunas, Spas and Hot Baths

Some women are concerned about using saunas and spas and having hot baths during pregnancy. They want to know if it is OK to relax in this way.

We recommend that you don't take a chance with a sauna, spa or hot bath. Your baby relies on you to maintain correct body temperature. If your body temperature is elevated high enough, and stays there for an extended period, it may damage the baby if it occurs at various critical times in its development. Wait until more medical research determines that it is not harmful to your baby.

ঔ *Electric Blankets*

There has been controversy about using electric blankets to keep you warm during pregnancy. There is still much disagreement and discussion about their safety. Some experts question whether these blankets can cause health problems.

Tip for Week 9 It's an old wives' tale that your hair won't curl if you have a perm during pregnancy. Our only precaution is that if odours affect you, the fumes from a perm or hair colouring could make you feel ill.

Electric blankets produce a low-level electromagnetic field. The developing foetus may be more sensitive than an adult to these electromagnetic fields.

Because researchers are uncertain about 'acceptable levels' of exposure for a pregnant woman and her baby, the safest alternative at this time is not to use an electric blanket during pregnancy. There are many other ways to keep warm, such as duvets and wool blankets. One of these is a better choice.

ঔ *Microwave Ovens*

Some women wonder about the safety of microwave ovens. Are they exposed to radiation? Microwave ovens are helpful to busy people who prepare meals. However, we don't know if there is danger to you if you use a microwave oven during pregnancy. More research is needed.

Initial research indicates tissues developing in the body, which would include the human foetus, may be particularly sensitive to the effects of microwaves. A microwave oven heats tissues from the inside. Follow the directions provided with your microwave oven, and don't stand next to or directly in front of it while it is in use.

Your Nutrition

Fruits and vegetables are important during pregnancy. Because different kinds of produce are available in different seasons, you can add variety to your diet quite easily with them. They are excellent sources of vitamins, minerals and fibre. Eating a variety can supply you with iron, folic acid, calcium and vitamin C.

Tasty, Low-Cal Sources of Vitamin C

Five excellent sources of vitamin C are easy to add to your diet, and if you're watching your weight, they're low in calories, too! Try the following:

- strawberries—170 g (6 oz) contains 94 mg of vitamin C
- orange juice—240 ml (8 fl oz) contains 82 mg of vitamin C
- kiwi fruit—1 medium contains 74 mg of vitamin C
- broccoli—45 g (1½ oz) cooked, contains 58 mg of vitamin C
- red peppers—¼ of a medium red pepper contains 57 mg of vitamin C

↗ *Vitamin C Is Important*

Vitamin C can be very important during pregnancy. It is important for foetal-tissue development and the absorption of iron. Recent research indicates vitamin C may help prevent pre-eclampsia. Deficiencies in the vitamin have also been linked to premature delivery; vitamin C helps build the amniotic sac. The recommended daily dose is 85 mg—a bit more than what is contained in a prenatal vitamin. You can get some of the extra vitamin C you need by eating fruits and vegetables rich in the vitamin.

Each day, eat one or two servings of fruit high in vitamin C and at least one dark-green or deep-yellow vegetable for extra iron, fibre and folic acid. Fruits and vegetables you may choose, and their serving sizes, include the following:

- grapes—85 g (3 oz)
- banana, orange, apple—1 medium
- dried fruit—45 g (1½ oz)
- fruit juice—120 ml (4 fl oz)
- canned or cooked fruit—115 g (4 oz)
- broccoli, carrots or other vegetable—150 g (2 oz)
- potato—1 medium
- leafy green vegetables—185 g (3 oz)
- vegetable juice—180 ml (6 fl oz)

Don't take more than the recommended dose of vitamin C; too much may cause you stomach cramps and diarrhoea. It can also negatively affect your baby's metabolism.

Dad Tip Ask your partner which visits to the doctor she'd like you to attend. Some couples attend every visit together, when possible. Ask her to let you know the date and time of each appointment.

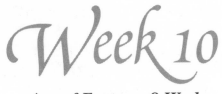

Week 10

Age of Foetus—8 Weeks

If you've just found out you're pregnant, you might want to begin by reading the previous chapters.

How Big Is Your Baby?

By the 10th week of pregnancy, the crown-to-rump length of your growing baby is about 3.1 to 4.2 cm (1¼ to 1¾ in). At this time, we can start measuring how much the baby weighs. Before this week, weight was too small to measure weekly differences. Now that the baby is starting to put on a little weight, weight is included in this section. The baby weighs close to 5 g (0.18 oz) and is the size of a small plum.

How Big Are You?

Changes are gradual, and you still may not show much. You may be thinking about and looking at maternity clothes, but you probably don't need them just yet.

☞ *Molar Pregnancy*

A condition that can make you grow too big too fast is a molar pregnancy, sometimes called *gestational trophoblastic neoplasia* (GTN) or *hydatidiform mole*. The occurrence of GTN is easily monitored by checking HCG levels (see Week 5). Molar pregnancy is treated with surgery.

When a molar pregnancy occurs, an embryo does not usually develop. Other tissue grows, which is abnormal placental tissue. The most common symptom is bleeding during the first trimester. Another symptom is the discrepancy between the size of the mother-to-be and how far along she is supposed to be in pregnancy. Half the time, a woman is too large. Twenty-five per cent of the time, she is too small. Excessive nausea and vomiting are other symptoms. Cysts may occur on the ovaries.

The most effective way to diagnose a molar pregnancy is by ultrasound. The ultrasound picture has a 'snowflake' appearance. A molar pregnancy is usually found when ultrasound is done early in pregnancy to determine the cause of bleeding or rapid growth of the uterus.

When a molar pregnancy is diagnosed, a dilatation and curettage (D&C) is usually done as soon as possible. After a molar pregnancy occurs, effective birth control is important to be sure the molar pregnancy is completely gone. Most doctors recommend using reliable birth control for at least 1 year before attempting pregnancy again.

How Your Baby Is Growing and Developing

The end of week 10 is the end of the embryonic period. At this time, the foetal period begins. It is characterized by rapid growth of the foetus when the three germ layers are established. (See Week 4 for further information.) During the embryonic period, the embryo is most susceptible to things that could interfere with its development. Most congenital malformations occur before the end of week 10. It is encouraging to know that a critical part of your baby's development is safely behind you.

Few malformations occur during the foetal period. However, drugs and other harmful exposures, such as severe stress or radiation (X-ray), can destroy foetal cells at any time during pregnancy. Continue to avoid them.

By the end of week 10, development of foetal organ systems and the body are well under way. Your baby is beginning to look more human.

Changes in You

✑ *Emotional Changes*

When your pregnancy is confirmed by an exam or a pregnancy test, you may be affected in many ways. Pregnancy can change many of your expectations. Some women see pregnancy as a sign of womanhood. Some consider it a blessing. Still others feel it is a problem to be dealt with.

You will experience many changes in your body. You may wonder if you are still attractive. Will your partner still find you desirable? (Many men believe pregnant women are beautiful.) Will your partner help you? Clothing may become an issue. Will you look attractive? Can you learn to adapt?

If you aren't immediately excited about pregnancy, don't feel alone. You may question your condition—that's common. Some of this reaction is because you're not sure of what lies ahead.

When and how you begin to regard the foetus as a person is different for everyone. Some women say it is when their pregnancy test is positive. Others say it occurs when they hear the foetal heartbeat, usually at around 12 weeks. For still others, it happens when they first feel their baby move, at between 16 and 20 weeks.

You may find you are emotional about many things. You may feel moody, cry at the slightest thing or drift off in daydreams. Emotional swings are normal and continue to some degree throughout your pregnancy.

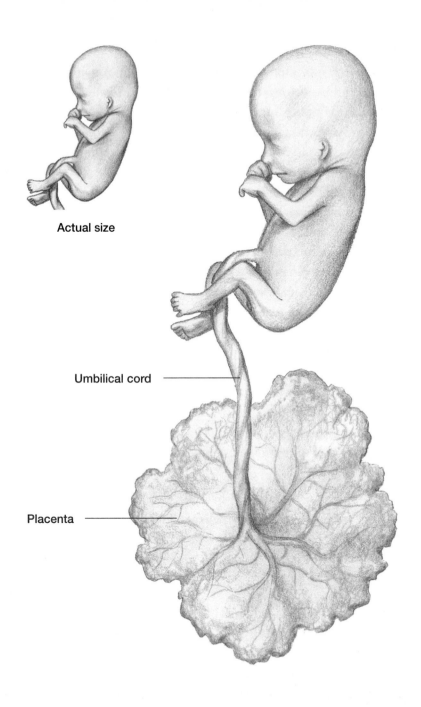

Actual size

Umbilical cord ————

Placenta ————

Baby is shown attached to the placenta by its umbilical cord. Eyelids are fused and remain closed until week 27 (foetal age—25 weeks).

How can you help yourself deal with emotional changes? One of the most important things you can do is get good antenatal care. Follow your doctor's/midwife's recommendations. Keep all your antenatal appointments. Establish good communication with your doctor/midwife and his or her surgery staff. Ask questions. If something bothers you or worries you, discuss it with someone reliable.

How Your Actions Affect Your Baby's Development

᠅ Vaccinations and Immunizations

Many vaccines are available to help prevent illness. A vaccine is given to provide you with protection against infection and is usually given by injection or taken orally.

Many women of childbearing age in the UK have been immunized against measles, mumps, rubella, tetanus and diphtheria. Your family doctor should have a record of your immunizations. In addition, your parents may remember if you had German measles as a child. If there is any doubt, immunity to German measles can be checked with a simple blood test.

Vaccination for measles, mumps and rubella (MMR) should be administered *only* when a woman is practising birth control. She must continue to use contraception for at least 4 weeks after receiving this immunization. Other vaccinations are also important, such as the tetanus or DPT (diphtheria, pertussis [whooping cough], tetanus) vaccine.

Risk of Exposure. It's important to consider your risk of exposure to various diseases when you are deciding whether to have a particular vaccination. During pregnancy, try to decrease your chance of exposure to disease and illness. Avoid visiting areas known to have prevalent diseases. Avoid people (usually children) with known illnesses.

It's impossible to avoid all exposure to all diseases. If you have been exposed, or if exposure is unavoidable, the risk of the disease must be balanced against the potential harmful effects of vaccination.

Then the vaccine must be evaluated in terms of its effectiveness and its potential for complicating pregnancy. There is little information available on harmful effects on the developing foetus from vaccines. In general, killed vaccines are safe. Live-measles vaccine should *never* be given to a pregnant woman.

The only immunizing agents recommended for use during pregnancy are the DPT vaccine and the flu vaccine. The flu vaccine is one you can take during pregnancy. If there are no contraindications, it should be taken by every pregnant woman who will be past the 3rd month of pregnancy during the flu season. This is usually from November through March, although the season has gone beyond March in some years. Talk to your doctor about it.

MMR vaccine should be given before pregnancy or after delivery. Immunization cannot be given during pregnancy as the vaccine is live and could also potentially cause problems for the baby. After being immunized, it is essential to use effective birth control for 3 months.

A pregnant woman should receive primary vaccination against polio only if her risk of exposure to the disease is high. Only inactivated polio vaccine should be used.

❧ Rubella during Pregnancy

It's a good idea to be checked for immunity to rubella before you get pregnant. Rubella (German measles) during pregnancy can be responsible for miscarriage or foetal malformation. Because there is no known treatment for rubella, the best approach is prevention.

If you're not immune, you can receive a vaccination while you take reliable birth control. Do not have a vaccination shortly before or during pregnancy because of the possibility of exposing the baby to the rubella virus.

❧ Chicken Pox during Pregnancy

Did you have chicken pox when you were a child? If not, you may be one of the 1 in 2000 women who will develop the infection during pregnancy. Chicken pox is a childhood disease; only 2 per cent of cases occur in the 15-to-49 age group.

If you contract chicken pox during pregnancy, take very good care of yourself. In about 15 per cent of those adults who contract chicken pox, a form of pneumonia develops—it can be especially serious for a pregnant woman. If you get chicken pox during pregnancy, just before delivery, your baby may get it, too, which can be serious in a newborn.

If you are exposed to the infection while you are pregnant, contact your doctor/midwife immediately! A pregnant woman with a significant exposure to this highly infectious herpes virus should receive varicella-zoster immune globulin (VZIG). If you receive VZIG within 72 hours of exposure, it can help prevent infection or it can lessen the severity of symptoms. If you do contract chicken pox, your doctor will probably treat you with aciclovir to lessen symptoms.

If you are exposed during pregnancy, and you're lucky enough not to get this infection, be sure to get vaccinated before your next pregnancy!

✕ Effects of Infections on Your Baby

Some infections and illnesses a woman contracts can also affect her baby's development during this growth period. See the box to the left for a list of some infections and diseases and the effects they may have on a developing baby.

Infections	Effects on Foetus
Cytomegalovirus (CMV)	microcephaly, brain damage, hearing loss
Rubella (German measles)	cataracts, deafness, heart lesions, can involve all organs
Syphilis	foetal death, skin defects
Toxoplasmosis	possible effects on all organs
Varicella	possible effects on all organs

Your Nutrition

Protein supplies you with amino acids, which are critical for the growth and repair of the embryo/foetus, placenta, uterus and breasts. Pregnancy increases your protein needs. Try to eat 50 g of protein each day during the first trimester and 60 g a day during the second and third trimesters. However, protein should only make up about 15 per cent of your total calorie intake.

Many protein sources are high in fat. If you need to watch your calories, choose low-fat protein sources. Some protein foods you may choose, and their serving sizes, include the following:

- chickpeas—170 g (6 oz)
- cheese, mozzarella—55 g (1 oz)
- chicken, roasted, skinless—½ breast (about 4 oz)
- eggs—1
- hamburger, grilled, lean—100 g (3½ oz)
- milk—240 ml (8 fl oz)
- peanut butter—2 tablespoons
- tuna, canned in water—85 g (3 oz)
- yoghurt—240 ml (8 fl oz)

✎ Brain Builders

Choline and docosahexaenoic acid (DHA) can help build baby's brain cells during foetal development and after birth, if baby breastfeeds. Choline is found in milk, eggs, peanuts, whole-wheat bread and beef. DHA is found in fish, egg yolks, poultry, meat, rapeseed oil, walnuts and wheat germ. If you eat these foods during pregnancy and while you're breastfeeding, you can help your baby obtain these important supplements.

Tip for Week 10 It's common for your breasts to tingle and to feel sore early in pregnancy. In fact, it may be one of the first signs of pregnancy.

✎ You Need to Gain Weight

You should be gaining weight slowly now; it can be harmful to your baby if you don't. A woman of normal weight can expect to gain between 11 and 16 kg (25 and 35 lb) total while pregnant. Your weight gain gives your doctor an indication of your well-being and that of your baby, too.

Pregnancy is not a time to experiment with different diets or cut down on calories. However, this doesn't mean you have the go-ahead to eat anything you want, any time you want. Exercise and a proper nutrition plan, without 'junk food,' will help you manage your weight. Be smart about food choices. It's true you're eating for two—however, you must eat wisely for both of you!

You Should Also Know

ᢒ *Chorionic Villus Sampling*

Chorionic villus sampling (CVS) is a test used to detect genetic abnormalities. Sampling is done early in pregnancy, usually between the 9th and 11th weeks.

CVS is done for many reasons. The test helps identify problems related to genetic defects, such as Down's syndrome. This test offers an advantage over amniocentesis because it is done much earlier in pregnancy; results are available in about 1 week. If a pregnancy will be terminated, it can be done earlier and may carry fewer risks to the woman.

Chorionic villus sampling involves placing an instrument through the cervix or abdomen to remove foetal tissue from the placenta. The test should be performed only by someone experienced in the technique.

If your doctor recommends you have CVS, ask about its risks. The risk of miscarriage is small—between 1 and 2 per cent. If you have CVS and are Rh-negative, you should receive Anti-D after the procedure.

ᢒ *Foetoscopy*

Foetoscopy provides a view of the baby and placenta inside your uterus. In some cases, abnormalities and problems can be detected and corrected.

The goal of foetoscopy is to correct a defect before the problem worsens, which could prevent a foetus from developing normally. A doctor can see some problems more clearly with foetoscopy than with ultrasound.

The test is done by placing a scope, like the one used in laparoscopy or arthroscopy, through the abdomen. The procedure is similar to amniocentesis, but the foetoscope is larger than the needle used for amniocentesis.

If your doctor suggests foetoscopy to you, discuss possible risks, advantages and disadvantages of the procedure with him or her. The test should be done only by someone experienced in the technique. Risk of miscarriage is 3 to 4 per cent with this procedure. It is not available everywhere. If you have foetoscopy and are Rh-negative, you should receive Anti-D after the procedure.

Dad Tip Are you concerned about sex during pregnancy? You both may have questions, so talk about them together and with your partner's doctor. Occasionally during a pregnancy you'll need to avoid intercourse. However, pregnancy is an opportunity for increased closeness and intimacy for you as a couple. Sex can be a positive part of this experience.

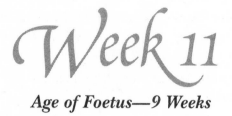

Week 11

Age of Foetus—9 Weeks

How Big Is Your Baby?

By this week, the crown-to-rump length of your baby is 4.4 to 6 cm (1½ to 2½ in). Fetal weight is about 8 g (0.3 oz). Your baby is about the size of a large lime.

How Big Are You?

While big changes are occurring in your baby, changes are probably happening more slowly with you. You are almost at the end of the first trimester; your uterus has been growing along with the foetus inside it. It is almost big enough to fill your pelvis and may be felt in your lower abdomen, above the middle of your pubic bone.

You won't be able to feel your baby moving yet. If you think you feel your baby move at this time, you either have gas or are further along in your pregnancy than you thought.

How Your Baby Is Growing and Developing

Foetal growth is rapid now. The crown-to-rump length of your baby doubles in the next 3 weeks. As you can see in the illustration on page 126, the head is almost half the baby's entire length. As the head extends (uncurls or tips backwards towards the spine), the chin rises from the chest, and the neck develops and lengthens. Fingernails appear.

External genitalia are beginning to show distinguishing features. Development of the foetus into a male or female is complete in another 3 weeks. If a miscarriage occurs after this point, it may be possible to tell if it is male or female.

All embryos begin life looking the same, as far as outward appearances are concerned. Whether the embryo develops into a male or female is determined by the genetic information contained within the embryo.

Changes in You

Some women notice changes in their hair, fingernails or toenails during pregnancy. This doesn't happen to everyone, but if it happens to you, don't worry about it. Some fortunate women notice an increase in hair and nail growth during pregnancy. Others find they lose some hair during this time.

Some doctors believe these changes occur during pregnancy because of increased circulation throughout your body. Others credit the hormonal changes occurring in you. Still others

Dad Tip Remember that despite morning sickness, headaches and a changing waistline, pregnancy is a miracle! Pregnancy and childbirth happen only a limited number of times in your life. Enjoy this special time together. You'll look back fondly at the challenge of becoming parents and probably even say, 'That wasn't so bad.' We know that because couples get pregnant again and have more kids!

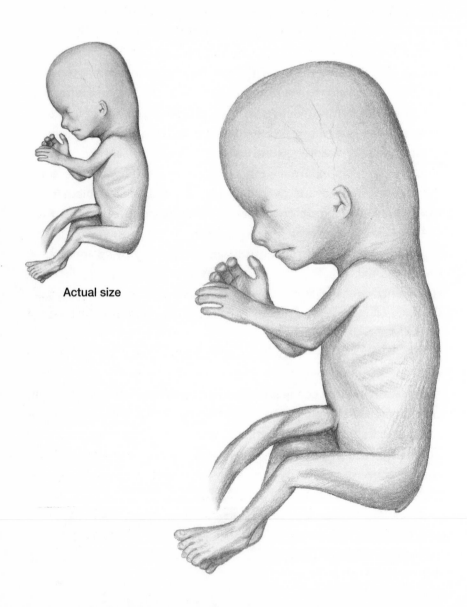

Actual size

By week 11 of gestation (foetal age—9 weeks), fingernails are beginning to appear.

explain these differences with a change in 'phase' of the growth cycle of the hair or nails. In any event, these differences are rarely permanent. There is little or nothing you can do about them.

How Your Actions Affect Your Baby's Development

✑ *Travelling during Pregnancy*

Pregnant women frequently ask whether travel during pregnancy can hurt their baby. If your pregnancy is uncomplicated and you are not at high risk, travel is usually acceptable. Ask your doctor/midwife about any travel you are considering *before* making firm plans or buying tickets.

Whether you travel by car, bus, train or aeroplane, it's wise to get up and walk at least every hour. Regular visits to the bathroom may take care of this requirement.

The biggest risk of travelling during pregnancy is development of a complication while you are away from those who know your medical and pregnancy history. If you do decide to take a trip, be sensible in your planning. Don't overdo it. Take it easy!

Travelling by Air. Air travel is safe for most pregnant women. Most airlines allow women to fly up to 35 weeks of pregnancy, though be sure to check with your particular carrier.

Pregnant women who are at significant risk for premature labour or who have placental abnormalities should avoid all air travel. You may want to keep the following things in mind if you're considering flying during pregnancy.

• Avoid flights that are high altitude (particularly long-haul flights) because they cruise at a higher altitude and oxygen levels are lower. This increases your heartbeat, as well as your baby's; your baby also receives less oxygen.

- If you have problems with swelling, wear loose-fitting shoes and clothes. (This is good advice for every traveller.) Avoid tights, tight clothes, knee-high socks or stockings, and tight waistlines.
- You can order special meals, such as low-sodium or vegetarian, if you want to avoid some foods that might cause you problems.
- Drink lots of water to keep you hydrated.
- Get up and move around when you can during the flight. Try to walk at least 10 minutes every hour. Sometimes just standing up helps your circulation.
- Try to get an aisle seat, close to the toilets. If you have to go to the bathroom a lot, it's easier if you don't have to crawl over someone to get out.
- Be careful of any X-ray devices in the airport.

ᔔ *Car Safety during Pregnancy*

Many women are concerned about driving and using seat belts during pregnancy. Wearing safety restraints dramatically decreases the incidence of injury in an accident. More than 3,400 deaths and 320,000 injuries are directly related to car accidents every year. Wearing a seat belt can decrease these losses. There is no reason not to drive while you're pregnant, if your pregnancy is normal and you feel OK.

Some women believe using a safety restraint might be harmful to their pregnancy. Here are some common excuses (and our responses) for not using seat belts in pregnancy.

- *'Using a safety belt will hurt my baby.'* There is no evidence that seat-belt use will increase the chance of foetal or uterine injury. Your chance of survival with a seat belt is better than without one. Your survival is important to your unborn baby.
- *'I don't want to be trapped in my car if there is a fire.'* Few car accidents result in fires. Even if a fire did occur, you could probably undo the restraint and escape if you were conscious. Ejection

from a car accounts for about 25 per cent of all deaths in car accidents. Seat-belt use prevents this.

- *'I'm a good driver.'* Defensive driving helps, but it doesn't prevent an accident.
- *'I don't need to use a safety belt; I'm just going a short distance.'* Most injuries occur within 40 km (25 miles) of home.

We know the lap/shoulder seat-belt system is safe to wear during pregnancy, so buckle up for you *and* your baby.

The Proper Way to Wear a Seat Belt

There is a proper way for you to wear a seat belt during pregnancy. Place the lap-belt portion under your abdomen and across your upper thighs. It should be as snug as is comfortably possible. The shoulder belt should also be snug but comfortable. Adjust your position so the belt crosses your shoulder without cutting into your neck. Position the shoulder belt between your breasts. Do not slip this belt off your shoulder. If it's a long trip, adjust the belt as needed for comfort.

Your Nutrition

Carbohydrate foods provide the primary source of energy for your developing baby. These foods also ensure that your body uses protein efficiently. Foods from this group are almost interchangeable, so it should be easy to get all the servings you need. Some carbohydrate foods you may choose, and their serving sizes, include the following:

- tortilla (wrap)—1 large
- pasta, cereal or rice, cooked—85 g (3 oz)
- cereal, ready-to-eat—25 g (1 oz)
- bagel—½ small

• bread—1 slice
• roll—1 medium

You Should Also Know

ᴦ Ultrasound in Pregnancy

By this point, you may have discussed ultrasound with your doctor. Or you may already have had an ultrasound test. Ultrasound (also called *sonography* or *sonogram*) is one of our most valuable methods for evaluating a pregnancy. Although doctors don't agree as to when ultrasound should be done or if every pregnant woman should have an ultrasound test during pregnancy, it definitely has its place. The test has proved useful in improving the outcome in pregnancy. It is a non-invasive test, and there are no known risks associated with it. In the UK thousands of obstetrical ultrasounds are performed each year.

Tip for Week 11 You may be able to get a 'picture' of your baby before birth from an ultrasound test. Some facilities can even make a videotape for you. Ask about it before the test, if you're scheduled to have one. You may be advised to bring a new, unused videotape.

Ultrasound involves the use of high-frequency sound waves made by applying an alternating current to a transducer. A lubricant is placed on the skin to improve contact with the transducer. The transducer passes over the abdomen above the uterus. Sound waves are projected from the transducer through the abdomen, into the pelvis. As sound waves bounce off tissues, they are directed towards and back to the transducer. The reflection of sound waves can be compared to 'radar' used by aeroplanes or ships.

Different tissues of the body reflect ultrasound signals differently, and we can distinguish among them. Motion can be distinguished, so we can detect motion of the baby or parts of the baby, such as the heart. With ultrasound, a foetal heart can be seen beating as early as 5 or 6 weeks into the pregnancy.

Ultrasound can detect foetal motion. Your baby's body and limbs can be seen moving as early as 4 weeks of embryonic growth (6th week of pregnancy).

Your doctor can use ultrasound in many ways in relation to your pregnancy, such as:

- helping in the early identification of pregnancy
- showing the size and growth rate of the embryo or foetus
- identifying the presence of two or more foetuses
- measuring the foetal head, abdomen or femur to determine the stage of pregnancy
- identifying some foetuses with Down's syndrome
- identifying foetal abnormalities, such as hydrocephalus and microcephaly
- identifying abnormalities of internal organs, such as the kidneys or bladder
- measuring the amount of amniotic fluid to help determine foetal well-being
- identifying the location, size and maturity of the placenta
- identifying placental abnormalities
- identifying uterine abnormalities or tumours
- determining the position of an IUD
- differentiating between miscarriage, ectopic pregnancy and normal pregnancy
- in connection with various tests, such as amniocentesis, percutaneous umbilical-cord blood sampling (PUBS) and chorionic villus sampling (CVS), to select a safe place to do each test

You may be asked to drink a lot of water before an ultrasound examination. If you have had an ultrasound exam during a previous pregnancy, one of the main things you may remember is how uncomfortable you were with your bladder full to overflowing!

Your bladder is in front of your uterus. When your bladder is empty, your uterus is harder to see because it is farther down inside the pelvic bones. Bones disrupt ultrasound signals and make the picture harder to interpret. With your bladder full, your uterus rises out of the pelvis and can be seen more easily. The bladder acts as a window to look through to see the uterus and the foetus inside.

Various Ultrasound Tests. There's a 3-dimensional ultrasound now available in some areas of the UK that provides detailed, clear pictures of the foetus in the womb. They're so clear the image almost looks like a picture. For the pregnant woman, the test is almost the same. The difference is that computer software 'translates' the picture into a 3-D image. This ultrasound may be used when there is suspicion of foetal abnormalities and the doctor wants to take a closer look. One use of the 3-D ultrasound is to help diagnose and evaluate cleft lip and cleft palate in a developing foetus. It helps medical personnel define the extent of the defect so a treatment programme to implement immediately after birth can be planned.

The ultrasound vaginal probe, also called the *transvaginal ultrasound*, can be used in early pregnancy for a better view of the baby and placenta. A probe is placed inside the vagina, and the pregnancy is viewed from this angle. You don't have to have your bladder full for this one!

Can Ultrasound Determine the Baby's Sex? Some couples ask for ultrasound to determine whether they are carrying a boy or girl. If the baby is in a good position and it is old enough for the genitals to have developed and they can be seen clearly, determination may be possible. However, many doctors feel this reason alone is not a good reason to do an ultrasound exam. Discuss it with your doctor. Understand ultrasound is a test, and tests can occasionally be wrong.

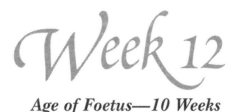

Week 12

Age of Foetus—10 Weeks

How Big Is Your Baby?

Your baby weighs between 8 to 14 g (⅓ and ½ oz), and crown-to-rump length is almost 6.1 cm (2½ in). As you can see on page 135, your baby's size has almost doubled in the past 3 weeks! Length of the baby is still a better measure at this time than foetal weight.

How Big Are You?

By the end of 12 weeks, your uterus is too large to remain completely in your pelvis. You may feel it above your pubic bone (pubic symphysis). The uterus has a remarkable ability to grow while you're pregnant. During pregnancy, it grows upwards to fill the pelvis and abdomen, and returns to its normal, pre-pregnancy size within a few weeks after delivery.

Before pregnancy, your uterus is almost solid. It holds about 10 ml (⅓ fl oz) or less. The uterus changes during pregnancy into a comparatively thin-walled, muscular container big enough to hold the foetus, placenta and amniotic fluid. The uterus increases its capacity 500 to

1000 times during pregnancy! The weight of the uterus also changes. When your baby is born, your uterus weighs almost 1.1 kg (40 oz) compared to 70 g (2½ oz) before pregnancy.

The uterine wall grows during the first few months of pregnancy due to hormonal stimulation by oestrogen and progesterone. Later in pregnancy, the growth of the baby and the placenta stretch and thin the uterine wall.

How Your Baby Is Growing and Developing

Few, if any, structures in the baby are formed after this week in pregnancy. However, the structures already formed continue to grow and to develop. At your 12-week visit (or close to that time), you'll probably be able to hear your baby's heartbeat! It can be heard with *doppler*, a special listening machine (not a stethoscope). It magnifies the sound of your baby's heartbeat so you can hear it.

The skeletal system now has centres of bone formation (ossification) in most bones. Fingers and toes have separated, and nails are growing. Scattered rudiments of hair appear on the body. External genitalia are beginning to show distinct signs of male or female sex characteristics.

Dad Tip At this doctor's/midwife's visit, it may be possible to hear the baby's heartbeat. If you can't be there, send a tape recorder with your partner so she can record the baby's heartbeat for you to listen to later.

The digestive system (small intestine) is capable of producing contractions that push food through the bowels. It is also able to absorb glucose (sugar).

At the base of your baby's brain, the pituitary gland is beginning to make many hormones. Hormones are chemicals that are made in one part of the body, but their action is exerted on another part of the body.

Other things are also happening. The foetal nervous system has developed further. Your baby is moving inside your uterus, but you probably

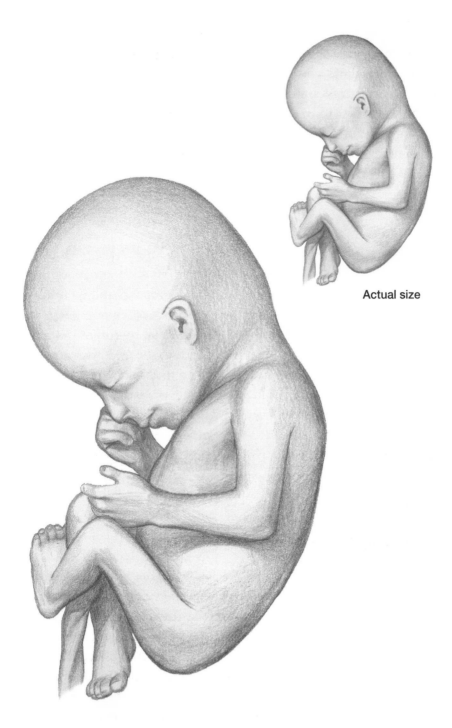

Actual size

Your baby is growing rapidly. It has doubled its length in the past 3 weeks.

won't feel it for a while yet. Stimulating the foetus in certain spots may cause it to squint, open its mouth and move its fingers or toes.

The amount of amniotic fluid is increasing. Total volume is now about 50 ml (1½ fl oz). At this time, the fluid is similar to maternal plasma (the non-cellular portion of your blood), except it contains much less protein.

Changes in You

You are probably starting to feel better than you have for most of your pregnancy. Around this time, morning sickness often begins to improve. You aren't extremely big and are probably still quite comfortable.

If it's your first pregnancy, you may still be wearing normal clothes. If you've had other pregnancies, you may start to show earlier and to feel more comfortable in looser clothing, such as maternity clothes.

You may be getting bigger in places besides your tummy. Your breasts are probably getting larger. They may have been sore for some time. You may also notice weight gain in your hips, legs and at your sides.

ᗌ Skin Changes

Your skin may change in various ways during pregnancy. In many women, skin down the middle of the abdomen becomes markedly darker or pigmented with a brown-black colour. It forms a vertical line called the *linea nigra*.

Occasionally irregular brown patches of varying size appear on the face and neck, called *chloasma* or *mask of pregnancy*. These disappear or get lighter after delivery. Oral contraceptives may cause similar pigmentation changes.

Vascular spiders (called *telangiectasias* or *angiomas*) are small red elevations on the skin, with branches extending outwards. The condition develops in about 65 per cent of white women and 10 per cent of black women during pregnancy.

A similar condition is redness of the palms, called *palmar erythaema*. It is seen in 65 per cent of white women and 35 per cent of black women.

Vascular spiders and palmar erythaema often occur together. Symptoms are temporary and disappear shortly after delivery. The occurrence of either condition is probably caused by high levels of oestrogen during pregnancy.

⌒ *Entering Pregnancy with High Blood Pressure*

If you have high blood pressure before you begin your pregnancy, you have an increased risk of pre-eclampsia. If left untreated during your pregnancy, hypertension reduces blood flow to the uterus and increases the risk of intrauterine-growth restriction (IUGR). In the mum-to-be, high blood pressure can cause seizures, kidney disease, liver disease, heart damage and brain damage.

Most blood-pressure medications are safe to use during pregnancy. However, ACE inhibitors should be avoided.

If your blood pressure is high when you begin your pregnancy, you may have more ultrasounds during pregnancy to monitor the baby's growth.

Tip for Week 12 If you have diarrhoea that doesn't go away in 24 hours, or if it keeps returning, call your doctor. You can take milk of magnesia for 24 hours to help deal with the problem, but don't self-medicate for longer than this time.

How Your Actions Affect Your Baby's Development

⌒ *Physical Injury during Pregnancy*

Trauma (physical injury) occurs in about 6 to 7 per cent of all pregnancies. Accidents involving motor vehicles account for about two-thirds of these cases; falls and assaults account for the remaining third. More than 90 per cent of these are minor injuries.

If you experience trauma during pregnancy, you may be taken care of by emergency-medicine personnel, trauma surgeons, general surgeons and your obstetrician. Most experts recommend observing a pregnant woman for a few hours after an accident. This provides adequate time to monitor the baby. Longer monitoring may be necessary in a more serious accident.

Your Nutrition

Some women misunderstand the concept of increasing their caloric intake during pregnancy. They think they can eat all they want. Don't fall into this trap! It's unhealthy for you and your baby if you gain too much weight during pregnancy, especially early in pregnancy. It makes carrying your baby more uncomfortable, and delivery may be more difficult. It may also be hard to shed the extra weight after pregnancy. After baby's birth, most women are anxious to return to 'normal' clothes and to look the way they did before pregnancy. Having to deal with extra weight can interfere with reaching this goal.

๛ Junk Food

Is junk food your kind of food? Do you eat it several times a day? Pregnancy is the time to break that habit! Now that you're pregnant, your dietary habits affect someone besides just yourself—your growing baby. If you're used to skipping breakfast, getting something 'from a machine' for lunch, then eating dinner at a fast-food restaurant, it doesn't help your pregnancy.

What and when you eat become more important when you realize how your actions affect your baby. Proper nutrition takes some planning on your part, but you can do it. Avoid foods that contain a lot of sugar and/or fat. Instead, choose healthy alternatives. If you work, take healthy foods with you for lunches and snacks. Stay away from fast food and junk food.

✧ Late-Night Snacks

Late-night nutritious snacks are beneficial for some women. However, for many women, snacking at night is unnecessary. If you're used to ice cream or other goodies before bed, you may pay for it during pregnancy with excessive weight gain. Food in your stomach late at night may also cause you more distress if you suffer from heartburn, indigestion or nausea and vomiting.

✧ Fats and Sweets

You may need to be cautious with fats and sweets, unless you're underweight and need to gain some weight. Many of these foods are high in calories and low in nutritional value. Eat them sparingly. Instead of selecting a food with little nutritional value, like crisps or biscuits, choose a piece of fruit, some cheese or a slice of whole-wheat bread with a little peanut butter. You'll satisfy your hunger and your nutritional needs at the same time! Some fats and sweets you may choose, and their serving sizes, include the following:

- sugar or honey—1 tablespoon
- oil—1 tablespoon
- margarine or butter—1 pat
- jam or jelly—1 tablespoon
- salad dressing—1 tablespoon

You Should Also Know

✧ Fifth Disease

Fifth disease, or *parvo virus B19*, which is also sometimes called 'slapped cheek' was the fifth disease to be described with a certain kind of rash. (It is *not* related to the parvo virus common in dogs.) Fifth disease is a mild, moderately contagious airborne infection. It spreads easily through groups, such as classrooms or day-care centres.

The rash looks like reddened skin caused by a slap (hence its common name). The reddening fades and recurs, and lasts from 2 to 34 days. There is no treatment.

This virus is important during pregnancy because it interferes with the production of red blood cells in the woman and the foetus. If you believe you have been exposed to fifth disease during pregnancy, contact your doctor. A blood test can determine whether you have previously had the virus. If you haven't, your doctor can monitor you to detect foetal problems. Some foetal problems can be dealt with before the baby is born.

⌁ Cystic Fibrosis Screening

Cystic fibrosis (CF) is a genetic disorder that causes digestive and breathing problems. Those with the disorder are usually diagnosed early in life. With modern technology and new screening tests, today we are able to determine whether there is a risk of delivering a child with CF. The screening test uses a blood sample or a saliva sample.

Your chances for carrying the gene are quite low. For a baby to have CF, *both* parents must carry the gene. Whites have a 3 per cent chance of carrying the CF gene; those of African descent a 1½ per cent chance and Asians about a 1 per cent chance. However, a family history of CF increases your chances of carrying the gene.

Testing for Cystic Fibrosis. Testing for cystic fibrosis is becoming more widespread. It is often offered to couples before pregnancy, as part of genetic counselling. One test available is called *Cystic Fibrosis (CF) Complete Test;* it can identify more than 1000 mutations of the CF gene. This identification process lets doctors offer accurate detection in carriers, which can lead to antenatal counselling and diagnosis.

If both you and your partner carry the CF gene, your baby will have a 25 per cent chance of having cystic fibrosis, even if you have other children who do not have the problem. Your developing baby can be tested during your pregnancy with chorionic villus sampling (see Week 10) around the 10th or 11th week of pregnancy. Amniocentesis (see pages 171–172) may also be used to test the foetus.

If you believe cystic fibrosis is a serious concern or if you have a family history of the disease, talk to your doctor about this test. Screening is recommended for those at higher risk for CF, such as Caucasians, including Ashkenazi Jews. Testing is a personal decision that you and your partner must make based on the information provided to you by your health-care team.

Many couples choose not to have the test because it would not change what they would do during the pregnancy. In addition, they do not want to expose the mother-to-be or the developing foetus to the risks of CVS or amniocentesis.

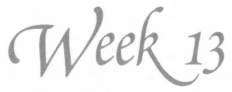

Week 13

Age of Foetus—11 Weeks

How Big Is Your Baby?

Your baby is growing rapidly! Its crown-to-rump length is 6.5 to 7.8 cm (2½ to 3 in), and it weighs between 13 to 20 g (½ and ¾ oz). It is about the size of a peach.

How Big Are You?

Your uterus has grown quite a bit. You can probably feel its upper edge above the pubic bone in the lowest part of your abdomen, about 10 cm (4 in) below your bellybutton. At 12 to 13 weeks, your uterus fills your pelvis and starts growing upwards into your abdomen. It feels like a soft, smooth ball.

Tip for Week 13 When cutting down on caffeine during pregnancy, read labels. More than 200 foods, beverages and over-the-counter medications contain caffeine!

You have probably gained some weight by now. If morning sickness has been a problem and you've had a hard time eating, you may not have gained much weight. As you feel better and as your baby rapidly starts to gain weight, you'll also gain weight.

How Your Baby Is Growing and Developing

Foetal growth is particularly striking from now through about 24 weeks of pregnancy. The baby has doubled in length since the 7th week. Changes in foetal weight have also been tremendous during the last 8 to 10 weeks of your pregnancy.

One interesting change is the relative slowdown in the growth of your baby's head compared to the rest of its body. In week 13, the head is about half the crown-to-rump length. By week 21, the head is about ⅓ of the baby's body. At birth, your baby's head is only ¼ the size of its body. Foetal body growth accelerates as foetal head growth slows.

Your baby's face is beginning to look more human-like. Eyes, which started out on the side of the head, move closer together on the face. The ears come to lie in their normal position on the sides of the head. External genitalia have developed enough so a male can be distinguished from a female if examined outside the womb.

Intestines initially develop within a large swelling in the umbilical cord outside the foetal body. About this time, they withdraw into the foetal abdominal cavity. If this doesn't occur and the intestines remain outside the foetal abdomen at birth, a condition called an *omphalocele* occurs. It is rare (occurs in 1 of 10,000 births). The condition can usually be repaired with surgery, and babies do well afterwards.

Changes in You

You are losing your waist! Clothing fits snugly. It's time to start wearing loose-fitting garments.

✐ Stretch Marks

Stretch marks, called *striae distensae*, are seen often, and in varying degrees, during pregnancy. They may appear early or later in your pregnancy, usually on the abdomen, breasts, and hips or buttocks. After pregnancy, they may fade to the same colour as the rest of your skin, but they won't go away. To help avoid the occurrence of stretch marks, gain weight slowly and steadily. Any large increases in weight can cause stretch marks to appear more readily.

If you use steroid creams, such as hydrocortisone, to treat stretch marks during pregnancy, you absorb some of the steroid into your system. The substance can then pass to your developing baby. *Don't use steroid creams during pregnancy without first checking with your doctor!*

Some Actions to Take. Although the formation of stretch marks may occur during pregnancy, there are some things you can do that may help reduce their severity. Try the following.

- Drink lots of water, and eat healthy foods. Foods high in antioxidants—fruits and vegetables that are bright red, orange or yellow—provide nutrients essential for tissue repair and healing.
- Maintain skin's elasticity by eating adequate amounts of protein and smaller amounts of fats. Flaxseed, flaxseed oil, fish and fish oils are all good sources. Be careful with your fish consumption—you don't want to eat *too* much. See the discussion of fish in Week 26.
- Stay out of the sun!
- Keep up with your exercise programme.
- Ask your doctor about using creams with alpha-hydroxy acid, citric acid or lactic acid. Some of these creams and lotions improve the quality of the skin's elastic fibres.

Treatment after Pregnancy. Many women want to know what they can do for the stretch marks they develop during pregnancy. After pregnancy, you have quite a few options for treatment. Some new treatments being used today seem to help a lot.

The use of Retin-A or Retinova, in combination with glycolic acid, has been shown to be fairly effective. Prescriptions are needed for Retin-A and Retinova. Another cream that has successfully been used to treat stretch marks is called StriVectin-SD. It is available directly from the manufacturer at www.StriVectin.com.

The most effective treatment is laser treatment, but it can be very costly. It is often done in combination with the medication methods described above. With *Nd:YAG laser treatment,* beams of laser light are directed into the collagen in the second layer of skin to help smooth wrinkles. *Pulsed dye laser treatment* can improve new and old stretch marks. However, lasers don't work for everyone.

Massage has proved effective—it increases blood flow to the area to stimulate the healing process and gets rid of dead surface cells. Various creams may also help. Discuss these treatments with your doctor if your stretch marks bother you.

✑ Changes in Your Breasts

You have probably noticed your breasts are changing. (See the illustration on page 146.) The mammary gland (another name for the breast) got its name from the Latin term for breast—*mamma.*

Your breast is made up of glands, connective tissue to provide support and fatty tissue to provide protection. Milk-producing sacs connect with the ducts leading to the nipple.

Before pregnancy, the average breast weighs about 200 g (7 oz). During pregnancy, breasts increase in size and weight. Near the end of pregnancy, each breast may weigh 400 to 800 g (14 to 28 oz). During nursing, each breast may weigh 800 g (28 oz) or more.

The size and shape of women's breasts vary greatly. Breast tissue usually projects under the arm. Glands that make up the breast open into ducts in the nipple. Each nipple contains nerve endings, muscle fibres, sebaceous glands, sweat glands and about 20 milk ducts.

Ðad Ꞇip Ask the doctor if there is some exercise you can do together on a regular basis during pregnancy, such as walking, swimming or playing golf or tennis.

The nipple is surrounded by the *areola,* a circular, pigmented area. During pregnancy, the areola darkens and grows larger. A darkened areola may act as a visual signal for the breastfeeding infant.

Breasts undergo many changes during pregnancy. In the early weeks, a common symptom of pregnancy is tingling or soreness of the

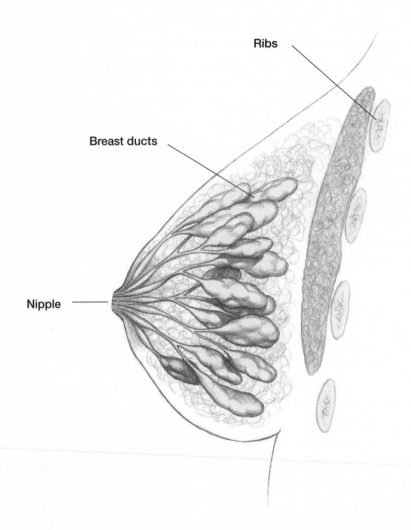

Ribs

Breast ducts

Nipple

Development of the maternal breast by end of the first trimester (13 weeks of pregnancy).

breasts. After about 8 weeks of pregnancy, your breasts may grow larger and become nodular or lumpy as glands and ducts inside the breasts grow and develop. As your breasts change during pregnancy, you may notice veins appear just beneath the skin.

During the second trimester, a thin yellow fluid called *colostrum* begins to form. It can sometimes be expressed from the nipple by gentle massage. If your breasts have grown, you may notice stretch marks on your breasts similar to those on your abdomen.

Mammary glands begin to develop in the 6-week-old embryo. By the time of birth, milk ducts are present. After birth, a newborn's breasts may be swollen and may even secrete a small amount of milk. This can occur in both male and female infants and is caused by the secretion of oestrogen.

How Your Actions Affect Your Baby's Development

✤ Working during Pregnancy

Today, many women work outside the home, and many continue to work during pregnancy. It is common for employers and patients to ask doctors about work and pregnancy.

'*Is it safe to work while I'm pregnant?*'

'*Can I work my entire pregnancy?*'

'*Am I in danger of harming my baby if I work?*'

Nearly 40 per cent of all women work or are seeking work. In the UK, thousands of babies are born to women who have been employed at some time during pregnancy. These women have understandable concerns about safety and occupational health.

Legislation that May Affect You. Pregnant women are entitled to certain rights and benefits depending on their circumstances, income and national insurance contributions. You also get free prescriptions and dental treatment, and you may get free milk and vitamins for yourself and any children under five.

If you work, your job has to be kept open for you irrespective of your length of service. In addition, all employed women are entitled to ordinary maternity leave which, in April 2003, was increased from 18 to 26 weeks, regardless of how long you have worked for your present employer. Women who have completed 26 weeks' continuous service with their employer by the beginning of the 14th week before their expected week of childbirth (EWC) can take additional maternity leave. Additional maternity leave starts immediately after ordinary maternity leave and continues for a further 26 weeks. Additional maternity leave is usually unpaid, although a woman may have contractual rights to pay during her period of additional maternity leave.

A pregnant employee must notify her employer of her intention to take maternity leave by the end of the 15th week before her EWC, unless this is not reasonably practicable. She must tell her employer:

• that she is pregnant
• the week her baby is expected to be born
• when she wants her maternity leave to start.

A woman can change her mind about when she wants to start her leave providing she tells her employer at least 28 days in advance (unless this is not reasonably practicable). The earliest date a woman can start her maternity leave continues to be the 11th week before her baby is due.

In terms of payment, you will receive Statutory Maternity Pay from your employer worth 90 per cent of your earning for 6 weeks, followed, currently, by 20 weeks at £100 (or 90 per cent of earnings for the full 26 weeks if this is less than £100 a week).

Since April 2003, fathers have also been entitled to paternity leave and pay. Eligible employees can take up to 2 weeks' paid leave to care for their new baby and support the mother.

Employees—both mothers and fathers—who have completed one year's service with their employers are entitled to 13 weeks' (unpaid) parental leave to care for their child. Parental leave can usually be taken up to 5 years from the date of birth. All employees are also entitled to take a reasonable amount of (unpaid) time off work to deal with an emergency or unexpected situation involving a dependant.

For more information, contact either the Department of Trade and Industry (DTI) or the Maternity Alliance (see Resources).

Some Risks If You Work during Pregnancy. It may be difficult to know the exact risk of a particular job. In most cases, we don't have enough information to know all the specific substances that can harm a developing baby.

The goal is to minimize the risk to the mother and baby while still enabling a woman to work. A normal woman with a normal job should be able to work throughout her pregnancy. However, she may need to modify her job somewhat. For example, she may need to spend less time standing. Studies show that women who stand in the same position for prolonged periods are more likely to give birth to premature babies and babies with low birthweight.

Work with your doctor and your employer. If problems arise, such as premature labour or bleeding, listen to your doctor. If bed rest at home is suggested, follow that advice. As your pregnancy progresses, you may have to work fewer hours or do lighter work. Be flexible. It doesn't help you or your baby if you wear yourself out and make complications of pregnancy worse.

Take Care of Yourself If You Work. If you work, you should take some precautions for you and your growing baby.

- Don't participate in anything that is dangerous for you or baby.
- Don't stand for long periods of time.
- Sit up straight at your desk.
- Place a low footstool under your desk to rest your feet on.
- Rest at breaks and during lunch.
- Get up and walk a little every 30 minutes. Going to the bathroom may be a good reason to get up and move around.

- Don't wear clothes that are tight around the waist, especially if you sit most of the day.
- Drink lots of water.
- Listen to soothing music, if you can.
- Bring healthy lunch and snack foods to help you keep tabs on your calorie intake. Fast foods are loaded with empty calories.
- Try to keep stress to a minimum.
- Don't take on new projects or ones that demand a lot of time and attention.

Your Nutrition

Caffeine is a central-nervous-system stimulant found in many beverages and foods, including coffee, tea, cola drinks and chocolate. Research shows that you may be more sensitive to caffeine during pregnancy. The stimulant is also found in some medications, such as diet aids and headache medications. For over 20 years, doctors have recommended that pregnant women avoid caffeine. To date, no benefits to you or your unborn baby have been found with its use.

A Caffeine Warning

High levels of caffeine in a pregnant woman—400 mg a day—may affect a baby's developing respiratory system. One study showed this exposure before birth might be linked to sudden infant death syndrome (SIDS).

High intake of caffeine has been associated with a decreased birthweight and a smaller head size in newborns. Some researchers also believe there is an association between caffeine use and miscarriage, stillbirth and premature labour.

Cut down on caffeine, or eliminate it from your diet. It crosses the placenta to the baby. It can affect your calcium metabolism and your baby's, too. If you're jittery, your baby may suffer from the same effects. Increased caffeine consumption may increase the chances of breathing problems in a newborn. Caffeine passes to breast milk, which can cause irritability and sleeplessness in a breastfed baby. An infant metabolizes caffeine slower than an adult, and caffeine can collect in the infant.

Effects of caffeine on you during pregnancy may include irritability, headaches, stomach upset, sleeplessness and jitters. Smoking may compound the stimulant effect of caffeine.

Eliminate caffeine from your diet, or limit the amount of caffeine you consume. Read labels on over-the-counter medications for caffeine. Most professionals agree that up to two cups *(not mugs)* of regular coffee or its equivalent each day is probably OK. That's less than 200 mg a day.

It may be a good idea to eliminate as much caffeine as you can from your diet. It's healthier for your baby, and you'll probably feel better, too. The list below details the amounts of caffeine from various sources:

- coffee, 150 ml (5 fl oz)—from 60 to 140 mg and higher
- tea, 150 ml (5 fl oz)—from 30 to 65 mg
- baking chocolate, 25 g (1 oz)—25 mg
- chocolate confectionary, 25 g (1 oz)—6 mg
- soft drinks, 350 ml (12 fl oz)—from 35 to 55 mg
- pain-relief tablets, standard dose—40 mg
- allergy and cold remedies, standard dose—25 mg

You Should Also Know

⌇ *Lyme Disease*
Lyme disease refers to an infection transmitted to humans by ticks. There are several stages of the illness. About 80 per cent of those bitten have a skin lesion with a distinctive look, called a *bull's eye*. There may be flu-like symptoms. After 4 to 6 weeks, symptoms may become more serious.

At the beginning of the illness, blood tests may not diagnose Lyme disease. A blood test done later in the illness can establish the diagnosis.

We know Lyme disease can cross the placenta. However, at this time we don't know if it is dangerous to the baby. Researchers are studying the situation.

Treatment for Lyme disease requires long-term antibiotic therapy and sometimes intravenous antibiotic therapy. Many medications used to treat Lyme disease are safe to use during pregnancy.

Avoid exposure to Lyme disease, if possible. Stay out of areas known to have ticks, especially heavily wooded areas. If you can't avoid these areas, wear long-sleeved shirts, long trousers, a hat or scarf, socks and boots or closed shoes. Be sure to check your hair when you come in; ticks often attach themselves there. Check your clothing to make sure no ticks remain in folds, cuffs or pockets.

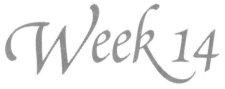

Week 14

Age of Foetus—12 Weeks

How Big Is Your Baby?

The crown-to-rump length is 8 to 9.3 cm (3¼ to 4 in). Your baby is about the size of your fist and weighs almost 25 g (1 oz).

How Big Are You?

Maternity clothes may be a 'must' by now. Some women try to get by for a while by not buttoning or zipping their trousers all the way or by using rubber bands or safety pins to increase the size of their waistbands. Others wear their partner's clothing, but that usually works for only a short time. You're going to get even bigger. You'll enjoy your pregnancy more and feel better with clothing that fits comfortably and provides you with room to grow.

How your body responds to this growth is influenced by any previous pregnancies and the changes your body experienced then. Your skin and muscles stretched to accommodate your uterus, placenta and baby, and that changed them permanently. Skin and muscles may give way faster to accommodate your growing uterus and baby. This means you may show sooner and feel bigger.

How Your Baby Is Growing and Developing

As you can see in the illustration on the opposite page, by this week your baby's ears have moved from the neck to the sides of the head. Eyes have been moving gradually from the side of the head to the front of the face. The neck continues to get longer, and the chin no longer rests on the chest.

> If you enjoy listening to your baby's heartbeat, devices are now available so you can listen at home! Some people believe this activity helps a couple bond with their child. If you are interested in a use-at-home doppler device, check with your doctor/midwife at your next visit. Or check out these devices on the Internet. See the Resource section, page 430.

Sexual development continues. It is becoming easier to determine male from female by looking at external genitalia, which are more developed.

Changes in You

✑ Skin Tags and Moles

Pregnancy can make skin tags and moles change and grow. Skin tags are small tags of skin that may appear for the first time or may grow larger during pregnancy. Moles may appear for the first time during pregnancy, or existing moles may grow larger and darken. If a mole changes, it must be checked. If you notice any change, show it to your doctor!

✑ Do You Have Haemorrhoids?

Haemorrhoids, dilated blood vessels around or inside the anus, are a common problem during or following pregnancy. They are caused during pregnancy by the decreased blood flow in the area around the uterus and the pelvis because of the weight of the uterus, causing congestion or

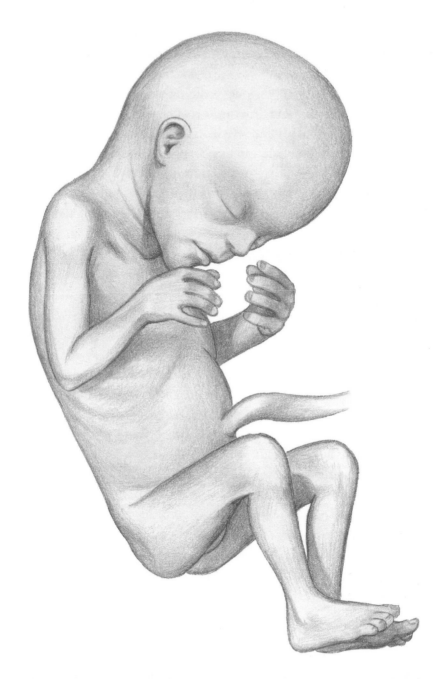

Your baby continues to change. Ears and eyes move to a more normal position by this week.

blockage of circulation. Haemorrhoids may worsen towards the end of pregnancy. They may also get worse with each succeeding pregnancy.

Haemorrhoid treatment includes avoiding constipation by eating adequate amounts of fibre and drinking lots of fluid. You may avoid haemorrhoids by using stool softeners. Other measures include sitz baths and suppository medications. You can buy suppositories without a prescription. Rarely, haemorrhoids are treated during pregnancy with surgery.

After pregnancy, haemorrhoids usually improve, but they may not go away completely. You can use the treatment methods mentioned above when pregnancy is over.

If haemorrhoids cause you a great deal of discomfort, discuss it with your doctor. He or she will know what treatment method is best for you.

Relieving the Discomfort of Haemorrhoids. If haemorrhoids are a problem, try any of the following suggestions for relief.

- Rest at least 1 hour every day with your feet and hips elevated.
- Lie with your legs elevated and knees slightly bent (Sims position) when you sleep at night.
- Eat adequate amounts of fibre, and drink lots of fluid.
- Take warm (not hot) baths for relief.
- Suppository medications, available without a prescription, may help.
- Apply ice packs, or cotton wool balls soaked in witch hazel, to the affected area.
- Don't sit or stand for long periods.

How Your Actions Affect Your Baby's Development

↷ X-Rays, CT Scans and MRIs during Pregnancy
Some women are concerned about tests that use radiation during pregnancy. Can these tests hurt the baby? Can you have them at any time in pregnancy?

No known amount of radiation is safe for a developing baby. Dangers to your baby include an increased risk of mutations and an increased risk of cancer later in life. Some doctors believe the only safe amount of X-ray during pregnancy is none.

Researchers have become more aware of the potential dangers of radiation to a developing foetus. At present, they believe the foetus is at greatest risk between 8 and 15 weeks gestation (between the foetal ages of 6 weeks and 13 weeks).

Problems, such as pneumonia or appendicitis, can and do occur in pregnant women and may require an X-ray for proper diagnosis and treatment. Discuss the need for X-rays with your doctor. It is your responsibility to let your doctor and others involved in your care know you are pregnant or may be pregnant before you undergo any medical test. It's easier to deal with the questions of safety and risk *before* a test is performed.

If you have an X-ray or series of X-rays, then discover you are pregnant, ask your doctor about the possible risk to your baby. He or she will be able to advise you.

Computerized tomographic scans, also called *CT scans,* are a form of specialized X-ray. This technique combines X-ray with computer analysis. Many researchers believe the amount of radiation received by a foetus from a CT scan is much lower than that received from a regular X-ray. However, these tests should be undertaken with caution until we know more about the effects even this small amount of radiation has on a developing foetus.

Magnetic resonance imaging, also called *MRI,* is another diagnostic tool widely used today. At this time, no harmful effects in pregnancy have been reported from the use of MRI. However, it is probably best to avoid MRI during the first trimester of pregnancy.

ᴥ *Dental Care*
In the UK, dental treatment is free for pregnant women (and for a year after you have given birth), so you have no reason to avoid your dentist or ignore your teeth while you're pregnant. See your dentist at least once during pregnancy. Tell your dentist you're pregnant. If you need dental work, postpone it until after the first 12 weeks, if possible. You

may not be able to wait if you have an infection. An untreated infection could be harmful to you and your baby.

Antibiotics or pain medications may be necessary. If you need medication, consult your doctor before taking anything. Many antibiotics and pain medications are OK to take during pregnancy.

Be careful with regard to anaesthesia for dental work during pregnancy. Local anaesthesia is OK. Avoid gas and general anaesthesia when possible. If general anaesthesia is necessary, make sure an experienced anaesthesiologist who knows you are pregnant administers it.

Dental Emergencies. Dental emergencies do occur. Emergencies you might face include root canal, tooth extraction, a large cavity, an abscessed tooth or problems resulting from an accident or injury. Any of these emergencies can occur during pregnancy. A serious dental problem must be treated. Problems that could result from not treating it are more serious than the risks you might be exposed to with treatment.

Tip for Week 14 If you must have dental work or diagnostic tests, tell your dentist or your doctor you are pregnant so they can take extra care with you. It may be helpful for your dentist and doctor to talk before any decisions are made.

Dental X-rays are sometimes necessary and can be done during pregnancy. Your abdomen must be shielded with a lead apron before X-rays are taken. If possible, wait until after the end of the first trimester to have any dental work done.

Your Nutrition

Being overweight when pregnancy begins may present special problems for you. Your doctor may advise you to gain less weight than the average 11 to 16 kg (25 to 35 lb) recommended for a normal-weight woman. You will probably have to choose lower-calorie, lower-fat foods to eat. A visit with a nutritionist may be necessary to help you develop a healthy food plan. You will be advised *not* to diet during pregnancy.

Extra weight may cause more problems, including gestational diabetes or high blood pressure. Backaches, varicose veins and fatigue may also be more troublesome. If you gain too much weight during your pregnancy—beyond the amount of weight your doctor recommends— you may have a greater chance of needing a Caesarean delivery.

Ðad Tip If you go out of town, call your partner at least once every day. Let her know you are thinking about her and the baby.

If you're overweight, your doctor may want to see you more often during your pregnancy. Ultrasound may be needed to help establish your due date because it's harder to determine the position and size of the foetus. Extra layers of abdominal fat may make manual examination difficult. Your doctor may order tests for gestational diabetes. Other diagnostic tests may also be necessary as your due date nears.

You Should Also Know

๛ *Pregnancy in the Armed Forces and Police Force*
Women serving in the Armed Forces and Police are entitled to Statutory Maternity Pay (described on page 148), and can claim sex discrimination, but are not entitled to the other rights for pregnant women workers.

Some General Cautions. We know that women who get pregnant while they are on active duty face many challenges. The pressure to meet military body-weight standards can have an effect on your health. Work hard to eat healthy foods so your iron stores and folic-acid levels are adequate. Examine your job for any hazards you may be exposed to, such as standing for prolonged periods, heavy lifting and exposure to toxic chemicals. Before receiving any vaccinations or inoculations, discuss them with your doctor. All of these factors can impact on your pregnancy.

If you are concerned about any of the above, discuss it with a superior. Changes beyond those described above may have to be made.

ᘍ *Taking Others to Your Doctor Visits*

Take your partner with you to as many antenatal appointments as possible. It's nice for your partner and doctor to meet before labour begins. Maybe your mother or the other grandmother-to-be would like to go with you to hear their grandchild's heartbeat. Or you may want to take a tape recorder and record the heartbeat for others to hear. Things have changed since your mother carried you; many grandmothers-to-be enjoy this type of visit.

It's a good idea to wait until you have heard your baby's heartbeat before bringing other people. You don't always hear it the first time, and this can be frustrating and disappointing.

Bringing Children to a Clinic Visit. Some women bring their children with them to a antenatal appointment. Most doctors and hospital staff don't mind if you bring your children with you occasionally. They understand it may not always be possible to find someone to watch your children. However, if you are having problems or have a lot to discuss with your doctor/midwife, don't bring your child or children.

If a child is sick, has just got over chicken pox or is getting a cold, leave him or her at home. Don't expose everyone else in the waiting room.

Some women like to bring one child at a time to a visit if they have more than one. That makes it special for the expectant mum and for them. Crying or complaining children can create a difficult situation, however, so ask your doctor/midwife when it's good to bring family members with you before you come in with them.

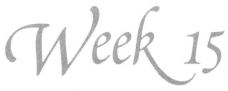

Week 15

Age of Foetus—13 Weeks

How Big Is Your Baby?

The foetal crown-to-rump length by this week of pregnancy is 9.3 to 10.3 cm (4 to 4½ in). The foetus weighs about 50 g (1¾ oz). It's close to the size of an orange.

How Big Are You?

You can easily tell you're pregnant by the changes in your lower abdomen, which change the way your clothes fit. You may be able to feel your uterus about 7.6 to 10 cm (3 or 4 in) below your bellybutton (also called the *umbilicus* or *navel*).

Dad Tip When you need to be away or out of touch, ask friends and family members to check on your partner and to be available to help out.

Your pregnancy may not be obvious to other people when you wear regular street clothes. But it may become obvious if you start wearing maternity clothes or put on a swim suit.

How Your Baby Is
Growing and Developing

It's still a little early to feel movement, although you should feel your baby move in the next few weeks!

Your baby's rapid growth continues. Its skin is thin. At this point in its development, you can see blood vessels through the skin. Fine hair, called *lanugo hair,* covers the baby's body.

By this time, your baby may be sucking its thumb. This has been seen with ultrasound examination. Eyes continue to move to the front of the face but are still widely separated.

Ears continue to develop externally. As you can see in the illustration on page 163, they now look more like normal ears. In fact, your baby looks more human with each passing day.

Bones that have already formed are getting harder and retaining calcium (ossifying) rapidly. If an X-ray were done at this time, the baby's skeleton would be visible.

✺ *Alpha-foetoprotein Testing*
As your baby grows inside you, it produces *alpha-foetoprotein.* This protein is found in increasing amounts in the amniotic fluid. Some alpha-foetoprotein crosses foetal membranes and enters your circulation. It is possible to measure the amount of alpha-foetoprotein by drawing your blood.

The level of this protein can be meaningful during pregnancy. An alpha-foetoprotein (AFP) test is usually done between 16 and 18 weeks of gestation. The timing of the test is important and must be correlated to the gestational age of your pregnancy and to your weight.

An elevated level of alpha-foetoprotein can indicate problems with the foetus, such as spina bifida (spinal-cord problem) or anencephaly (serious central-nervous-system defect). Some researchers have even found an association between a low level of alpha-foetoprotein and Down's syndrome. In the past, amniocentesis was the only way to test for Down's syndrome.

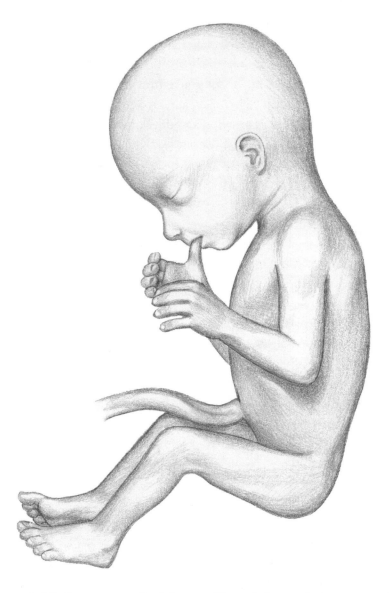

By week 15 of pregnancy (foetal age—13 weeks), your baby may suck its thumb. Eyes are at the front of the face but are still widely separated.

If the level of alpha-foetoprotein is abnormal, a careful ultrasound examination is done to look for spina bifida, anencephaly and Down's syndrome. This ultrasound may help determine how far along in pregnancy you are.

The AFP test is not done on all pregnant women. If the test isn't offered to you, ask about it. There is relatively little risk, and it tells your doctor how your foetus is growing and developing.

Changes in You

↷ *Cervical Smears during Pregnancy*

A cervical smear may be carried out if there is any concern when the cervix is visualised during a speculum examination. However, cervical smears are not routine practise in the U.K.

The pap (or cervical) smear (short for *Papanicolaou smear*) is a screening test done at the time of a pelvic exam. It identifies cancerous or precancerous cells coming from the cervix, which is located at the top of the vagina. This test has contributed to a significant decrease in mortality from cervical cancer because of early detection and treatment.

An Abnormal Cervical Smear. Cervical smears are screening tests. If you have an abnormal cervical smear, your doctor must verify the findings and decide on treatment. Continue to get checked as your doctor advises.

An abnormal cervical smear during pregnancy must be handled individually. When abnormal cells are 'not too bad' (premalignant or not as serious), it may be possible to watch them during pregnancy with colposcopy or cervical smears; biopsies are not usually done at this time. The cervix bleeds easily during pregnancy because of changes in circulation. This situation must be handled carefully.

Women who deliver vaginally may see a change in abnormal cervical smears. One study showed that 60 per cent of a group of women who were diagnosed with high-grade squamous intra-epithelial lesions in the cervix before giving birth had normal Pap smears after their baby was born.

How Your Actions Affect Your Baby's Development

∾ *Change Sleeping Positions Now*

Some women have questions and concerns about their sleeping positions and sleep habits while they're pregnant. Some want to know if they can sleep on their stomachs. Others want to know if they should stop sleeping on their waterbed. (It's OK to continue to sleep on a waterbed.)

As you grow larger during pregnancy, finding comfortable sleeping positions will become more difficult. Don't lie on your back when you sleep. As your uterus gets larger, lying on your back can place the uterus on top of important blood vessels (the aorta and the inferior vena cava) that run down the back of your abdomen. This can decrease circulation to your baby and parts of your body. Some pregnant women also find it harder to breathe when lying on their backs.

Lying on your stomach puts extra pressure on your growing uterus. This is another reason to learn to sleep on your side. For some women, their favourite thing after delivery is to be able to sleep on their stomach again!

Tip for Week 15 Start now to learn to sleep on your side; it will pay off later as you get bigger. Sometimes it helps to use a few extra pillows. Put one behind you so if you roll onto your back, you won't lie flat. Put another pillow between your legs, or rest your 'top' leg on a pillow. Some manufacturers make a 'pregnancy pillow' that supports your entire body.

Your Nutrition

About this time, you'll probably need to start adding an extra 300 calories to your meal plan to meet the needs of your growing foetus and your changing body. Below are some choices of extra food for one day to get those 300 calories. Be careful—300 calories is *not* a lot of food.

- Choice 1—2 thin slices pork, 50 g (2 oz) cabbage, 1 carrot
- Choice 2—85 g (3 oz) cooked brown rice, 115 g (4 oz) strawberries, 240 ml (8 fl oz) orange juice, 1 slice fresh pineapple
- Choice 3—125-g (4½ oz) salmon steak, 3–4 asparagus spears, 115 g (4 oz) Romaine (Cos) lettuce
- Choice 4—85 g (3 oz) cooked pasta, 1 slice fresh tomato, 240 ml (8 fl oz) skimmed milk, 50 g (2 oz) cooked green beans, ¼ cantaloupe
- Choice 5—1 small carton of yoghurt, 1 medium apple

You Should Also Know

✂ *Getting a Good Night's Sleep*
Sleeping soundly may be difficult for you now or later in pregnancy. Try some of the following suggestions to ensure a restful sleep.

- Go to bed and wake up at the same time each day.
- Don't drink too much fluid at night. Slow down after 6 pm so you don't have to get up to go to the bathroom all night long.
- Avoid caffeine after late afternoon.
- Get regular exercise.
- Sleep in a cool bedroom; 21.1°C (70°F) is about the highest temperature for comfortable sleeping.
- If you experience heartburn at night, sleep propped up.

You may experience shortness of breath due to your enlarging abdomen, which can interfere with your sleep. If you do, try lying on your left side. Prop up your head and shoulders with extra pillows. If this measure doesn't provide relief, light exercise followed by a warm shower or a soak in a warm (not hot) bath and a glass of warm milk might be beneficial. If you just can't get comfortable in bed, try sleeping partially sitting up in a recliner.

Were You Hard to Live with When You Had Morning Sickness?

If you suffered with morning sickness and you're starting to feel better, you may want to take stock of your relationship with your partner and others close to you. Were you hard to get along with when you weren't feeling good? Your partner needs your support as your pregnancy progresses, just as you need his support. You may need to make an effort to work very hard at treating each other well—you're both in this together!

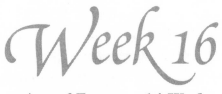

Week 16

Age of Foetus—14 Weeks

How Big Is Your Baby?

The crown-to-rump length of your baby by this week is 10.8 to 11.6 cm (4⅓ to 4⅔ in). Weight is about 80 g (2¾ oz).

How Big Are You?

As your baby grows, your uterus and placenta are also growing. Six weeks ago, your uterus weighed about 140 g (5 oz). Today, it weighs about 250 g (8¾ oz). The amount of amniotic fluid around the baby is also increasing. There is now about 220 ml (7½ fl oz) of fluid. You can easily feel your uterus about 7.5 cm (3 in) below your bellybutton.

How Your Baby Is Growing and Developing

Fine lanugo hair covers your baby's head. The umbilical cord is attached to the abdomen; this attachment has moved lower on the body of the foetus.

Fingernails are well formed. The illustration on page 170 shows soft hair, called *lanugo,* beginning to grow. At this stage, legs are longer than arms, and arms and legs are moving. You can see this movement during an ultrasound examination. You may also be able to feel your baby move at this point in your pregnancy.

Many women describe feelings of movement as a 'gas bubble' or 'fluttering.' Often, it's something you have noticed for a few days or more, but you didn't realize what you were feeling. Then you realize you're feeling the baby moving inside you!

Changes in You

ᵔ *Quickening*

If you haven't felt your baby move yet, don't worry. Foetal movement, also called *quickening,* is usually felt between 16 and 20 weeks of pregnancy. The time is different for every woman. It can also be different from one pregnancy to another. One baby may be more active than another and move more. The size of the baby or the number of foetuses can also affect what you feel.

ᵔ *Triple-Screen Test*

Tests are now available that go beyond alpha-foetoprotein testing in helping your doctor determine if you might be carrying a child with Down's syndrome. With the triple-screen test, your alpha-foetoprotein level is checked, along with the amounts of human chorionic gonadotropin (HCG) and unconjugated oestriol (a form of oestrogen produced by the placenta).

The levels of these three chemicals in your blood may indicate an increased chance your baby has Down's syndrome. For older mothers, the detection rate of the problem is better than 60 per cent, with a false-positive rate of nearly 25 per cent.

If you have an abnormal result with a triple-screen test, an ultrasound and amniocentesis may be recommended. An elevated alpha-foetoprotein level can indicate an increased risk of a neural-tube

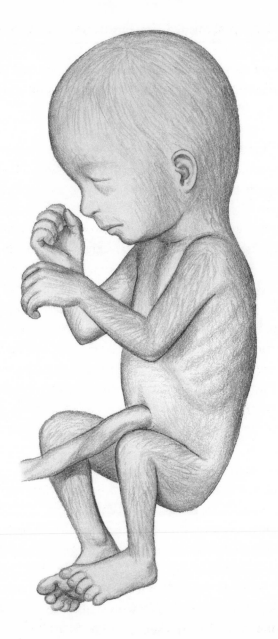

By this week, soft lanugo hair covers the baby's body and head.

defect (such as spina bifida). HCG and oestriol are normal in this case.

These blood tests are used to find *possible* problems. They are *screening* tests. A *diagnostic* test will usually be done to confirm any diagnosis.

How Your Actions Affect Your Baby's Development

ᴈ *Amniocentesis*

If it is necessary, an amniocentesis test is usually performed for prenatal evaluation around 16 to 18 weeks of pregnancy. By this point, your uterus is large enough and there is enough fluid surrounding the baby to make the test possible. Doing the procedure at this time allows a woman enough time to make decisions about terminating the pregnancy, if that is what she desires.

With amniocentesis, ultrasound is used to locate a pocket of fluid where the foetus and placenta are not in the way. The part of the abdomen above the uterus is cleaned. Skin is numbed, and a needle is passed through the abdominal wall into the uterus. Fluid is withdrawn from the amniotic cavity (area around the baby) with a syringe. About 30 ml (1 fl oz) of amniotic fluid is needed to perform various tests.

Foetal cells that float in the amniotic fluid can be grown in cultures and can be used to identify foetal abnormalities. We know of more than 400 abnormalities a child can be born with—amniocentesis identifies about 40 (10 per cent) of them, including the following:

- chromosomal problems, particularly Down's syndrome
- foetal sex, if sex-specific problems such as haemophilia or Duchenne muscular dystrophy must be identified
- skeletal diseases, such as osteogenesis imperfecta
- foetal infections, such as herpes or rubella
- central-nervous-system diseases, such as anencephaly

• haematologic (blood) diseases, such as erythroblastosis foetalis
• inborn errors of metabolism (chemical problems or deficiencies of enzymes), such as cystinuria or maple-syrup-urine disease

Risks from amniocentesis include injury to the foetus, placenta or umbilical cord, infection, miscarriage or premature labour. The use of ultrasound to guide the needle helps avoid complications but doesn't eliminate all risk. There can be bleeding from the foetus to the mother, which can be a problem because foetal and maternal blood are separate and may be different types. This is a particular risk to an Rh-negative mother carrying an Rh-positive baby (see the discussion on page 176). This type of bleeding can cause isoimmunization. An Rh-negative woman should receive Anti-D at the time of amniocentesis to prevent isoimmunization.

Foetal loss from amniocentesis complications is estimated to be less than 3 per cent. The procedure should be done only by someone who has experience doing it.

ᛘ *Are You an Older Mother-to-Be?*

More women every year are getting pregnant in their 30s or 40s. If you waited to start a family, you are not alone. The fertility rate in the UK for women aged 35 to 39 has risen at the fastest rate over the last 20 years, nearly doubling between 1981 and 1997. Women aged 25 to 29 are still the most likely to give birth, but since 1992 those in the 30 to 34 age group have been more likely to give birth than those aged 20 to 24.

When you are older, your partner may also be older. You may have married late or you may be in a second marriage and are starting a family together. Some couples have experienced infertility and do not achieve a pregnancy until they have gone through a major workup and testing or even surgery. Or you may be a single mother who has chosen donor insemination to achieve pregnancy.

Today, many healthcare professionals gauge pregnancy risk by the pregnant woman's health status, not her age. Pre-existing medical conditions are the most significant indicator of a woman's well-being during pregnancy. For example, a healthy 39-year-old is less likely to develop pregnancy problems than a woman in her 20s who suffers from diabetes. A woman's fitness can have a greater effect on her pregnancy than her age.

Most women who become pregnant in their 30s and 40s are in good health. A woman in good physical condition who has been exercising regularly may go through pregnancy as easily as a woman 15 to 20 years younger. An exception—women in a first pregnancy who are over 40 may encounter more complications than women the same age who have previously had children. But most healthy women will have a safe delivery.

Some health problems are age related—the risk of developing a condition increases with age. High blood pressure and some forms of diabetes are age related. You may not know you have these conditions unless you see your doctor regularly. Either condition can complicate a pregnancy and should be brought under control before pregnancy, if possible.

Genetic Counselling May Be a Wise Choice. If either you or your partner is over 35, genetic counselling may be recommended; this can raise many questions. The risk of chromosome abnormalities exceeds 5 per cent for this age group. The father's age can also impact on a pregnancy.

Genetic counselling brings together a couple and professionals who are trained to deal with the questions and problems associated with the occurrence, or risk of occurrence, of a genetic problem. With genetic counselling, information about human genetics is applied to a particular couple's situation. Information is interpreted so the couple can understand it and make informed decisions about childbearing. For further information on genetic counselling, see Preparing for Pregnancy.

Tip for Week 16 Some of the foods you normally love to eat may make you sick to your stomach during pregnancy. You may need to substitute other nutritious foods you tolerate better.

When a mother is older, the father is often older, too. It can be difficult to determine whose age—the mother's or the father's—matters the most in pregnancy. Some studies have demonstrated that men

55 or older are more likely to father babies with Down's syndrome. These studies indicate the risk increases with an older mother. We estimate that at the age of 40, a man's risk of fathering a child with Down's syndrome is about 1 per cent; that rate doubles at age 45 but is still only 2 per cent.

Some researchers now recommend that men father children before they are 40. This is a conservative viewpoint, and not everyone agrees with it. More data and research are needed before we can make definitive statements about a father's age and its effect on pregnancy.

Will Your Pregnancy Be Different If You're Older? As an older pregnant woman, your doctor may see you more often or you may have more tests performed. You may be advised to have amniocentesis or CVS, to determine whether your child will have Down's syndrome. This may be advisable, even if you would never terminate your pregnancy. Knowing these facts helps you prepare for the birth of your baby.

You may be watched more closely during pregnancy for signs and symptoms of gestational diabetes or hypertension. Both can be troublesome during pregnancy, but with good medical care, they can usually be handled fairly well. Older women are also more likely to have twins.

As far as physical effects, you may gain more weight, see stretch marks where there were none before, notice your breasts sag lower and feel a lack of tone in your muscles. Pregnancy and being older takes its toll. Attention to your lifestyle—nutrition and exercise—can help a great deal.

Because of demands on your time and energy, fatigue may be one of your greatest problems. It's a pregnant woman's most common complaint. Rest is essential to your health and to your baby's. Seize every opportunity to rest and nap. Don't take on more tasks or new roles. Don't volunteer for a big project at work or anywhere else. Learn to say 'No.' You'll feel better!

Moderate exercise can help boost your energy level and may eliminate or alleviate some discomforts. However, check first with your doctor before starting any exercise programme.

Stress can also be a problem. To alleviate feelings of stress, exercise, eat healthily and get as much rest as possible. Take time for yourself.

Some women find a pregnancy support group is an excellent way to deal with difficulties they may experience. Check with your doctor/midwife for further information.

Through research, we know that labour and delivery for an older woman may be different. Your cervix may not dilate as easily as in a younger woman, so labour may last longer. Older women also have a higher rate of Caesarean sections. One cause may be that older women often have larger babies, which may necessitate a C-section. After baby's birth, your uterus may not contract as quickly either. Postpartum bleeding may last longer and be heavier.

For an in-depth look at pregnancy for women over age 35, read our book *Your Pregnancy after 35*.

Your Nutrition

Good news—pregnant women should snack often, particularly during the second half of pregnancy! You should have three or four snacks a day, in addition to your regular meals. There are a couple of catches, though. Firstly, snacks must be nutritious. Secondly, meals may need to be smaller so you can eat those snacks. One nutritional goal in pregnancy is to eat enough so important nutrients are always available for your body's use and for use by the growing foetus.

Usually you want a snack to be quick and easy. It may take some planning and effort on your part to make sure nutritious foods are available for snacking. Prepare things in advance. Cut up fresh vegetables for later use in salads and for munching with low-calorie dip. Keep some hard-boiled eggs on hand. Peanut butter (reduced-fat or regular), pretzels and plain popcorn are good choices. Low-fat cheese and cottage cheese provide calcium. Fruit juice can replace fizzy drinks. If juice has more sugar than you need, cut it with water. Herbal teas can be healthy. (See the discussion of herbal teas in Week 30.)

You Should Also Know

✣ *Don't Lie on Your Back*

Week 16 is the turning point—no more lying flat on your back in bed while resting or sleeping or lying flat on the floor while exercising or relaxing. This position puts extra pressure on the aorta and vena cava, which can reduce blood flow to your baby.

Blood flow from mother to growing baby supplies the nutrients the foetus needs to develop and to grow. Don't endanger your baby's health and well-being by forgetting this important action.

Reclining in a chair or propped against pillows is OK. Just don't lie flat on your back!

✣ *Rh-sensitivity*

The lab tests you've had determined your blood type and Rh-factor. You may know this information by now. Your blood type (such as O, A, B, AB) and the Rh-factor are important. The Rh-factor is a protein in the blood; it is a genetic trait. Rh-positive means you have the factor; Rh-negative means the factor is missing. In the past, an Rh-negative woman who carried an Rh-positive child faced a complicated pregnancy, which could result in a very sick baby.

Your blood is separate from your baby's blood. If you are Rh-positive, you don't have to worry about any of this. If you are Rh-negative, you need to know about it.

If you are Rh-negative and your baby is Rh-positive or if you have had a blood transfusion or received blood products of some kind, there's a risk you could become Rh-sensitized or isoimmunized. *Isoimmunized* means you make antibodies that circulate inside your system, which don't harm you but can attack the Rh-positive blood of your growing baby. (If your baby is Rh-negative, there is no problem.) Your antibodies can cross the placenta and attack your baby's blood. This can cause blood disease of the foetus or newborn. It can make your baby anaemic while still inside the uterus, and it can be serious. Exposure to antibodies does not cause problems for the mother-to-be.

Fortunately, this reaction is preventable. The use of Rh-immune globulin (Anti-D) has alleviated many problems. It is given at 28 weeks gestation to prevent sensitization before delivery. Few women today are sensitized. If you are Rh-negative and pregnant, an Anti-D injection should be part of your pregnancy. Anti-D is a product that is extracted from human blood. If you have religious, ethical or personal reasons for not using blood or blood products, consult your doctor or minister.

An injection of Anti-D may be given to you if you are exposed to your baby's blood, which is more likely to happen during the last 3 months of pregnancy and at delivery. An injury to the abdomen may expose you to foetal blood. Multiple doses of Anti-D may also be given following delivery if blood tests show that a larger than normal number of Rh-positive blood cells (from the baby) have entered your bloodstream.

Anti-D is also given to you within 72 hours after delivery, if your baby is Rh-positive. If your baby is Rh-negative, you don't need Anti-D after delivery and you didn't need the shot during pregnancy. But it's better not to take that risk and to have the Anti-D injection during pregnancy.

If you have an ectopic pregnancy and are Rh-negative, you should receive Anti-D. This applies to miscarriages and abortions as well. If other procedures are performed that can cause the baby's blood and the mother's blood to mix, such as with amniocentesis or CVS, and you are Rh-negative, you should receive Anti-D.

Dad Tip Do you have concerns that you haven't shared with anyone? Are you concerned about your partner's health or the baby's? Do you wonder about your role in labour and delivery? Are you worried about being a good father? Share your thoughts with your partner. You won't burden her. In fact, she'll probably be relieved to know she's not alone in feeling a little overwhelmed by this monumental life change.

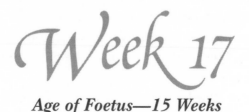

Week 17

Age of Foetus—15 Weeks

How Big Is Your Baby?

The crown-to-rump length of your baby is 11 to 12 cm (4½ to 4¾ in). Foetal weight has doubled in 2 weeks and is about 100 g (3½ oz). By this week, your baby is about the size of your hand spread open wide.

How Big Are You?

Your uterus is 3.8 to 5 cm (1½ to 2 in) below your bellybutton. You are showing more now and have an obvious swelling in your lower abdomen. By this time, expanding or maternity clothing is a must for comfort's sake. When your partner gives you a hug, he may feel the difference in your lower abdomen.

The rest of your body is still changing. A total 2.25- to 4.5-kg (5- to 10-lb) gain by this point in your pregnancy is normal.

How Your Baby Is Growing and Developing

If you look at the illustration on page 180 and then look at earlier chapters, you'll see the incredible changes that are occurring in your baby. Fat begins to form during this week and the weeks that follow. Also called *adipose tissue,* fat is important to the body's heat production and metabolism.

At 17 weeks of development, water makes up about 85 g (3 oz) of your baby's body. In a baby at term, fat makes up about 2.4 kg (5¼ lb) of the total average weight of 3.5 kg (7¾ lb).

You have felt your baby move, or you will soon. You may not feel it every day. As pregnancy progresses, movements become stronger and probably more frequent.

Changes in You

Feeling your baby move can reassure you that things are going well with your pregnancy. This is especially true if you've had problems.

As your pregnancy advances, the top of the uterus becomes almost spherical. It increases more rapidly in length (upwards into your abdomen) than in width, so the uterus becomes more oval than round. The uterus fills the pelvis and starts to grow into the abdomen. Your intestines are pushed upwards and to the sides. The uterus eventually reaches almost to your liver. The uterus doesn't float around, but neither is it firmly attached to one spot.

When you stand, your uterus touches your abdominal wall in the front. You may feel it most easily in this position. When you lie down, it can fall backwards onto your spine and blood vessels (vena cava and aorta).

ᴖ *Round-ligament Pain*
Round ligaments are attached to each side of the upper uterus and to the pelvic side wall. During pregnancy and the growth of the uterus,

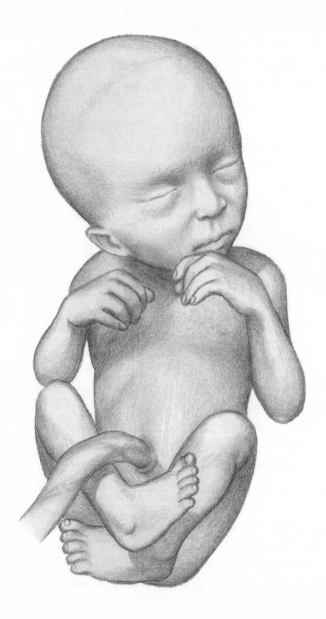

Your baby's fingernails are well formed. The baby is beginning to accumulate a little fat.

these ligaments are stretched and pulled. They become longer and thicker. Your movements can stretch and pull these ligaments, causing pain or discomfort called *round-ligament pain*. It doesn't signal a problem; it indicates your uterus is growing. Pain may occur on one side only or both sides, or it may be worse on one side than another. This pain does not harm you or the baby.

If you experience this pain, you may feel better if you lie down and rest. Talk to your doctor/midwife if pain is severe or if other symptoms arise. Warning signs of serious problems include bleeding from the vagina, loss of fluid from the vagina or severe pain.

How Your Actions
Affect Your Baby's Development

∿ Increased Vaginal Discharge
During pregnancy, it is normal to have an increase in vaginal discharge or vaginal secretions, called *leucorrhoea*. This discharge is usually white or yellow and fairly thick. It is not an infection. We believe it is caused by the increased blood flow to the skin and muscles around the vagina, which causes a violet or blue coloration of the vagina. This appearance, visible to your doctor early in pregnancy, is called *Chadwick's sign.*

You may have to wear sanitary pads if you have a heavy discharge. Avoid wearing tights and nylon underwear; choose underwear with a cotton crotch to allow more air circulation.

Tip for Week 17 If you experience leg cramps during pregnancy, don't stand for long periods. Rest on your side as often as possible. Careful stretching exercises may help. You may also use a heating pad on the cramped area, but don't use it for longer than 15 minutes at a time. Add potassium to your diet to help deal with leg cramps *before* they start—raisins and bananas are excellent sources of potassium.

Vaginal infections can and do occur during pregnancy. The discharge that accompanies these infections is often foul-smelling. It is yellow or green, and causes irritation or itching around or inside the vagina. If you have any of these symptoms, call your doctor. Many creams and antibiotics used to treat vaginal infections are safe to use during pregnancy.

↗ *Douching during Pregnancy*
Most doctors/midwives agree you should not douche during pregnancy. Bulb-syringe douches are definitely out!

Using a douche may cause you to bleed or may cause more serious problems, such as an air embolus. An air embolus results when air gets into your bloodstream from the pressure of the douche. It is rare, but it can cause serious problems for you.

Your Nutrition

Some women choose to eat a vegetarian diet because of personal or religious preferences. Some women are nauseated by meat during pregnancy. Is it safe to eat vegetarian while you're pregnant? It can be, if you pay close attention to the types and combinations of foods you eat.

If you eliminate meat from your diet, you need to eat enough calories to meet your energy needs. These need to be the right kind of calories, such as fresh fruits and vegetables. Avoid empty calories that have little or no nutritional value. Your goal is to eat enough different sources of protein to provide energy for the foetus and for you.

It's important to get the vitamins and minerals you need. If you eat a wide variety of whole grains, dried beans and peas, dried fruit and wheat germ, you should be able to meet your body's demands for iron, zinc and other trace minerals. You must find other sources of calcium and vitamins B_2, B_{12} and D.

Dad Tip Offer your partner tension-relieving, muscle-relaxing head, back and foot massages.

If you're not eating meat because it makes you ill, ask your doctor for a referral to a nutritionist. You'll probably need help developing a good eating plan. If you're a vegetarian by choice, and have been for a while, you may know how to get many of the nutrients you need. However, if you have questions, be sure to discuss them with your doctor.

You Should Also Know

↭ *Quad-screen Test*

The quad-screen test can help your doctor determine if you might be carrying a baby with Down's syndrome. This blood test can also help rule out other problems in your pregnancy, such as neural-tube defects.

The quad-screen test is the same as the triple-screen, with the addition of a fourth measurement—your inhibin-A level. This fourth measurement raises the sensitivity of the standard triple-screen test by 20 per cent in determining whether a foetus has Down's syndrome.

The quad-screen test is able to identify 79 per cent of those foetuses with Down's syndrome. It has a false-positive result 5 per cent of the time.

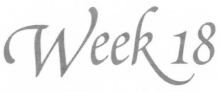

Week 18

Age of Foetus—16 Weeks

How Big Is Your Baby?

The crown-to-rump length of your growing baby is 12.5 to 14 cm (5 to 5½ in) by this week. Weight of the foetus is about 150 g (5¼ oz).

How Big Are You?

You can feel your uterus just below your bellybutton. If you put your fingers sideways and measure, it is about two finger-widths (2.5 cm/ 1 in) below your bellybutton. Your uterus is the size of a cantaloupe melon or a little larger.

Your total weight gain to this point should be 4.5 to 5.8 kg (10 to 13 lb). However, this can vary widely. If you have gained more weight than this, talk to your doctor/midwife. You may need to see a nutritionist. You still have more than half of your pregnancy ahead of you, and you're going to gain more weight.

Gaining more than the recommended weight can make pregnancy and delivery harder on you. And extra weight may be hard to lose afterwards.

Keep watching what you eat. Choose food for the nutrition it provides you and your growing baby.

How Your Baby Is Growing and Developing

Your baby is continuing to grow and to develop, but now the rapid growth rate slows down a little. As you can see in the illustration on page 187, your baby has a human appearance now.

ᴄ᷉ *Development of the Heart and Circulatory System*
At about the 3rd week of foetal development, two tubes join to form the heart. The heart begins to contract by day 22 of development or about the beginning of the 5th week of gestation. A beating heart is visible as early as 5 to 6 weeks of pregnancy during an ultrasound examination.

The heart tube divides into bulges. These bulges develop into heart chambers, called *ventricles* (left and right) and *atria* (left atrium and right atrium). These divisions occur between weeks 6 and 7. During week 7, tissue separating the left and right atria grows, and an opening between the atria called the *foramen ovale* appears. This opening lets blood pass from one atrium to the other, allowing it to bypass the lungs. At birth, the opening closes.

The ventricles, the lower chambers of the heart (lying below the atria), also develop a partition. The ventricle walls are muscular. The left ventricle pumps blood to the body and brain, and the right ventricle pumps blood to the lungs.

Heart valves develop at the same time as the chambers. These valves fill and empty the heart. Heart sounds and heart murmurs are caused by blood passing through these valves.

Blood from your baby flows to the placenta through the umbilical cord. In the placenta, oxygen and nutrients

Ɖad Ƭip Offer to run errands. Take her dry cleaning in, and pick it up when it's done. Stop by the bank for her. Take her car to a car wash. Return her library books or rented videos.

are transported from your blood to the foetal blood. Although the circulation of your blood and that of your baby come close, there is no direct connection. These circulation systems are completely separate.

At birth, the baby has to go rapidly from depending entirely on you for oxygen to depending on its own heart and lungs. The foramen ovale closes. Blood goes to the right ventricle, the right atrium and the lungs for oxygenation for the first time. It is truly a miraculous conversion.

At 18 weeks of gestation, ultrasound can detect some abnormalities of the heart. This can be helpful in identifying some problems, such as Down's syndrome. A skilled ultrasonographer looks for specific heart defects. If an abnormality is suspected, further ultrasound exams may be ordered to follow a baby's development as pregnancy progresses.

Changes in You

ᔆ *Does Your Back Ache?*

Nearly every pregnant woman experiences backache at some time in pregnancy. You may have felt it already, or it may come later as you get bigger. Some women have severe back pain following excessive exercise, walking, bending, lifting or standing. It is more common to have mild backache than severe problems. Some women need to take special care getting out of bed or getting up from a sitting position. In severe instances, some women find it difficult to walk.

Tip for Week 18 During exercise, your oxygen demands increase. Your body is heavier, and your balance may change. You may also tire more easily. Keep these points in mind as you adjust your fitness programme.

A change in joint mobility may contribute to the change in your posture and may cause discomfort in the lower back. This is particularly true in the latter part of pregnancy.

The growth of the uterus moves your centre of gravity forward, over your legs, which can affect the joints around the pelvis. All your joints are looser. Hormonal increases are potential causes; however,

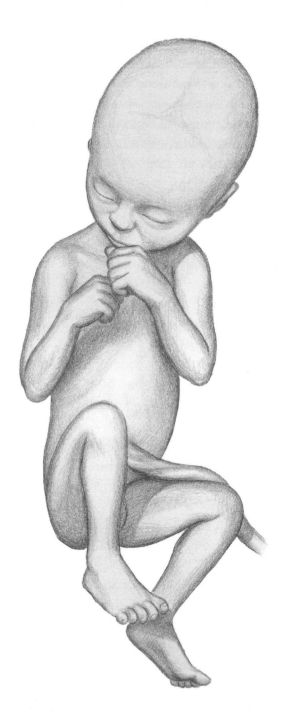

Your baby continues to grow. By this week, it is about 12.5 cm (5 in) from crown to rump. It looks much more human now.

discomfort may also be an indication of more serious problems, such as pyelonephritis or a kidney stone (see page 192). Check with your doctor if back pain is a chronic problem for you.

What can you do to prevent or lessen your pain? Try some or all of the following tips as early in your pregnancy as possible, and they will pay off as your pregnancy progresses.

- Watch your diet and weight gain.
- Continue exercising within guidelines during pregnancy.
- Get in the habit of lying on your side when you sleep.
- Find time during the day to get off your feet and lie down for 30 minutes on your side.
- If you have other children, take a nap when they take theirs.
- It's OK to take paracetamol for back pain.
- Use heat on the area that is painful.
- If pain becomes constant or more severe, talk to your doctor about it.

How Your Actions Affect Your Baby's Development

ᥐ *Exercise in the Second Trimester*

Everyone has heard stories of women who continued with strenuous exercise or strenuous activities until the day of delivery without problems. Stories are told of Olympic athletes who were pregnant at the time they won medals in the Olympic games. This kind of training and physical stress isn't a good idea for most women during pregnancy.

As your uterus grows and your abdomen gets larger, your sense of balance may be affected. You may feel clumsy. This isn't the time for contact sports or sports where you might fall easily, injure yourself or be struck in the abdomen.

Pregnant women can participate safely in many sports and exercise activities throughout their pregnancy. This is a different attitude from those held 20, 30 and 40 years ago. Bed rest and decreased activity were common then. Today, we believe exercise and activity can benefit you and your growing baby.

Discuss your particular activities at an antenatal visit. If your pregnancy is high risk or if you have had several miscarriages, it's particularly important to discuss exercise with your doctor *before* starting an activity. Now is not the time to train for any sport or to increase activity. In fact, this may be a good time to decrease the amount or intensity of exercise you are doing. Listen to your body. It will tell you when it's time to slow down.

What about the activities you are already involved in or would like to begin? Below is a discussion of various activities and how they will affect you in your second and third trimester. (See Week 3 for additional information on exercise in pregnancy.)

Swimming. Swimming can be good for you when you're pregnant. The support and buoyancy of the water can be relaxing. If you swim, swim throughout pregnancy. If you can't swim and have been involved in water exercises (exercising in the shallow end of a swimming pool), you can continue this throughout your pregnancy as well. This is an exercise you can begin at any time during pregnancy, if you don't overdo it.

Bicycling. Now is not the time to learn to ride a bike. If you're comfortable riding and have safe places to ride, you can enjoy this exercise with your partner or family.

Your balance will change as your body changes. This can make getting on and off a bicycle difficult. A fall from a bicycle could injure you or your baby.

A stationary bicycle is good for bad weather and for later in pregnancy. Many doctors suggest you ride a stationary bike in the last 2 to 3 months of pregnancy to avoid the danger of a fall.

Walking. Walking is a desirable exercise during pregnancy. It can be a good time for you and your partner to talk. Even when the weather is bad, you can walk in many places, such as an enclosed shopping mall, to get a good workout. Two miles of walking at a good pace is adequate. As pregnancy progresses, you may need to decrease your speed and distance. Walking is an exercise you can begin at any time during pregnancy, if you don't overdo it.

Jogging. Some women continue to jog during pregnancy. Jogging may be permitted during pregnancy, but check with your doctor first. If your pregnancy is high risk, jogging may not be a good idea.

Pregnancy is not the time to increase mileage or to train for a race. Wear comfortable clothing and supportive athletic shoes with good cushioning. Allow plenty of time to cool down.

During the course of your pregnancy, you'll probably need to slow down and to decrease the number of miles you run. You may even change to walking. If you notice pain, contractions, bleeding or other symptoms during or after jogging, call your doctor immediately.

Other Sports Activities.

- Tennis and golf are safe to continue in the second and third trimesters but may provide little actual exercise.
- Horse riding is not advisable during pregnancy at any time.
- Avoid water skiing while you're pregnant.
- Bowling is OK, although the amount of exercise you get varies. Be careful in late pregnancy; you could fall or strain your back. As your balance changes, bowling could become more difficult for you.
- Talk to your doctor about skiing before you hit the slopes. Again, in the latter part of pregnancy, your balance changes significantly. A fall could be harmful to you and your baby. Most doctors agree that skiing in the second half of pregnancy is not a good idea. Some doctors may allow skiing in early pregnancy, but only if there are no complications with this or a previous pregnancy.
- Riding snowmobiles, jet skis or motorcycles is not advised. Some doctors may allow you to ride if it is not strenuous. However, most believe the risk is too great, especially if you have had problems during this or a previous pregnancy.

Your Nutrition

Iron is important to you while you're pregnant. You need about 30 mg a day to meet the increased needs of pregnancy, due to the increase in your blood volume. During your pregnancy, your baby draws on your iron stores to create its own stores for its first few months of life. This protects baby from iron deficiency if you breastfeed.

Most prenatal vitamins contain enough iron to meet your needs. If you must take iron supplements, take your iron pill with a glass of orange juice or grapefruit juice to increase its absorption. Avoid drinking milk, coffee or tea when you take an iron supplement or eat iron-rich foods. They prevent the body from absorbing the iron it needs.

If you feel tired, have trouble concentrating, suffer from headaches, dizziness or indigestion, or if you get sick easily, you may have an iron deficiency. An easy way to check is to examine the inside of your lower eyelid. If you're getting enough iron, it should be dark pink. Your nail beds should be pink, too.

Only 10 to 15 per cent of the iron you consume is absorbed by the body. Your body stores it efficiently, but you need to eat iron-rich foods on a regular basis to maintain those stores. Foods that are rich in iron include chicken, red meat, organ meats (liver, heart, kidneys), egg yolks, dried fruit, spinach, kale and tofu. Combining a vitamin-C food and an iron-rich food ensures better iron absorption by the body. A spinach salad with orange or grapefruit sections is a good example.

Your prenatal vitamin contains about 60 mg of iron. If you eat a well-balanced diet and take your prenatal vitamin every day, you may not need additional iron. Discuss it with your doctor if you are concerned.

You Should Also Know

↳ *Bladder Infections*
One of the most common problems of pregnancy is frequent urination. Urinary-tract infections (UTIs) may cause you to urinate even more frequently while you're pregnant. A UTI is the most common

problem involving your bladder or kidneys during pregnancy. As the uterus grows larger, it sits directly on top of the bladder and on the ureters, the tubes leading from the kidneys to the bladder. This blocks the flow of urine. Other names for urinary-tract infections are *bladder infections* and *cystitis.*

Symptoms of a bladder infection include the feeling of urgency to urinate, frequent urination and painful urination, particularly at the end of urination. A severe urinary-tract infection may cause blood to appear in the urine.

Your doctor/midwife may do a urinalysis and urine culture at your first prenatal visit. He or she may check your urine for infection at other times during pregnancy and when bothersome symptoms arise.

You can help avoid infection by not holding your urine. Empty your bladder as soon as you feel the need. Don't wait to go to the bathroom; it could lead to a urinary-tract infection. Drink plenty of fluid; cranberry juice may help you avoid infections. For some women, it helps to empty the bladder after having intercourse.

If you have a urinary-tract infection (UTI) during pregnancy, call your doctor, and take care of it. Research has found that risks of giving birth to a child who is mentally retarded or who will exhibit developmental delays increases when UTIs are left untreated. UTIs during pregnancy might also be a cause of premature labour or a low-birthweight infant.

If you feel uncomfortable taking medication for the problem, understand that there are many safe antibiotics available. If you have a UTI, take the full course of antibiotics prescribed for you. It may be harmful to your baby if you don't treat the problem!

If left untreated, urinary-tract infections can get worse. They can even lead to pyelonephritis, a serious kidney infection (see the discussion below).

Pyelonephritis. A more serious problem resulting from a bladder infection is pyelonephritis. This type of infection occurs in 1 to 2 per cent of all pregnant women.

Symptoms include frequent urination, a burning sensation during urination, the feeling you need to urinate and nothing will come out, high fever, chills and back pain. Pyelonephritis may require hospital-ization and treatment with intravenous antibiotics.

If you have pyelonephritis or recurrent bladder infections during pregnancy, you may have to take antibiotics throughout pregnancy to prevent reinfection.

Kidney Stones. Another problem involving the kidneys and bladder is kidney stones (*renal calculi*). They occur about once in every 1500 pregnancies. Kidney stones cause severe pain in the back or lower ab-domen. They may also be associated with blood in the urine.

A kidney stone during pregnancy can usually be treated with pain medication and by drinking lots of fluids. In this way, the stone may be passed without surgical removal or lithotripsy (an ultrasound procedure).

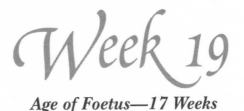

Week 19

Age of Foetus—17 Weeks

How Big Is Your Baby?

Crown-to-rump length of the growing foetus is 13 to 15 cm (5¼ to 6 in) by this week. Your baby weighs about 200 g (7 oz). It's incredible to think your baby will increase its weight more than 15 times between now and delivery!

How Big Are You?

You can feel your uterus about 1.3 cm (½ in) below your umbilicus. The illustration on page 196 gives you a good idea of the relative size of you, your uterus and your developing baby. A side view really shows the changes in you!

Your total weight gain at this point is between 3.6 and 6.3 kg (8 and 14 lb). Of this weight, only about 200 g (7 oz) is your baby! The placenta weighs about 170 g (6 oz); the amniotic fluid weighs another 310 g (11 oz). The uterus weighs 310 g (11 oz). Your breasts have each increased in weight by about 185 g (6½ oz). The rest of the weight you have gained is your increased blood volume and other maternal stores.

How Your Baby Is Growing and Developing

❧ *Your Baby's Nervous System*

The beginning of the baby's nervous system (brain and other structures, such as the spinal cord) is seen as early as week 4 as the neural plate begins to develop. By week 6, the main divisions of the central nervous system are established.

These divisions consist of the forebrain, midbrain, hindbrain and spinal cord. In week 7, the forebrain divides into the two hemispheres that will become the two cerebral hemispheres of the brain.

❧ *Hydrocephalus*

Organization and development of the brain continues from this early beginning. Cerebral spinal fluid (CSF), which circulates around the brain and the spinal cord, is made by the choroid plexus. Fluid must be able to flow without restriction. If openings are blocked and flow is restricted for any reason, it can cause *hydrocephalus* (water on the brain).

Hydrocephalus causes enlargement of the head. Occurring in about 1 in 2000 babies, it is responsible for about 12 per cent of all severe birth defects found at birth.

Hydrocephalus is often associated with spina bifida and occurs in about 33 per cent of those cases. It can also be associated with meningomyelocele and omphalocele (hernias of the spine and navel). Between 440 to 1300 ml (15 and 45 fl oz) of fluid can accumulate, but much more than that has been found. Brain tissue is compressed by all this fluid, which is a major concern.

Ultrasound is the best way to diagnose the problem. Hydrocephalus can usually be seen on ultrasound by 19 weeks of pregnancy. Occasionally it is found by routine exams and by 'feeling' or measuring your uterus.

In the past, nothing could be done about hydrocephalus until after delivery. Today, intrauterine therapy—treatment while the foetus is still in the uterus—can be performed in some cases.

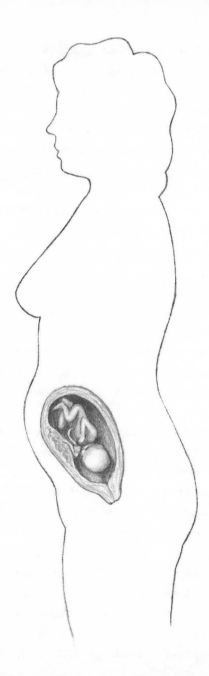

Comparative size of the uterus at 19 weeks of pregnancy (foetal age—
17 weeks). The uterus can be felt just under the umbilicus (bellybutton).

There are two methods of treating hydrocephalus in utero (inside the uterus). In one method, a needle passes through the mother's abdomen into the area of the baby's brain where fluid is collecting. Some fluid is removed to relieve pressure on the baby's brain. In another method, a small plastic tube is placed into the area where fluid collects in the baby's brain. This tube is left in place to drain fluid continuously.

Hydrocephalus is a high-risk problem. These procedures are highly specialized and should be performed only by someone experienced in the latest techniques. This requires consultation with a perinatologist specializing in high-risk pregnancies.

Changes in You

✎ *Feeling Dizzy*

Feeling dizzy during pregnancy is a fairly common symptom, often caused by hypotension (low blood pressure). It usually doesn't appear until the second trimester but may occur earlier.

There are two common reasons for hypotension during pregnancy. It can be caused by the enlarging uterus putting pressure on your aorta and vena cava. This is called *supine hypotension* and occurs when you lie down. You can alleviate or prevent it by not sleeping or lying on your back.

The second cause of hypotension is rising rapidly from a sitting, kneeling or squatting position. This is called *postural hypotension*. Your blood pressure drops when you rise rapidly as blood leaves your brain because of gravity. This problem is cured by rising slowly.

If you are anaemic, you may feel dizzy, faint or tired, or you may fatigue easily. Your blood is checked routinely during pregnancy. Your doctor/midwife will tell you if you have anaemia. (See Week 22 for more information about anaemia.)

Pregnancy also affects your blood-sugar level. High blood sugar (hyperglycaemia) or low blood sugar (hypoglycaemia) can make you feel dizzy or faint. Many doctors routinely test pregnant women for problems with blood sugar during pregnancy, particularly if they have problems with dizziness or a family history of diabetes. Most women can avoid or improve the problem by eating a balanced diet, not skipping meals and not going a long time without eating. Carry a piece of fruit or several crackers with you for a quick boost in blood sugar when you need it.

Eat More Meals Every Day!

Researchers have found that pregnant women who eat frequent, small meals during the day may provide better nutrition to their growing babies than women who eat three large meals. Though they are eating the same amount of calories, there is a difference.

Studies have found that keeping the blood level of maternal nutrients constant (by eating frequent, small meals) is better for foetal development than the mother-to-be eating a large meal, then not eating again for quite a while. Three larger meals means that nutrient levels rise and fall during the day, which isn't as beneficial for the growing baby. Eating small meals frequently can also help alleviate or avoid some other problems associated with pregnancy, such as nausea, heartburn and indigestion.

How Your Actions
Affect Your Baby's Development

∿ *Warning Signs during Pregnancy*

Many women are nervous because they don't think they would know if something important or serious happened during pregnancy. Most women have few, if any, problems during pregnancy. If you are concerned, read the list below of the most important symptoms to be aware of. Call your doctor/midwife if you experience any of the following:

- vaginal bleeding
- severe swelling of the face or fingers
- severe abdominal pain

- loss of fluid from the vagina, usually a gush of fluid, but sometimes a trickle or continuous wetness
- a big change in the baby's movement or a lack of movement
- high fever (more than 38.7°C; 101.6°F) or chills
- severe vomiting or an inability to keep food or liquid down
- blurring of vision
- painful urination
- a headache that won't go away or a severe headache
- an injury or accident, such as a fall or car accident, that causes you concern about the well-being of your baby

One way to get to know your doctor/midwife better is to ask his or her opinion about your concerns. Don't be embarrassed to ask questions about anything; your doctor has probably heard it before. And he or she would rather know about problems while they are easier to deal with.

Referral to a Consultant Obstetrician. If problems warrant it, your care may be referred to a consultant obstetrician.

You may not have a high-risk pregnancy at the beginning of your pregnancy. However, if problems develop with you (such as premature labour) or your baby (such as spina bifida), you may be referred to a consultant for an evaluation and possible care during your pregnancy. You may be able to return to your regular doctor/midwife for your delivery.

If you are under consultant care, you may have to deliver your baby at a hospital other than the one you had chosen. This is usually because the hospital has specialized facilities or can administer specialized tests to you or your baby.

Your Nutrition

✑ *Herbal Use in Pregnancy*
In the past, have you used herbs and botanicals, in the forms of teas, tinctures, pills or powders, to treat various medical and health problems?

We advise you *not* to treat yourself with an herbal remedy during pregnancy *without checking first with your doctor/midwife!*

You may believe an herbal remedy is OK to use, but it could be dangerous during pregnancy. For example, if you are constipated, you may decide to use senna as a laxative. However, senna stimulates uterine muscles and may cause a miscarriage. Some herbs may irritate your bowels and baby's bowels, too. So play it safe—be extremely careful with any substance your doctor/midwife has not specifically recommended for you. Always check with him or her first before you take anything!

↣ Pay Attention to Your Calcium Intake

It's very important for you to get enough calcium every day. You need 1200 mg each day during pregnancy—50 per cent more than before pregnancy. For information on calcium and some tips on ways to add it to your food plan, see the nutrition discussion in Week 7.

You Should Also Know

↣ Allergies during Pregnancy

Allergies sometimes get a little worse during pregnancy. If you have allergy medication, don't assume it's safe to take. Some types of allergy medication may not be advised. Many allergy medicines are combinations of several medicines that you should be careful about using during pregnancy. Ask your doctor about your medicine, whether prescription or non-prescription. This advice also applies to nasal sprays.

Medications that are OK to use during pregnancy include antihistamines and decongestants. Decongestants that contain oxymetazoline, such as Afrazine, may be recommended. Some allergy-blocking nasal sprays are also safe to use. Ask your doctor which brands are

Dad Tip When you can, take some time off from work or other obligations to spend time with your partner. Together, focus on planning your pregnancy and preparing for the birth of your baby.

safest for you to use if your allergy problems interfere with your normal lifestyle.

To help deal with allergies, try to avoid anything that triggers them. For example, if dust bothers you, keep windows closed and avoid outdoor activities in the morning, when the pollen is usually at its worst. Wear a mask when you vacuum. Use a humidifier if you live in a very dry climate. To help deal with the problem, drink plenty of fluid.

Tip for Week 19 Fish can be a healthy food choice during pregnancy, but don't eat shark, swordfish or tuna (fresh or frozen) more than once a week.

Some fortunate women notice their allergies get better during pregnancy, and symptoms improve. Certain things they had trouble with before pregnancy are no longer a problem.

᥍ Will You Be a Single Mother?

Many women choose to have a child without a spouse; situations vary from woman to woman. Some women are deeply involved with their partner, the baby's father, but have chosen not to marry. Some women are pregnant without their partner's support. Still other single women have chosen donor (artificial) insemination as a means of getting pregnant.

No matter what the personal situation, many concerns are shared by all of them. This discussion reflects some of the issues they have raised.

In most situations—whether a mother is single, widowed or divorced—a child's overall environment is more important than the presence of a man in the household. The vast majority of single-parent households in the UK are headed by women. Recent studies indicate that if a woman has other supportive adults to depend on, a child can fare well in a home headed by a single woman.

Some people may think your choice is unwise and tell you so. However, it's no one's business but your own. If someone is intent on giving you a hard time, change the subject. Don't discuss your reasons for having a baby with anyone unless you *want* to.

Even if you are 'alone,' you're not really alone. Seek support from family and friends. Mothers of young children can identify with your experiences—they have had similar ones recently. If you have friends or family members with young children, talk with them. You would probably share your concerns with these people even if you were married. Try not to let your particular situation alter this.

Finding people you can count on for help during your pregnancy and after your baby arrives is important. One woman said she thought about whom she would call at 2 am if her baby were crying uncontrollably. When she answered that question, she had the name of someone she believed she could count on in any type of emergency—during and after pregnancy!

It may help to choose someone to be with you when you labour and deliver, and who will be there to help afterwards. The only part of labour and delivery that might require special planning because you're single is your plan to get to the hospital when you go into labour. One woman wanted her friend to drive, but couldn't reach her when the time came. Her next option (all part of the plan) was to call a taxi, which got her to the hospital in plenty of time.

Legal Questions. Because your situation is unique, it's important to have answers to questions. The following questions have been posed by women who chose to be single mothers. We repeat them here without answers because they are legal questions that should be reviewed with a solicitor who specializes in family law. These can help you clarify the kinds of questions you need to consider as a single mother.

- A friend who's had a baby by herself told me I'd better consider the legal ramifications of this situation. What was she talking about?
- I'm having my baby alone, and I'm concerned about who can make medical decisions for me and my expected baby. Can I do anything about this concern?
- I'm not married, but I am deeply involved with my baby's father. Can my partner make medical decisions for me if I have problems during labour or after the birth?
- If anything happens to me, can my partner make medical decisions for our baby after it is born?

- What are the legal rights of my baby's father if we are not married?
- Do my partner's parents have legal rights in regard to their grandchild (my child)?
- My baby's father and I went our separate ways before I knew I was pregnant. Do I have to tell him about the baby?
- I chose to have donor (artificial) insemination. If anything happens to me during my labour or delivery, who can make medical decisions for me? Who can make decisions for my baby?
- I got pregnant by donor insemination. What do I put on the birth certificate under 'father's name'?
- Is there a way I can find out more about my sperm donor's family medical history?
- Will the sperm bank send me notices if medical problems appear in my sperm donor's family?
- As my child grows up, she may need some sort of medical help (such as a donor kidney) from a sibling. Will the sperm bank supply family information?
- I had donor insemination, and I'm concerned about the rights of the baby's father to be part of my child's life in the future. Should I be concerned?
- What type of arrangements must I make for my child in case of my death?
- Someone joked to me that my child could marry its sister or brother some day and wouldn't know it because I had donor insemination. Is this possible?
- Are there any other things I should consider because of my unique situation?

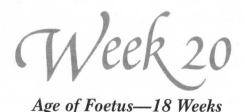

Week 20

Age of Foetus—18 Weeks

How Big Is Your Baby?

At this point in development, the crown-to-rump length is 14 to 16 cm (5½ to 6½ in). Your baby weighs about 255 g (9 oz).

How Big Are You?

Congratulations—20 weeks marks the midpoint. You're halfway through your pregnancy! Remember, the entire pregnancy is 40 weeks from the beginning of your last period if you go full term.

Your uterus is probably about even with your bellybutton. Your doctor has been watching your growth and the enlargement of your uterus. Growth to this point may have been irregular but usually becomes more regular after the 20th week.

✑ *Measuring the Growth of Your Uterus*
Your uterus is measured often to keep track of your baby's growth. Your doctor may use a measuring tape or his or her fingers and measure by finger breadth.

Your doctor/midwife needs a point of reference against which to measure your growth. This measurement is taken from the pubic symphysis. The *pubic symphysis* is the place where the pubic bones meet in the middle-lower part of your abdomen. This bony area is just above your urethra (where urine comes out), 15.2 to 25.4 cm (6 to 10 in) below the bellybutton, depending on how tall you are. It may be felt 2.5 to 5 cm (1 or 2 in) below your pubic hairline.

Measurements are made from the pubic symphysis to the top of the uterus. After 20 weeks of pregnancy, you should grow almost 1 cm (½ in) each week. If you are 20 cm (8 in) at 20 weeks, at your next visit (4 weeks later), you should measure about 24 cm (10 in).

If you measure 28 cm (11¼ in) at this point in pregnancy, you may require further evaluation with ultrasound to determine if you are carrying twins or to see if your due date is correct. If you only measure 15 cm (6 in) at this point, it may be a reason to do further evaluation by ultrasound. Your due date could be wrong, or there may be a concern about intrauterine-growth restriction or some other problem.

Not every doctor/midwife measures the same way, and not every woman is the same size. Babies vary in size. If pregnant friends ask, 'How much did you measure?' don't worry if their measurements are different. Measurements differ among women and are often different for a woman from one pregnancy to another.

If you see a doctor/midwife you don't normally see or if you see a new doctor/midwife, you may measure differently. This does not indicate a problem or that someone is measuring incorrectly. It's just that everyone measures a little differently.

Tip for Week 20 An ultrasound test done at this point in pregnancy may make it possible to determine the sex of the baby, but the baby must cooperate. Sex is recognized by seeing the genitals. Even if the sex looks obvious, ultrasound operators have been known to be mistaken about a baby's sex.

Having the same person measure you on a regular basis can be helpful in following the growth of your baby. Within limits, changing measurements are a sign of foetal well-being and foetal growth. If they appear abnormal, it can be a warning sign. If you're concerned about your size and the growth of your pregnancy, discuss it with your doctor/midwife.

How Your Baby Is Growing and Developing

✂ *Your Baby's Skin*

The skin covering your baby begins growing from two layers. These layers are the *epidermis,* which is on the surface, and the *dermis,* which is the deeper layer. By this point in your pregnancy, the epidermis is arranged in four layers. One of these layers contains epidermal ridges, which are responsible for surface patterns on fingertips, palms and soles. They are genetically determined.

The dermis lies below the epidermis. It forms projections that push upward into the epidermis. Each projection contains a small blood vessel (capillary) or a nerve. This deeper layer also contains large amounts of fat.

When a baby is born, its skin is covered by a white substance that looks like paste. Called *vernix,* it is secreted by the glands in the skin beginning around 20 weeks of pregnancy. Vernix protects your growing baby's skin from amniotic fluid.

Hair appears at around 12 to 14 weeks of pregnancy. It grows from the epidermis; hair ends (hair papillae) push down into the dermis. Hair is first seen on the foetus on the upper lip and eyebrow. It is usually shed around the time of birth and is replaced by thicker hair from new follicles.

Ðad Tip **Around 20 weeks of pregnancy, your partner may have an ultrasound exam. Try to be present for this test. Ask your partner to consider your schedule when making the appointment for her ultrasound.**

✂ *Ultrasound Pictures*

The illustration on the opposite page shows an ultrasound exam (and an interpretive illustration of the ultrasound) in a pregnant woman at about 20 weeks gestation. An ultrasound is often easier to understand

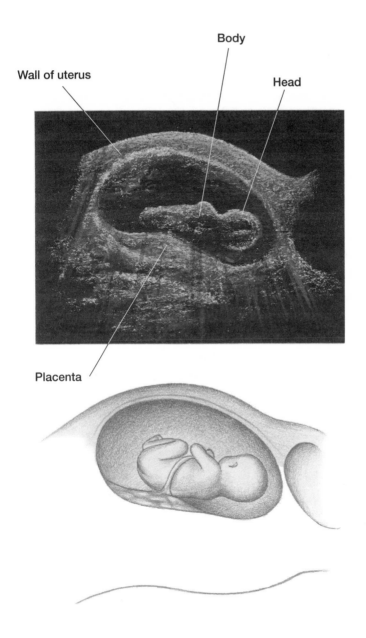

Ultrasound of a baby at 20 weeks gestation (foetal age—18 weeks). The interpretive illustration may help you see more detail.

when it is actually being done. The pictures you see are more like motion pictures.

If you look closely at the illustration, it may make sense to you. Read the labels, and try to visualize the baby inside the uterus. An ultrasound picture is like looking at a slice of an object. The picture you see is 2-dimensional.

An ultrasound done at this point in pregnancy is helpful for confirming your due date. If the ultrasound is done very early or very late (first or last 2 months), the accuracy of dating a pregnancy is not as good. If two or more foetuses are present, they can usually be seen. Some foetal problems can also be seen at this time.

∽ *Percutaneous Umbilical-Cord Blood Sampling*
Percutaneous umbilical-cord blood sampling (PUBS), also called *cordocentesis,* is a test done on the foetus while it is still developing inside your uterus. The advantage of the test is that results are available in a few days. The disadvantage is that it carries a slightly higher risk of miscarriage than amniocentesis does.

Guided by ultrasound, a fine needle is inserted through the mother's abdomen into a tiny vein in the umbilical cord. A small sample of the baby's blood is removed for analysis. PUBS detects blood disorders, infections and Rh-incompatibility.

The baby's blood can be checked before birth, and the baby can be given a blood transfusion, if necessary. This procedure can help prevent life-threatening anaemia that may develop if the mother is Rh-negative and has antibodies that are destroying her baby's blood. If you are Rh-negative, you should receive Anti-D after this procedure.

Changes in You

∽ *Stretching Abdominal Muscles*
Your abdominal muscles are being stretched and pushed apart as your baby grows. Muscles are attached to the lower portion of your ribs and

run vertically down to your pelvis. They may separate in the midline. These muscles are called the rectus muscles; when they separate, it is a hernia called a *diastasis recti.*

You will notice the separation most often when you are lying down and you raise your head, tightening your abdominal muscles. It will look like there is a bulge in the middle of your abdomen. You might even feel the edge of the muscle on either side of the bulge. It isn't painful and doesn't harm you or your baby. What you feel in the gap between the muscles is the uterus. You may feel the baby's movement more easily here.

If this is your first baby, you may not notice the separation at all. With each pregnancy, separation is often more noticeable. Exercising can strengthen these muscles, but you may still have the bulge or gap.

Following pregnancy, these muscles tighten and close the gap. The separation won't be as noticeable, but it may still be present. A girdle probably won't help get rid of the bulge or gap.

How Your Actions Affect Your Baby's Development

✧ Sexual Relations

Pregnancy can be an important time of growing closer to your partner. As you get larger, sexual intercourse may become difficult because of discomfort for you. With some imagination and with different positions (ones in which you are not on your back and your partner is not directly on top of you), you can continue to enjoy sexual relations during this part of your pregnancy.

If you feel emotional pressure from your partner—either his concern about the safety of intercourse or requests for frequent sexual relations—discuss it openly with him. Don't be afraid to invite your partner to antenatal visits to discuss these things with your doctor/midwife.

If you're having problems with contractions, bleeding or complications, you and your partner should talk with your doctor/midwife.

Together you can decide whether you should continue to have sexual relations during your pregnancy.

Your Nutrition

Many women use artificial sweeteners to help cut calories. Aspartame and saccharin are the two most common artificial sweeteners added to foods and beverages. Aspartame (sold under the brand names Canderel and Hermesetas) may be the most popular artificial sweetener. It is used in many foods and beverages to help reduce calorie content. Saccharin is also added to many foods and beverages. A fairly new product, Splenda, is also being marketed.

ᴕ *Aspartame*
Aspartame is a combination of phenylalanine and aspartic acid, two amino acids. There has been controversy as to its safety. We advise you to substitute foods that do not contain the sweetener. At this point, we're unsure about its safety for pregnant women and their developing babies. If you suffer from phenylketonuria, you must follow a low-phenylalanine diet or your baby may be adversely affected. Phenylalanine in aspartame contributes to phenylalanine in the diet.

ᴕ *Saccharin*
Saccharin is another artificial sweetener used in foods and beverages. Although it is not used as much today as in the past, it still appears in many foods, beverages and other substances. The Food Standards Agency limits the amount that is allowed and monitors its use. Nevertheless, it would probably be better to avoid using this product while you're pregnant.

ᴕ *Avoid Aspartame and Saccharin*
Don't use these artificial sweeteners or food additives during pregnancy, if you can avoid them. It's probably best to eliminate any sub-

stance you don't really need from the foods you eat and the beverages you drink. Do it for the good of your baby.

↬ *Splenda*

Splenda is a trade name for a low-calorie sweetener called *sucralose,* and it is made from sugar. It is available in granular form, and is also found in a variety of processed products. Sucralose passes through the body without being metabolized—your body does not recognize it as either a sugar or a carbohydrate, which makes it low calorie.

Sucralose is used in salad dressings, baked goods, desserts, dairy products beverages, jams and jellies, coffee and tea, syrups and chewing gum. **Splenda is safe for pregnant and nursing women to use.**

You Should Also Know

↬ *Hearing Your Baby's Heartbeat*

It may be possible to hear your baby's heartbeat with a Pinard stethoscope or sonicard machine at 20 weeks. Before doctors had doppler equipment that enabled them to hear the heartbeat and ultrasound to see the heart beating, a Pinard stethoscope helped the listener hear the baby's heartbeat. This usually occurred after quickening for most women.

If you can't hear your baby's heartbeat with a stethoscope, don't worry. It's not always easy for a doctor who does this on a regular basis!

If you hear a swishing sound (baby's heartbeat), you have to differentiate it from a beating sound (mother's heartbeat). A baby's heart beats rapidly, usually 110 to 160 beats every minute. Your heartbeat or pulse rate is slower, in the range of 60 to 80 beats a minute.

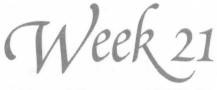

Week 21

Age of Foetus—19 Weeks

How Big Is Your Baby?

Your baby is getting larger in this first week of the second half of your pregnancy. It now weighs about 300 g (10½ oz), and its crown-to-rump length is about 18 cm (7¼ in). It is about the size of a large banana.

How Big Are You?

You can feel your uterus about 1 cm (½ in) above your bellybutton. At the doctor's surgery, your uterus measures almost 21 cm (8½ in) from the pubic symphysis. Your weight gain should be between 4.5 and 6.3 kg (10 and 15 lb).

Tip for Week 21 **A good way to add calcium to your diet is to cook rice and oatmeal in skim milk instead of water.**

By this week, your waistline is definitely gone. Your friends and relatives—and strangers, too—can tell you're pregnant. It would be hard to hide your condition!

How Your Baby Is
Growing and Developing

The rapid growth rate of your baby has slowed. However, the baby continues to grow and to develop. Different organ systems within the baby are maturing.

✌ *The Foetal Digestive System*

The foetal digestive system is functioning in a simple way. By the 11th week of pregnancy, the small intestine begins to contract and relax, which pushes substances through it. The small intestine is capable of passing sugar from inside itself into the baby's body.

By 21 weeks of pregnancy, development of the foetal digestive system enables the foetus to swallow amniotic fluid. After swallowing amniotic fluid, the foetus absorbs much of the water in it and passes unabsorbed matter as far as the large bowel.

✌ *Foetal Swallowing*

As mentioned above, your baby swallows before it is born. Using ultrasound, you can observe the baby swallowing at different stages of pregnancy. We have seen babies swallowing amniotic fluid as early as 21 weeks of pregnancy.

Dad Tip It's not too early to start thinking about baby names. Sometimes couples have very different ideas about names for their child. There are lots of books available to help you. Do you plan to honour a close friend or relative by using their name? Will you use a family name? What problems could arise if you choose a peculiar, difficult-to-say or hard-to-spell name? What do the initials spell out? What nicknames go with the name? Start thinking about it now, even if you decide you won't pick a name until after you meet your baby.

Why does a baby in the womb swallow? Researchers believe swallowing amniotic fluid may help growth and development of the foetal digestive system. It may also condition the digestive system to function after birth.

Studies have determined how much fluid a foetus swallows and passes through its digestive system. Evidence indicates babies at full-term may swallow large amounts of amniotic fluid, as much as 500 ml (17 fl oz) of amniotic fluid in a 24-hour period.

Amniotic fluid swallowed by the baby contributes a small amount to its caloric needs. Researchers believe it may contribute essential nutrients to the developing baby.

✣ *Meconium*

During your pregnancy, you may hear the term *meconium* and wonder what it means. It refers to undigested debris from swallowed amniotic fluid in the foetal digestive system. Meconium is made mostly of mucosal cells from the lining of the baby's gastrointestinal tract. It contains no bacteria, so it is sterile.

It is a greenish-black to light-brown substance that your baby passes from its bowels before delivery, during labour or after birth.

Passage of meconium into the amniotic fluid may be caused by distress in the foetus. Meconium seen during labour may be an indication of foetal distress.

If a baby has had a bowel movement before birth and meconium is present in the amniotic fluid, the foetus may swallow the fluid. If baby inhales meconium into the lungs, it could develop pneumonia or pneumonitis. For this reason, if meconium is seen at delivery, an attempt is made to remove it from the baby's mouth and throat with a small suction tube.

Changes in You

In addition to your growing uterus, other parts of your body continue to change and to grow. You may notice swelling in your lower legs and feet, particularly at the end of the day. If you're on your feet a lot, you may notice less swelling if you're able to get off your feet and rest for a while during the day.

ᔐ *Blood Clots in the Legs*

A serious complication of pregnancy is a blood clot in the legs or groin. Symptoms of the problem are swelling of the legs accompanied by leg pain and redness or warmth over the affected area in the legs.

This problem has many names, including *venous thrombosis, thromboembolic disease, thrombophlebitis* and *lower deep-vein thrombosis.* The problem is not limited to pregnancy, but pregnancy is a time when it is more likely to occur. This is due to the slowing of blood flow in the legs because of uterine pressure and changes in the blood and its clotting mechanisms.

The most probable cause of blood clots in the legs during pregnancy is decreased blood flow, also called *stasis.* If you have had a previous blood clot—in your legs or any other part of your body—tell your doctor at the beginning of your pregnancy. He or she needs to know this important information.

Deep-Vein Thrombosis. Superficial thrombosis and deep-vein thrombosis in the leg are different conditions. A blood clot in the superficial veins of the leg is not as serious. This condition is usually noted in veins close to the surface of the skin that can often be felt on the surface. This type of clot is treated with a mild pain reliever, such as paracetamol, elevation of the leg, the use of a support bandage or stockings, and occasionally heat. If the condition doesn't improve rapidly, deep-vein thrombosis must be considered.

Deep-vein thrombosis (DVT) is more serious; it requires diagnostic procedures and treatment. Symptoms of deep-vein thrombosis in the lower leg can differ greatly, depending on the location of the clot and how bad it is. The onset of deep-vein thrombosis can be rapid, with severe pain and swelling of the leg and thigh.

If you have had a blood clot in the past for any reason, pregnancy-related or not, see your doctor/midwife early in pregnancy. Tell him or her at your first antenatal visit about any previous problems you've had with blood clots.

The greatest danger from deep-vein thrombosis is a pulmonary embolism, in which a piece of the blood clot breaks off and travels from the legs to the lungs. This is a rare problem during pregnancy and is reported in only 1 in every 3000 to 7000 deliveries. Although it is a serious complication in pregnancy, it can often be avoided with early treatment.

Symptoms to Watch For. With deep-vein thrombosis (DVT), the leg may occasionally appear pale and cool, but usually a portion of the leg is tender, hot and swollen. Often skin over the affected veins is red. There may even be streaks of red on the skin over veins where blood clots have occurred.

Squeezing the calf or leg may be extremely painful, and it may be equally painful to walk. One way to tell if you have deep-vein thrombosis is to lie down and flex your toes towards your knee. If the back of the leg is tender, it is a positive indication of this problem; this is called *Homan's sign.* (This type of pain may also occur with a strained muscle or a bruise.) Check with your doctor if this occurs.

Diagnosing the Problem. Diagnostic studies of DVT may be different for a pregnant woman than for a non-pregnant woman. In the non-pregnant woman, an X-ray may be accompanied by an injection of dye into leg veins to look for blood clots. This test is not usually performed on a pregnant woman because of exposure to radiation and the dye. Ultrasound is used to diagnose this problem in pregnant women.

Treating DVT. Treatment of DVT usually consists of hospitalization and heparin therapy. Heparin (a blood thinner) must be given intravenously; it cannot be taken as a pill. It is safe during pregnancy and is not passed to the foetus. A woman may be required to take extra calcium during pregnancy if she receives heparin. While heparin is being administered, the woman is required to stay in bed. The leg may be elevated and heat applied. Mild pain medicine is prescribed.

Recovery time, including hospitalization, may be 7 to 10 days. After this time, the woman continues taking heparin until delivery. Following pregnancy, she will need to continue taking a blood thinner for up to several weeks, depending on the severity of the clot.

If a woman has a blood clot during one pregnancy, she will likely need heparin during subsequent pregnancies. If so, heparin can be given by daily injections the woman administers to herself under her doctor's or midwife's supervision.

Another medication used to treat deep-vein thrombosis is warfarin, an oral medication. Warfarin is not given during pregnancy because it crosses the placenta and can be harmful to the baby. Warfarin is usually given to the woman after pregnancy to prevent blood clots. It may be prescribed for a few weeks or a few months, depending on the severity of the clot.

How Your Actions Affect Your Baby's Development

ᔑ *Safety of Ultrasound*
On page 218 is an illustration of an ultrasound exam, accompanied by an interpretive illustration. These show a baby inside a uterus; the mother-to-be also has a large cyst in her abdomen.

Many women wonder about the safety of ultrasound exams. Most medical researchers agree ultrasound exams do not pose any risk to you or your baby. Researchers have looked for potential problems many times without finding evidence of any.

Ultrasound is an extremely valuable tool in diagnosing problems and answering some questions during pregnancy. Information that ultrasound testing provides can be reassuring to the doctor and the pregnant woman.

If your doctor has recommended ultrasound for you and you're concerned about it, discuss it with him or her. He or she may have an important reason for doing an ultrasound exam. It could affect the well-being of your developing baby.

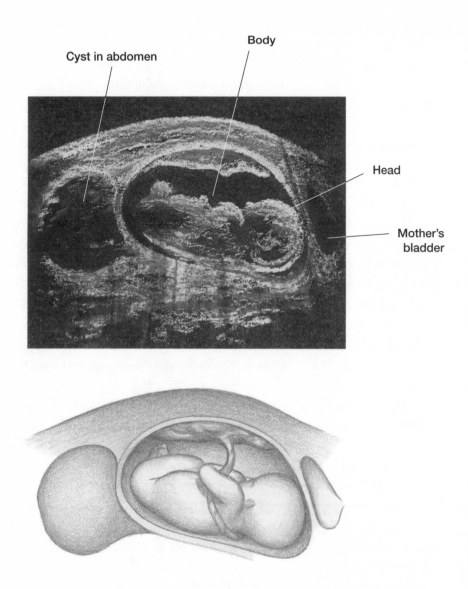

Ultrasound may be used to detect problems. In this ultrasound of a baby in-utero, there is a cyst in the mother-to-be's abdomen. The interpretive illustration clarifies the ultrasound image.

Your Nutrition

Some women experience food cravings during pregnancy. Food cravings have long been considered a non-specific sign of pregnancy. Craving a particular food can be both good and bad. If the food you crave is nutritious and healthy, eat it in moderation. Don't eat food that isn't good for you. If you crave foods that are high in fat and sugar or loaded with empty calories, be careful. Take a little taste, but don't let yourself go. Try eating another food, such as a piece of fresh fruit or some cheese, instead of indulging in your craving.

What Foods Do Pregnant Women Crave?

Recent research indicates three common cravings among pregnant women.

- 33% crave chocolate
- 20% crave sweets of some sort
- 19% crave citrus fruits and juices

We don't understand all the reasons a woman might crave a food while she's pregnant. We believe the hormonal and emotional changes that occur in pregnancy contribute to the situation.

On the opposite side of cravings is food aversion. Some foods that you have eaten without problems before pregnancy may now make you sick to your stomach. This is common. Again, we believe the hormones of pregnancy are involved. In this case, hormones affect the gastrointestinal tract, which can affect your reaction to some foods.

You Should Also Know

Ꮿ Will You Get Varicose Veins?

Varicose veins, also called *varicosities* or *varices,* occur to some degree in most pregnant women. There appears to be an inherited predisposition to varicose veins that can be made more severe by pregnancy, increased age and pressure caused by standing for long periods of time.

Varicose veins are blood vessels that are engorged with blood. They occur primarily in the legs but may also be present in the vulva and rectum. The change in blood flow and pressure from the uterus make varices worse, which causes discomfort.

In most instances, varicose veins become more noticeable and more painful as pregnancy progresses. With increasing weight (especially if you spend a lot of time standing), they may worsen.

Symptoms vary. For some, the main symptom is a blemish or purple-blue spot on the legs with little or no discomfort, except perhaps in the evening. Other women have bulging veins that require elevation at the end of the day.

Following pregnancy, swelling in the veins should go down, but varicose veins probably won't disappear altogether. Various methods, including laser treatment, injection and surgery, can get rid of these veins; the surgery is called *vein stripping*. It would be unusual to operate on varicose veins during pregnancy, although it is a treatment to consider when you are not pregnant.

Treating Varicose Veins. Following these measures may help keep veins from swelling as much.

- Wear medical support hose; many types are available. Ask your doctor for a recommendation.
- Wear clothing that doesn't restrict circulation at the knee or the groin.
- Spend as little time on your feet as you can. Lie on your side or elevate your legs when possible. This enables veins to drain more easily.
- Wear flat shoes when you can.
- Don't cross your legs. It cuts off circulation and can make problems worse.
- The type of exercise you choose may compound the problem. High-impact exercise, such as step aerobics or jogging, can cause trauma to the veins. Low-impact exercises, such as cycling, antenatal yoga or using an elliptical trainer, may be a better choice.

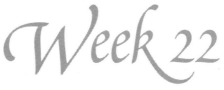

Week 22

Age of Foetus—20 Weeks

How Big Is Your Baby?

Your baby now weighs about 350 g (12¼ oz). Crown-to-rump length at this time is about 19 cm (7⅔ in).

How Big Are You?

Your uterus is now about 2 cm (¾ in) above your bellybutton or almost 22 cm (9 in) from the pubic symphysis. You may feel 'comfortably pregnant.' Your enlarging abdomen is not too large and doesn't get in your way much. You're still able to bend over and to sit comfortably. Walking shouldn't be an effort. Morning sickness has probably passed, and you're feeling pretty good. It's kind of fun being pregnant now!

Tip for Week 22 Drink extra fluids (water is best) throughout pregnancy to help your body keep up with the increase in your blood volume. You'll know you're drinking enough fluid when your urine looks almost like clear water.

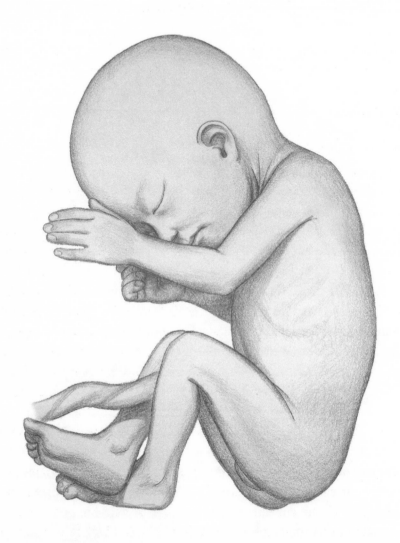

By the 22ⁿᵈ week of pregnancy (foetal age—20 weeks), your baby's eye-lids and eyebrows are well developed. Fingernails have grown and now cover the fingertips.

How Your Baby Is Growing and Developing

Your baby continues to grow; its body is getting larger every day. As you can see by looking at the illustration on the previous page, your baby's eyelids, and even the eyebrows, are developed. Fingernails are also visible.

✐ *Liver Function*

Your baby's organ systems are becoming specialized for their particular functions. Consider the liver. The function of the foetal liver is different from that of an adult. Enzymes (chemicals) are made in an adult liver that are important in various body functions. In the foetus, these enzymes are present but in lower levels than those present after birth.

An important function of the liver is the breakdown and handling of bilirubin. Bilirubin is produced by the breakdown of blood cells. The life span of a foetal red blood cell is shorter than that of an adult. Because of this, a foetus produces more bilirubin than an adult does.

The foetal liver has a limited capacity to convert bilirubin, then remove it from the foetal bloodstream. Bilirubin passes from foetal blood through the placenta to your blood. Your liver helps get rid of foetal bilirubin. If a baby is born prematurely, it may have trouble processing bilirubin because its own liver is too immature to get rid of bilirubin from the bloodstream.

A newborn baby with high bilirubin may exhibit *jaundice.* Jaundice in a newborn is typically triggered by the transition from bilirubin being handled by the mother's system to the baby handling it on its own. The baby's liver can't keep up. Jaundice is more likely to occur in an immature infant when the liver is not ready to take over this function.

A baby with jaundice has a yellow tint to the skin and eyes. Jaundice is usually treated with phototherapy. Phototherapy uses light that penetrates the skin and destroys the bilirubin.

(For detailed information about this and other situations that might occur with your newborn, read our book *Your Baby's First Year Week by Week.*)

Changes in You

∞ Foetal Fibronectin

In some cases, normal discomforts of pregnancy, such as lower-abdominal pain, dull backache, pelvic pressure, uterine contractions (with or without pain), cramping and a change in vaginal discharge may be confused with preterm labour. Until now, we have not had a reliable method of determining if a woman was truly at risk of delivering a preterm baby. A test is now available that can help doctors make this determination.

Foetal fibronectin (fFN) is a protein found in the amniotic sac and foetal membranes. However, after 22 weeks of pregnancy, fFN is not normally present until around week 38.

When it is present in the cervical-vaginal secretions of a pregnant woman after 22 weeks (and before week 38), it indicates increased risk for preterm delivery. If it is absent, risk of premature labour is low, and the woman probably won't deliver within the next 2 weeks.

The test is performed like a cervical smear. A swab of vaginal secretions is taken from the top of the vagina, behind the cervix. It is sent to the lab, and results are available within 24 hours.

∞ What Is Anaemia?

Anaemia is a common problem during pregnancy. If you suffer from anaemia, treatment is important for you and your baby. If you are anaemic, you won't feel well during pregnancy. You'll tire easily. You may experience dizziness.

There is a fine balance in your body between the production of blood cells that carry oxygen to the rest of your body and the destruction of these cells. Anaemia is the condition in which the number of red blood cells is low. If you are anaemic, you have an inadequate number of red blood cells.

During pregnancy, the number of red blood cells in your bloodstream increases. The amount of *plasma* (the liquid part of the blood) also increases but at a higher rate. Your doctor/midwife keeps track of these changes in your blood with a *haematocrit* reading. Your haematocrit is a measure of the percentage of the blood that is red blood cells. Your *haemoglobin* level is also tested. Haemoglobin is the protein component of red blood cells. If you are anaemic, your haematocrit is lower than 37 and your haemoglobin is under 12.

A haematocrit determination is usually made at the first antenatal visit along with other lab work. It may be repeated once or twice during pregnancy. It is done more often if you are anaemic.

There is always some blood loss at delivery. If you're anaemic when you go into labour, you are at higher risk of needing a blood transfusion after your baby is born. Follow your doctor's advice about diet and supplementation if you suffer from anaemia.

Iron-Deficiency Anaemia. The most common type of anaemia seen in pregnancy is *iron-deficiency anaemia*. During pregnancy, your baby uses some of the iron stores you have in your body. If you have iron-deficiency anaemia, your body doesn't have enough iron left to make red blood cells because the baby has used some of your iron for its own blood cells.

Most prenatal vitamins contain iron, but it is also available as a supplement. If you are unable to take a prenatal vitamin, you may be given 300 to 350 mg of ferrous sulphate or ferrous gluconate 2 or 3 times a day. Iron is the most important supplement to take. It is required in almost all pregnancies.

Even with supplemental iron, some women develop iron-deficiency anaemia during pregnancy. Several factors may make a woman more likely to have this condition in pregnancy, including:

- failure to take iron or failure to take a prenatal vitamin containing iron
- bleeding during pregnancy
- multiple foetuses
- previous surgery on the stomach or part of the small bowel (making it difficult to absorb an adequate amount of iron before pregnancy)
- antacid overuse that causes a decrease in iron absorption
- poor dietary habits

The goal in treating iron-deficiency anaemia is to increase the amount of iron you consume. Iron is poorly absorbed through the gastrointestinal tract and must be taken on a daily basis. It can be given as an injection, but it's painful and may stain the skin.

Side effects of taking iron supplements include nausea and vomiting, with stomach upset. If this occurs, you may have to take a lower dose. Taking iron may also cause constipation.

If you cannot take an oral iron supplement, an increase in dietary iron from foods, such as liver or spinach, may help prevent anaemia. Ask your doctor for information on what types of foods you should include in your diet.

Sickle-Cell Anaemia. For women who are dark-skinned and of Mediterranean or African descent, sickle-cell anaemia can cause significant problems during pregnancy. Anaemia occurs in these cases because the bone marrow, which produces the body's red blood cells, cannot replace red blood cells as quickly as they are destroyed. In sickle-cell anaemia, the red blood cells produced are also abnormal, which can cause severe pain because they become blocked in the blood vessels and cannot flow.

You may carry the trait for sickle-cell anaemia without having the disease. You could possibly pass the trait or the disease to your baby. Tell your doctor of any family history of the disease.

A blood test easily detects the sickle-cell trait. Sickle-cell anaemia can be diagnosed in the foetus with amniocentesis (discussed in Week 16) or chorionic villus sampling (discussed in Week 10).

Women with the sickle-cell trait are more likely to have pyelonephritis (see Week 18) and bacteria in the urine during pregnancy. They are also susceptible to developing sickle-cell anaemia during pregnancy.

A woman who has sickle-cell anaemia may have repeated episodes of pain (sickle crises) throughout her lifetime. Pain in the abdomen or limbs is caused by the blockage of blood vessels by abnormal red blood cells. Episodes of pain may be severe and may require hospitalization for treatment with fluids and pain medication.

Hydroxyurea has proved effective as a treatment, but its use carries some risks. Because we do not have research data on long-term effects, pregnant women are advised not to use it.

Risks to a pregnant woman with sickle-cell disease are those of painful sickle crisis, infections and even congestive heart failure. Risks to the foetus include a high incidence of miscarriage and stillbirth, estimated to be as high as 50 per cent. Even though the risks are greater, many women with sickle-cell anaemia have successful pregnancies.

Thalassaemia. Another type of anaemia encountered less frequently is thalassaemia, which occurs most often in Mediterranean populations. It is characterized by underproduction of part of the simple protein that makes up red blood cells, and anaemia results. If you have a family history of thalassaemia or know you have thalassaemia, discuss it with your doctor.

How Your Actions Affect Your Baby's Development

✧ When You Feel 'Under the Weather'

It's possible you could have diarrhoea or a cold during pregnancy, as well as other viral infections such as the flu. These problems may raise concerns for you.

- What can I do when I feel ill?
- What medication or treatment is acceptable?
- If I'm sick, should I take my prenatal vitamins?
- If I'm sick and unable to eat my usual diet, what should I do?

If you become sick during pregnancy, don't hesitate to call your GP's surgery or midwife's office. Get your doctor's or midwife's advice about a plan of action. He or she will be able to advise you about what medications you may be able to take to help you feel better. Even if it's only a cold or the flu, your doctor wants to know when you're feeling ill. If any further measures are needed, your doctor/midwife will recommend them.

Is there anything you can do to help yourself? Yes, there is. If you have diarrhoea or a possible viral infection, increase your fluid intake. Drink a lot of water, juice and other clear fluids, such as broth. You may find a bland diet without solid food helps you feel a little better.

Going off your regular diet for a few days won't be harmful to you or your baby, but you do need to drink plenty of fluids. Solid foods may be difficult for you to handle and can make diarrhoea a bigger problem. Milk products may also make diarrhoea worse.

Ðad Tip When you ride together in the car with your partner, ask if you can help her in any way. You may offer to assist her getting in and out of the car. You may propose trading vehicles (if you have more than one), if it's more comfortable for her to drive the other car. Ask if she needs help adjusting her seat belt or the car seat. Try to make riding and driving as easy and accessible as possible for her.

If diarrhoea continues beyond 24 hours, call your doctor. Ask which medications you can take for diarrhoea during pregnancy.

If you are sick, it's OK to skip your prenatal vitamin for a few days. However, begin taking it again when you are able to keep food down.

Don't take any medication without consulting your doctor first. Usually a viral illness with diarrhoea is a short-term problem and won't last more than a few days. You may have to stay home from work or rest in bed until you feel better.

Your Nutrition

You need to drink water and other fluids during pregnancy—lots of it! Fluid helps your body process nutrients, develop new cells, keep up your blood volume and regulate body temperature. You may feel better during your pregnancy if you drink more water than you normally do.

Studies show that for every 15 calories your body burns, you need about 1 tablespoon of water. If you burn 2000 calories a day, you need to drink about 1.1 litres (2 pints) of water! Because your calorie needs increase during pregnancy, so does your need for water. Six to eight glasses a day is a good target. You can meet your goal of at least 1.1 litres (2 pints) a day by sipping water and other fluids throughout the day. If you decrease your consumption later in the day, you may save yourself some trips to the bathroom at night.

Some women wonder if they can drink other beverages besides water. Water is the best source of fluid; however, other fluid sources help meet your needs. You can drink milk, vegetable juice, fruit juice and some herbal teas. Eating vegetables and fruits, other milk products, meat and grain products also help you meet your fluid-consumption target. Avoid tea, coffee and cola—they may contain sodium and caffeine, which act as diuretics. They essentially *increase* your water needs.

Some of the common problems women experience during pregnancy may be eased by drinking water. Headaches, uterine cramping and bladder infections may be less of a problem for you when you drink lots of water.

Check your urine to see if you're drinking enough. If it is light yellow to clear, you're getting enough fluid. Dark-yellow urine is a sign to increase your fluid intake. Don't wait till you get thirsty to drink something. By the time you get thirsty, you've already lost at least 1 per cent of your body's fluids.

You Should Also Know

✑ *Stress during Pregnancy*

Feeling stress is common during pregnancy. Your body is changing, you and your partner are facing the prospect of parenthood and you may not be feeling very well. You may feel stress from working or other obligations. Relax, and take it easy! Stress isn't good for anyone, especially a pregnant woman.

There are quite a few things you can do to help relieve stress in your life right now. Try them, and encourage your partner to try them, too, if he's also feeling stressed out.

- Get enough sleep each night. Lack of sleep can make you feel stressed.
- Rest and relax during the day. Read or listen to music during a quiet period.
- Exercise to help you work off stress. Take a walk or visit the gym. Put on an exercise video for pregnant women. Do something active and physical (but not too physical) to relieve stress. Ask your partner to join you.
- Eat nutritiously. Having enough calories available all through the day will help you avoid 'lows.'
- Do something you enjoy, and do it for you.
- Put on a happy face. Sometimes just changing how you think about something—deciding to be more positive—can have an effect on you. Smiling instead of frowning can help ease stress.
- If smells are important to you, make sure you include them in your life. Burn scented candles, or buy fragrant flowers to help you relax.
- Don't be the 'Lone Ranger.' Share your concerns with your partner, or find a group of pregnant women you can talk with.

༚ Appendicitis

Appendicitis can happen at any time, even during pregnancy. Pregnancy can make the diagnosis difficult because some of the symptoms are typical in a normal pregnancy, such as nausea and vomiting. Diagnosis is also difficult because as the uterus grows larger, the appendix moves upwards and outwards, so pain and tenderness are located in a different place than normal. See the illustration on page 231.

Treatment for appendicitis is immediate surgery. This is major abdominal surgery, with a 7.5- or 10-cm (3- or 4-in) incision, and it

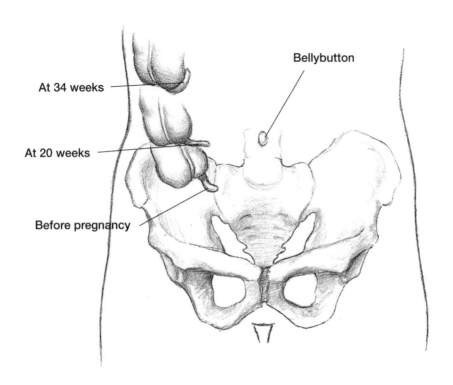

Location of the appendix at various times during pregnancy.

requires a few days in the hospital. Laparoscopy, or 'keyhole' surgery, which requires smaller incisions, is used in some situations, but laparoscopy may be more difficult to perform during pregnancy because of the enlarged uterus.

Serious complications can arise when an infected appendix ruptures. Most doctors believe it's better to operate and remove a 'normal' appendix than to risk infection of the abdominal cavity if the infected appendix ruptures. Antibiotics are administered; many antibiotics are safe to use during pregnancy.

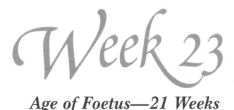

Week 23

Age of Foetus—21 Weeks

How Big Is Your Baby?

By this week, your baby weighs almost 450 g (1 lb)! Its crown-to-rump length is 20 cm (8 in). Your baby is about the size of a small doll.

How Big Are You?

Your uterus extends about 3.75 cm (1½ in) above your bellybutton or about 23 cm (9¼ in) from the pubic symphysis. The changes in your abdomen are progressing slowly, but you definitely have a round appearance now. Your total weight gain should be between 5.5 and 6.8 kg (12 and 15 lb).

How Your Baby Is Growing and Developing

Baby continues to grow. Its body is getting plumper but skin is still wrinkled; it will gain even more weight. See the illustration on page 234.

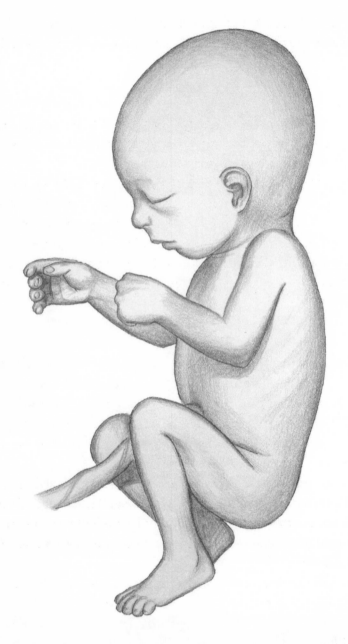

By the 23rd week of pregnancy (foetal age—21 weeks), your baby's eye-lids and eyebrows are well developed.

Lanugo hair on the body occasionally turns darker at this time. The baby's face and body begin to assume more of the appearance of an infant at birth.

∽ *Foetal Pancreas Function*

Your baby's pancreas is developing. This organ is important in hormone production, particularly insulin production; insulin is necessary for the body to break down and to use sugar.

When the foetus is exposed to high blood-sugar levels, the foetal pancreas responds by increasing the blood-insulin level. Insulin has been identified in a foetal pancreas as early as 9 weeks of pregnancy. Insulin in foetal blood has been detected as early as 12 weeks of pregnancy.

Insulin levels are generally high in the blood of babies born to diabetic mothers. That is one reason your doctor/midwife may monitor you for diabetes.

Changes in You

At this point, friends may comment on your size. They may say you must be carrying twins because you're so large. Or they may say you're too small for how far along you think you are. If these comments concern you, discuss them with your doctor.

Your doctor will measure you at every visit after this point. He or she is watching for changes in your weight gain and in the size of your uterus. Remember that women and babies are different sizes and grow at different rates. What's important for you is continual change and continual growth.

As your baby gets larger, the placenta gets larger. The amount of amniotic fluid also increases.

∽ *Loss of Fluid*

As your pregnancy progresses, your uterus grows larger and gets heavier. In early pregnancy, it lies directly behind the bladder, in front of the rectum and the lower part of the colon, which is part of the bowel.

Later in pregnancy, the uterus sits on top of the bladder. As it increases in size, it can put a great deal of pressure on your bladder. You may notice times when your underwear is wet.

You may be uncertain whether you have lost urine or if you are leaking amniotic fluid. It may be difficult to tell the difference between the two. However, when your membranes rupture, you usually experience a gush of fluid or a continual leaking from the vagina. If you experience this, call your doctor immediately!

ᔑ *Emotional Changes Continue*

Do you find your mood swings are worse? Are you still crying easily? Do you wonder if you'll ever be in control again?

Don't worry. These emotions are typical at this point in your pregnancy. Most authorities believe they occur from the hormonal changes that continue throughout pregnancy.

There is little you can do about periods of moodiness. If you think your partner or others are suffering from your emotional outbursts, talk about it with them. Explain that these feelings are common in pregnant women. Ask them to be understanding. Then relax, and try not to get upset about it. Feeling emotional is a normal part of being pregnant.

How Your Actions Affect Your Baby's Development

ᔑ *Diabetes and Pregnancy*

Once a very serious problem during pregnancy, diabetes continues to be an important complication. Today, however, many diabetic women go through pregnancy safely with proper medical care and good nutrition—and by following their doctor's instructions.

Before insulin was available, it was unusual for a diabetic woman to get pregnant. With the discovery of insulin and the development of various ways to monitor a foetus, it is uncommon to have a severe problem today. Survival rate of babies is good.

Diabetes is a condition defined as a lack of insulin in the bloodstream. Insulin is important for breaking down sugar and transporting it to the cells. If you do not have insulin, you will have high blood sugar and a high sugar content in your urine.

There are two types of diabetes. *Type 1* causes the body to stop making insulin; *Type 2* causes the body to use insulin ineffectively. Research has found that Type 2 diabetes is becoming more common in pregnant women. The result of either type is that too much sugar circulates in the woman's blood.

Diabetes during pregnancy can cause several medical problems, including kidney problems, eye problems and other blood or vascular problems, such as atherosclerosis or myocardial infarction (heart attack). These can be serious for you and your baby.

Dad Tip   Since April 2003, fathers who have worked continuously for their employer for 26 weeks, ending with the 15th week before the baby is due, are entitled to take either 1 or 2 consecutive weeks' paternity leave. If you plan to take time off, you need to make arrangements by the end of the 15th week before the baby is expected.

Controlling Diabetes during Pregnancy. If your diabetes is not controlled during pregnancy, you have a greater chance of giving birth to a large baby. This increases your chances of having a C-section. You also increase your risk of pre-eclampsia. In addition, the baby is at greater risk of hypoglycaemia (low blood sugar) and jaundice.

One way to maintain steady blood-sugar levels is never to skip meals and to get enough exercise, according to your finger sticks. You may have to adjust the amount of oral medication you usually take, and insulin may need to be added during pregnancy. If you already take insulin, you may need to adjust your dosage, the timing of your dosage or the amount of insulin you take. You may also have to check your blood-sugar levels 4 to 8 times a day.

Insulin is the safest way to control your diabetes during pregnancy. However, long-lasting insulin should be avoided by pregnant women.

Oral hypoglycaemic medications, such as metformin, are not recommended for use during pregnancy.

Diagnosing Diabetes in Pregnancy. Pregnancy is well known for its tendency to reveal women who are predisposed to diabetes. Women who have trouble with high blood-sugar levels during pregnancy are more likely to develop diabetes in later life. Symptoms of diabetes include the following:

* more frequent urination
* blurred vision
* weight loss
* dizziness
* increased hunger

It may be necessary to do blood tests to diagnose diabetes during pregnancy. In some areas, this testing is done routinely. If you have diabetes or know members of your family who have diabetes now or have had diabetes in the past, tell your doctor/midwife. He or she will decide what course of action is best for you.

Gestational Diabetes. Some women develop diabetes only during pregnancy; it is called *gestational diabetes.* Gestational diabetes affects about 10 per cent of all pregnancies. After pregnancy is over, nearly all women who experience this problem return to normal, and the problem disappears. However, if gestational diabetes occurs with one pregnancy, there is almost a 90 per cent chance it will recur in subsequent pregnancies.

We believe gestational diabetes occurs for two reasons. One is the mother's body produces less insulin during pregnancy. The second is the mother's body can't use insulin effectively. Both situations result in high blood-sugar levels.

A woman's weight when she was born may be an indicator of her chances of developing gestational diabetes. One study showed women who were in the *bottom 10th percentile* of weight when they were born were 3 to 4 times more likely to develop gestational diabetes during pregnancy.

If left untreated, gestational diabetes can be serious for you and your baby. You will both be exposed to a high concentration of sugar, which is not healthy for either of you. You might experience *polyhydramnios* (excessive amounts of amniotic fluid). This may cause premature labour because the uterus becomes overdistended.

A woman with gestational diabetes may have a long labour because the baby is quite large. Sometimes a baby cannot fit through the birth canal, and a Caesarean delivery is required.

If your blood-sugar level is high, you may experience more infections during pregnancy. The most common infections include those in the kidneys, the bladder, the cervix and the uterus.

Treatment of gestational diabetes includes regular exercise and increased fluid intake. Diet is essential in handling this problem. Your doctor will probably recommend a six-meal, 2000- to 2500-calorie per day eating plan. You may also be referred to a dietitian.

Your Nutrition

ᠵ *Your Sodium Intake*

You may need to be careful with your sodium intake during pregnancy. Consuming too much sodium may cause you to retain water, which can cause swelling and bloating. Avoid foods that contain lots of sodium or salt, such as salted nuts, crisps, pickles, canned foods and processed foods.

Tip for Week 23 Keep your consumption of sodium to 3 g (3000 mg) or less a day. This may help you reduce fluid retention.

Read food labels. They list the amount of sodium in a serving. Some books list the sodium content of foods without labels, such as fast foods. Check them out. You'll be surprised how many milligrams of sodium a fast-food hamburger contains!

Sodium Content of Various Foods

Food	Serving Size	Sodium Content (mg)
Asparagus	14.5-oz can	970
Bacon, back	100 g (3½ oz)	2700
Big Mac hamburger	1 regular	963
Chips	100 g (3½ oz)	850
Cola	240 ml (8 fl oz)	16
Cornflakes	100 g (3½ oz)	1100
Crisps	20 regular	400
Flounder	85 g (3 oz)	201
Gelatin, sweet	85 g (3 oz)	270
Gherkin	1 medium	928
Ham, baked	85 g (3 oz)	770
Honeydew melon	½	90
Lima beans	240 g (8½ oz)	1070
Processed cheese	1 slice	322
Salt	1 teaspoon	1938
Smoked salmon	100 g (3½ oz)	1880

Look at the chart above, which lists some common foods and their sodium content. You can see foods that contain sodium do not always taste salty. Read labels, and check other available information before you eat!

You Should Also Know

↗ *Sugar in Your Urine*

It is common for non-diabetic pregnant women to have a small amount of sugar in their urine. This occurs because of changes in sugar levels and how sugar is handled in the kidneys, which control the amount of sugar in your system. If excess sugar is present, you will lose it in your urine. Sugar in the urine is called *glucosuria*. It is common during pregnancy, particularly in the second and third trimesters.

Testing for diabetes is particularly important if you have a family history of diabetes. Blood tests used to diagnose diabetes are a fasting blood-sugar and glucose-tolerance test (GTT).

For a fasting blood-sugar test, you eat your normal meal the evening before the test. In the morning, before eating anything, you go to the lab and have a blood test done. A normal result indicates that diabetes is unlikely. An abnormal result is a high level of sugar in the blood, which needs further study.

Further study involves the glucose-tolerance test. You have to fast after dinner the night before this test. In the morning at the lab, you are given a solution to drink that has a measured amount of sugar in it. It is similar to a can of fizzy drink but doesn't taste as good. After you drink the solution, blood is drawn at predetermined intervals; usually at 30 minutes, 1 hour and 2 hours and sometimes even 3 hours. Drawing the blood at intervals gives an indication of how your body handles sugar.

If you need treatment, your doctor will devise a plan for you.

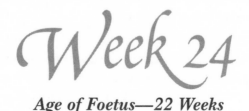

Week 24

Age of Foetus—22 Weeks

How Big Is Your Baby?

By this week, your baby weighs about 540 g (1¼ lb). Its crown-to-rump length is about 21 cm (8½ in).

How Big Are You?

Your uterus is now about 3.8 to 5.1 cm (1½ to 2 in) above the belly-button. It measures almost 24 cm (10 in) above the pubic symphysis.

How Your Baby Is Growing and Developing

Your baby is filling out. Its face and body look more like that of an infant at the time of birth. Although it weighs a little over 450 g (1 lb) at this point, it is still very tiny.

ᕼ *Role of the Amniotic Sac and Amniotic Fluid*

By about the 12th day after fertilization, there is an early beginning of the amniotic sac. The baby grows and develops in the amniotic fluid inside the amniotic sac. (See the illustration on page 244.) Amniotic fluid has several important functions.

- It provides an environment in which the baby can move easily.
- It cushions the foetus against injury.
- Amniotic fluid regulates temperature for the baby.
- It provides a way of assessing the health and maturity of the baby.

Amniotic fluid increases rapidly from an average volume of 50 ml (1½ fl oz) by 12 weeks of pregnancy to 400 ml (12 fl oz) at midpregnancy. The volume of amniotic fluid continues to increase as your due date approaches until a maximum of about 1.1 litres (2 pints) of fluid is reached at 36 to 38 weeks gestation.

Composition of amniotic fluid changes during pregnancy. During the first half of pregnancy, amniotic fluid is similar to maternal plasma (the fluid in your blood without blood cells), except it has a much lower protein content. As pregnancy advances, foetal urine makes an increasingly important contribution to the amount of amniotic fluid present. Amniotic fluid also contains old foetal blood cells, lanugo hair and vernix.

The foetus swallows amniotic fluid during much of pregnancy. If it can't swallow amniotic fluid, you will develop a condition of excess amniotic fluid, called *hydramnios* or *polyhydramnios*.

Tip for Week 24 Overeating and eating before going to bed at night are two major causes of heartburn. Eating five or six small, nutritious meals a day and skipping snacks before bedtime may help you feel better.

If the foetus swallows but doesn't urinate (for example, if the baby lacks kidneys), the volume of amniotic fluid surrounding the foetus may be very small. This is called *oligohydramnios*.

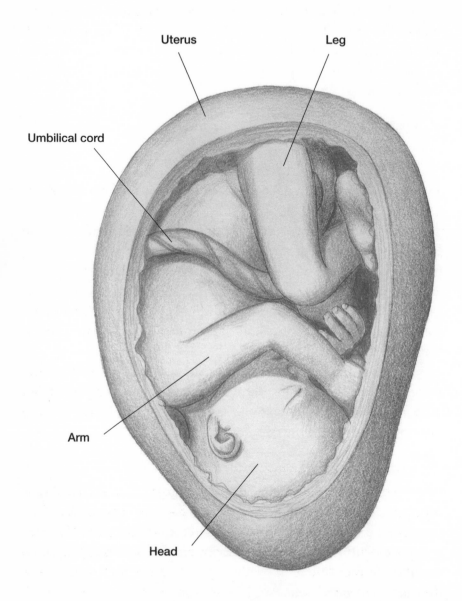

Uterus

Leg

Umbilical cord

Arm

Head

The foetus doesn't appear to have a great deal of room to move in the uterus by the 24th week. As the weeks pass, space gets even tighter.

Amniotic fluid is important. It provides the baby space to move and allows it to grow. If there is an inadequate amount of amniotic fluid, the baby usually shows decreased growth.

Changes in You

๛ *Nasal Problems*

Some women complain of stuffiness in their nose or frequent nose-bleeds during pregnancy. Some researchers believe these symptoms occur because of changes in circulation due to hormonal changes during pregnancy. This can cause the mucous membranes of your nose and nasal passageways to swell and to bleed more easily.

Some decongestants and nasal sprays have been proved safe for use during pregnancy. Some brands to consider include chlophenamine (Piriton) decongestants and oxymetazoline (Afrazine, Dristan Long-Lasting) nasal sprays. Before you begin using any product, discuss it with your doctor.

It may also help to use a humidifier, particularly during the winter months when heating may dry out the air. Some women get relief from increasing their fluid intake and/or using a gentle lubricant in their nose, such as petroleum jelly.

๛ *Depression during Pregnancy*

Many people have heard about postpartum depression (feeling blue or being depressed after baby's birth). There has been a great deal of information on the subject in the media in the last few years. However, you probably haven't heard much about depression *during* pregnancy, but it does occur. Studies show that up to 25 per cent of all mums-to-be experience some degree of depression, and nearly 10 per cent will experience a major depression.

When you are pregnant, your body goes through many changes. It may be hard to distinguish between some of the normal pregnancy changes and signs of depression. Many symptoms of depression are similar to those of pregnancy, including fatigue and sleeplessness. The difference is how intense the symptoms are and how long they last. Some common symptoms of depression include:

- overpowering sadness that lasts for days, without an obvious cause
- difficulty sleeping, or waking up very early
- wanting to sleep all the time or great fatigue (this can be normal early in pregnancy but usually gets better after a few weeks)
- no appetite (as distinguished from nausea and vomiting)
- lack of concentration
- thoughts of harming yourself

If you have these symptoms and they don't get better in a few weeks or every day seems to be bad, talk to your doctor. There are medications that can help, such as antidepressants; some are safe to use during pregnancy. If your depression is severe, medication may be necessary for your good health and the good health of your baby. In addition, counselling may be recommended.

Other suggestions for dealing with depression include getting enough exercise and being sure you get enough B vitamins, folic acid and omega-3 fatty acids (see the discussion of fish in Week 26). Additional therapies include massage and reflexology.

Another option for treating this type of depression is light therapy, similar to the type of treatment given to those who suffer from 'seasonal affective disorder.' When a person is depressed, exposure to bright-white fluorescent light for 60 minutes a day, up to 5 times a week, has proved beneficial. A recent study showed that moods improved in about 50 per cent of those who underwent the treatment. We believe that bright light influences your biorhythms and helps release certain hormones that help deal with depression.

If you believe you are depressed, bring it up at an antenatal visit. There are steps you and your doctor can take to help you feel better again. It's important to do it for yourself and your baby!

How Your Actions
Affect Your Baby's Development

⌒ *What Your Baby Can Hear*

Can a growing baby hear sounds while it's inside the uterus? From various research studies, we know that sounds can penetrate amniotic fluid and reach your baby's developing ears.

If you work in a noisy place, you may want to request a quieter area during your pregnancy. From data gathered in some studies, it is believed that chronic loud noise and short, intense bursts of sound may cause hearing damage to the foetus before and after birth.

It's OK to expose your growing baby to loud noises, such as a concert, every once in a while. But if you are repeatedly exposed to noise that is so loud it forces you to shout, there may be potential danger to your baby.

Your Nutrition

Many pregnant women are concerned about eating out. Some want to know if they can eat certain types of food, such as Indian, Chinese or Thai food. They're concerned that spicy or rich foods could be harmful to the baby. It's OK to eat out, but you might find certain foods don't agree with you.

The best types of food to eat at restaurants are those you tolerate well at home. Chicken, fish, fresh vegetables and salads are usually good choices. Restaurants that feature spicy foods or unusual cuisine may cause you stomach or intestinal distress. You may even notice an increase in weight from water retention after eating at a restaurant.

During pregnancy, avoid restaurants that serve highly

Ðad Tip Now is a good time to find out about antenatal classes in your area. Find out how many classes there are, when and where to register and the registration cost. You may be able to take classes at the hospital or birthing centre where you plan to deliver. Try to *complete* the classes at least 1 month *before* your baby is due.

salted food, food high in sodium or food loaded with calories and fat, such as gravies, fried food, junk food and rich desserts. It may be difficult to control your calorie intake at specialty restaurants.

Another challenge of eating out is maintaining a healthy diet if you work outside the home. It may be necessary to go to business lunches or to travel for your company. Be selective. If you can choose off the menu, look for healthy or low-fat choices. You may ask about preparation—maybe a dish can be steamed instead of fried. On a business trip, take along some of your own food. Choose healthy, non-perishable foods, such as fruits and vegetables, that don't need refrigeration.

You Should Also Know

ᎌ *How Pregnancy Affects You Sexually*

Pregnancy and sex. Are you interested? Is it just too much to think about right now? Has your sexual desire increased? Is sex the last thing on your mind?

Generally, women experience one of two sex-drive patterns during pregnancy. One is a lessening of desire in the first and third trimesters, with an increase in the second trimester. The second is a gradual decrease in desire for sex as pregnancy progresses.

During the first trimester, you may experience fatigue and nausea. During the third trimester, your weight gain, enlarging abdomen, tender breasts and other problems may make you desire sex less. This is normal. Tell your partner how you feel, and try to work out a solution that is satisfactory to you both.

Pregnancy actually enhances the sex drive for some women. In some cases, a woman may experience orgasms or multiple orgasms for the first time during pregnancy. This is due to heightened hormonal activity and increased blood flow to the pelvic area.

Some women feel less attractive during pregnancy because of their size and the changes in their bodies. Discuss your feelings with your partner. Tenderness and understanding can help you both.

You may find new positions for lovemaking are necessary as pregnancy progresses. Your abdomen may make some positions more uncomfortable than others. In addition, we advise you not to lie flat on your back after 16 weeks until the baby's birth because the weight of the uterus restricts circulation. You might try lying on your side or use a position that puts you on top.

When to Avoid Sexual Activity. Some situations should alert you to abstain from sexual activity. If you have a history of early labour, your doctor may warn against intercourse and orgasm; orgasm causes mild uterine contractions. Chemicals in semen may also stimulate contractions, so it may not be advisable for a woman's partner to ejaculate inside her.

If you have a history of miscarriage, your doctor may caution you against sex and orgasm. However, no data actually links sex and miscarriage. Avoid sexual activity if you have placenta previa or a low-lying placenta, an incompetent cervix, premature labour, ruptured bag of waters, pain with intercourse, unexplained vaginal bleeding or discharge, either partner has an unhealed herpes lesion or you believe labour has begun.

Sexual Practices to Avoid. Some sexual practices should be avoided when you're pregnant. Don't insert any object into the vagina that could cause injury or infection. Blowing air into the vagina is dangerous because it can force a potentially fatal air bubble into a woman's bloodstream. (This can occur whether or not you are pregnant.) Nipple stimulation releases oxytocin, which causes uterine contractions; you might want to discuss this practice with your doctor/midwife.

✂ *An Incompetent Cervix*

An incompetent cervix refers to the painless premature dilatation of the cervix, which usually results in delivery of a premature baby. It can be an important problem during pregnancy.

Dilatation (stretching of the cervix) goes unnoticed by the woman until the baby is delivering; it often occurs without warning. Diagnosis is usually made after one or more deliveries of a premature infant without any pain before delivery.

The cause of cervical incompetence is usually unknown. Some medical researchers believe it occurs because of previous injury or surgery to the cervix, such as dilatation and curettage (D&C) for an abortion or a miscarriage.

Usually the cervix doesn't dilate in this way before the 16th week of pregnancy. Before this time, the products of conception are not heavy enough to cause the cervix to dilate and to thin out.

A pregnancy that is lost from an incompetent cervix is completely different from a miscarriage. A miscarriage during the first trimester is common. Incompetent cervix is a relatively rare complication in pregnancy.

Treatment for an incompetent cervix is usually surgical. The weak cervix is reinforced with a suture that sews the cervix shut, called a *McDonald cerclage*.

If this is your first pregnancy, there is no way you can know whether you have an incompetent cervix. If you have had problems in the past or have had premature deliveries and have been told you might have an incompetent cervix, share this important information with your doctor/midwife.

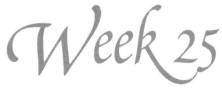

Week 25

Age of Foetus—23 Weeks

How Big Is Your Baby?

Your baby now weighs about 700 g (1½ lb), and crown-to-rump length is about 22 cm (8¾ in). Remember, these are average lengths and weights, and vary from one baby to another and from one pregnancy to another.

How Big Are You?

Look at the illustration on page 252. By this week of pregnancy, your uterus has grown quite a bit. When you look at a side view, you're obviously getting bigger.

The measurement from the pubic symphysis to the top of your uterus is about 25 cm (10 in). If you saw your doctor/midwife when you were 20 or 21 weeks pregnant, you have probably grown about 4 cm (1½ in). At this point, your uterus is about the size of a football.

The top of the uterus is about halfway between your bellybutton and the lower part of your sternum. (The sternum is the bone between your breasts where the ribs come together.)

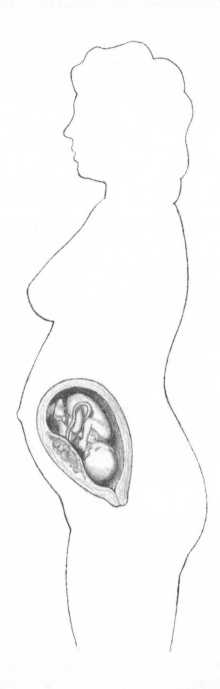

Comparative size of the uterus at 25 weeks of pregnancy (foetal age—
23 weeks). The uterus can be felt about 5 cm (2 in) above your
umbilicus (bellybutton).

How Your Baby Is Growing and Developing

∽ Survival of a Premature Baby

It may be hard to believe, but if your baby were delivered now, it would have a chance of surviving. Some of the greatest advances in medicine have been in the care of the premature baby. No one wants a baby to deliver this early, but with new treatment methods, such as ventilators, monitors and medication, a baby does have a chance of surviving.

The baby weighs less than 900 g (2 lb) and is extremely small. Survival is difficult for an infant delivered this early. The baby would probably spend several months in the hospital, with risks of infection and other possible complications. Also see the discussion in Week 29.

∽ Is It a Boy? Is It a Girl?

One of the most common questions parents-to-be ask is, 'What is the sex of our baby?' Amniocentesis can determine the sex of the baby by chromosome study. Ultrasound examination can also be used to reveal the sex of the baby but may be inaccurate. Don't get your heart set on a particular sex if ultrasound is used. For many people, not knowing is part of the fun of having a baby.

Some people believe a baby's heartbeat rate can indicate its sex. A normal heart rate for a baby ranges from 110 to 160 beats a minute. Some believe a fast heartbeat indicates a girl, and a slow heartbeat indicates a boy. Unfortunately, there is no scientific proof of this. Don't pressure your doctor to guess based on this method because it is *only* a guess.

A more reliable source might be a mother, mother-in-law or someone who can look at you and tell by how you're carrying the baby if it is a boy or girl. Although we make this statement with our tongues placed firmly in our cheeks, many people believe it's true. Some people claim they're never wrong about guessing or predicting the sex of a baby before birth. Again, there is no scientific basis for this method.

Your doctor is more concerned about your health and well-being, and that of your baby. He or she will concentrate on making sure you and your baby, whether it's a boy or girl, are progressing through pregnancy safely and that you both get through pregnancy, labour and delivery in good health.

Changes in You

⁓ *Itching*

Itching (*pruritus gravidarum*) is a common symptom during pregnancy. There are no bumps or lesions on the skin; it just itches. Nearly 20 per cent of all pregnant women suffer from itching, often in the last weeks of pregnancy, but it can occur at any time. It may occur with each pregnancy and may also appear when you use oral contraceptives. The condition doesn't present any risk to you or your baby.

Tip for Week 25

Pregnancy can be a time of communication and personal growth with your partner. Listen when he talks. Let him know he is an important source of emotional support for you.

As your uterus has grown and filled your pelvis, your abdominal skin and muscles have stretched. Itchiness is a natural consequence. Lotions are OK to use to help reduce itching. Try not to scratch and irritate your skin—that can make it worse! You might want to ask your doctor about taking antihistamines or using cooling lotions containing menthol or camphor. Often no treatment is needed.

⁓ *Stress Can Affect You*

Stress in your life can have an impact on your pregnancy. Research is showing an increasing connection between stress experienced by the mother-to-be and pregnancy problems, such as pre-eclampsia, miscarriage and premature labour.

If you have major stress in your life right now—you've lost your job or moved, or someone close to you has died—be sure to take good care of yourself. Eat well, get enough rest and try to de-stress. Talking about it can help—ask your doctor to recommend a support group.

How Your Actions
Affect Your Baby's Development

✑ Falling and Injuries from Falls

A fall is the most frequent cause of minor injury during pregnancy. Fortunately, a fall is usually without serious injury to the baby or mother. The uterus is well protected in the abdomen inside the pelvis. The baby is protected against injury by the cushion of amniotic fluid surrounding it. Your uterus and abdominal wall also offer some protection.

If You Fall. If you fall, contact your doctor/midwife; he or she may want to examine you. You may feel reassured if you are monitored and your baby's heartbeat is checked. The baby's movement after a fall can be reassuring.

Minor injuries to the abdomen are treated in the usual fashion, as though you were not pregnant. However, avoid X-rays if possible.

Ultrasound evaluation may be important after a fall. This is judged on an individual basis, depending on the severity of your symptoms and your injury.

Take Care to Avoid Falls. Remember your balance and mobility change as you grow larger during pregnancy. Be careful during the winter when car parks and pavements may be wet or icy. Many pregnant women also fall on stairs; always use the handrail. Walk in well-lit areas, and try to stay on pavements.

Slow down a little as you get larger; you won't be able to get around as quickly as you normally do. With the change in your balance, plus any dizziness you may experience, it's important to be vigilant to try to avoid falling.

Signs to Watch for after a Fall. Some signs can alert you to a problem after a fall:

- bleeding
- a gush of fluid from the vagina, indicating rupture of membranes
- severe abdominal pain

Placental abruption (discussed in Week 33) is one of the most serious events that can occur because of a fall or injury. With placental abruption, the placenta prematurely separates from the uterus. Another significant injury is a broken bone or an injury that immobilizes you. (See the discussion below.)

Treating Broken Bones. Sometimes a fall or accident causes a broken bone, which may require X-rays and surgery. Treatment cannot be delayed until after pregnancy; the problem must be dealt with immediately.

If X-rays are required, your pelvis and abdomen must be shielded. If they cannot be shielded, the need for the X-ray must be weighed against the risks it poses to the baby.

Anaesthesia or pain medication may be necessary with a simple break that requires setting or pinning. It is best for you and the baby to avoid general anaesthesia if possible. You may need pain medication, but keep its use to a minimum.

If general anaesthesia is required to repair a break, the baby should be monitored closely. You may not have a lot of choice in the matter. Your surgeon and obstetrician will work together to provide the best care for you and your baby.

Your Nutrition

Pregnancy increases your need for vitamins and minerals. It's best if you can meet most of these needs through the foods you eat. However, being realistic, we know that's difficult for many women. That's one reason your doctor prescribes a prenatal vitamin for you—to help you meet your nutritional needs.

Some women do need extra help during pregnancy—supplements are often prescribed for them. These pregnant women include teenagers (whose bodies are still growing), severely underweight women, women who ate a poor diet before conception and women who have previously given birth to multiples. Women who smoke or drink heav-

Some Alternative Food Choices

As you move through your pregnancy, you may find adding nutritious foods to your eating plan is getting harder. You may be bored with the foods you've been eating. The points below may help make it easier to choose different healthy foods.

- Complex carbohydrates that are high in fibre provide your body with a constant source of energy and help you feel full longer. Try wholemeal rolls, bagels, tortillas or risotto.
- Green leafy veggies, such as spinach and broccoli, contain different nutrients than orange vegetables, such as yams or carrots. Try to have a combination of these every day. One great dish that may satisfy your needs and taste great at the same time is a 'Squash Bake.' In a non-stick frying pan, heat a little water, then add cut up courgettes, tomatoes, yellow squash and onions. Cover and cook for 30 to 45 minutes.
- Foods high in nutrients, such as fruits and vegetables, provide a lot of vitamins and minerals but are not usually high in calories. For example, kiwi fruit has more vitamins C and E per serving than any other fruit. It's also a natural laxative.
- When choosing lettuce, darker is better. Romaine and spinach have a lot of vitamin A and folic acid. Iceberg lettuce has the most fibre and is a good source of potassium. Rocket and leaf lettuce add texture and vitamins A and C.
- To help control a sweet tooth, limit yourself to 100 calories of confectionary a day–a handful of jelly beans, half a packet of Maltesers or half a 40-g chocolate bar. Read labels!
- Looking for some different ways to get the nutrients you need? For a vegetable serving, try 120 ml (4 fl oz) spaghetti sauce. For a serving from the bread and cereal group, 3 cups popped popcorn meet your needs. And when you're looking for protein, choose from 45 g (1½ oz) egg substitute, 2 tablespoons of any kind of nut butter or 115 g (4 oz) textured vegetable protein.

ily need supplements, as do some who have a chronic medical condition, those who take certain medications and those who have problems digesting cow's milk, wheat and other essential foods. In some cases, vegetarians may need supplements.

Your doctor will discuss the situation with you. If you need more than a prenatal vitamin, he or she will advise you.

Caution: Never take *any* supplements without your doctor's OK! (See also the Nutrition discussion in Week 27.)

You Should Also Know

ᴈ *Thyroid Disease*

Thyroid problems and thyroid disease can affect your pregnancy. Thyroid hormone is made in the thyroid gland; this hormone affects your entire body and is important in your metabolism.

Thyroid-hormone levels may be high or low. High levels of thyroid cause a condition called *hyperthyroidism;* low levels cause *hypothyroidism.* Women who have a history of miscarriage or premature delivery or who have problems around the time of delivery may have problems with their thyroid-hormone levels.

> *Ɖad Tip* Offer to do the shopping. Even if you don't shop solo, go with your partner to lift and to carry her purchases.

Symptoms You May Notice. Symptoms of thyroid disease may be hidden by pregnancy. Or you may notice changes during pregnancy that cause you and your doctor to suspect the thyroid is not functioning properly. These changes could include an enlarged thyroid, changes in your pulse, redness of the palms and warm, moist palms. Because thyroid-hormone levels can change during pregnancy (*because* of pregnancy), your doctor must be careful interpreting lab results about this hormone while you're pregnant.

Thyroid Test. The thyroid is tested primarily by blood tests (a thyroid panel), which measure the amount of thyroid hormone produced. The tests also measure levels of another hormone, thyroid-stimulating hormone (TSH), made at the base of the brain. An additional test, an X-ray study of the thyroid (radioactive iodine scan), should not be done during pregnancy.

Treatment of Thyroid Disease. If you have hypothyroidism, thyroid replacement (thyroxin) is prescribed. It is believed to be safe during pregnancy. Your doctor may check the level during pregnancy with a blood test to make sure you are receiving enough of the hormone.

If you have hyperthyroidism, the medication propylthiouracil is used for treatment. It does pass through the placenta to the baby. Your doctor will prescribe the lowest possible amount to reduce risk to your baby. Blood testing during pregnancy is necessary to monitor the amount of medication needed. Iodide is another medication used for hyperthyroidism. Avoid iodide during pregnancy because of harmful effects to a developing baby.

After delivery, it's important to test the baby and to watch for signs of thyroid problems related to the medications prescribed during pregnancy. If you have a past history of problems with your thyroid, if you are now taking medication or if you have taken medication in the past for your thyroid, tell your doctor. Discuss treatment during pregnancy.

Week 26

Age of Foetus—24 Weeks

How Big Is Your Baby?

Your baby now weighs almost 900 g (2 lb). By this week, its crown-to-rump length is around 23 cm (9¼ in). See the illustration on page 262. Your baby is beginning to put on weight.

How Big Are You?

The measurement of your uterus is about 6 cm (2½ in) above your bellybutton or nearly 26 cm (10½ in) from your pubic symphysis. During this second half of pregnancy, you will grow nearly 1 cm (½ in) each week. If you have been following a nutritious, balanced meal plan, your total weight gain is probably between 7.2 to 9.9 kg (16 and 22 lb).

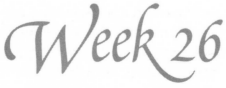

Tip for Week 26 Lying on your side (your left side is best) when you rest provides the best circulation to your baby. You may not experience as much swelling if you rest on your left side during the day.

How Your Baby Is Growing and Developing

By now you have heard your baby's heartbeat at several visits. Listening to your developing baby's heartbeat is reassuring.

The foetus now has distinct sleeping and waking cycles. You may find a pattern; at certain times of the day your baby is very active, while at other times he or she is asleep. In addition, all five senses are now fully developed.

✢ *Heart Arrhythmia*

When listening to your baby's heartbeat during pregnancy, you may be startled to hear a skipped beat. An irregular heartbeat is called an *arrhythmia.* This is best described by regular pulsing or pounding with an occasional skipped or missed heartbeat. Arrhythmias in a foetus are not unusual.

There are many causes of foetal arrhythmias. An arrhythmia may occur as the heart grows and develops. As the heart matures, the arrhythmia often disappears. It may occur in the foetus of a pregnant woman who has lupus.

If an arrhythmia is discovered before labour and delivery, you may require foetal heart-rate monitoring during labour. When an arrhythmia is detected during labour, it may be desirable to have a paediatrician present at the time of delivery. He or she will make sure the baby is all right or is treated right away if a problem exists.

Changes in You

You are getting bigger as your uterus, placenta and baby grow larger. Discomforts such as back pain, pressure in your pelvis, leg cramps and headaches may occur more frequently.

Time is passing quickly. You are approaching the end of the second trimester. Two-thirds of the pregnancy is behind you; it won't be long until your baby is born.

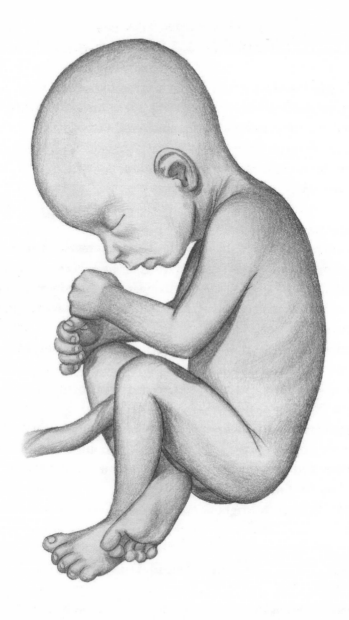

By this week, your baby weighs about 900 g (2 lb). It is now putting on some weight and filling out.

How Your Actions Affect Your Baby's Development

✣ *How to Have a Successful Labour and Delivery*

It's not too early to start thinking about your labour and delivery. One way to have a successful labour and delivery is to understand what elements contribute to that success. Below are some things you may want to consider as you progress through your pregnancy.

Become informed about pregnancy and the birth experience. Knowledge is power. When you understand what can and will occur during your pregnancy, you may be able to relax more. Read our other pregnancy books, discuss questions and concerns with your doctor/ midwife and share information and your knowledge with your partner.

The relationships you have with your doctor/midwife and other members of your healthcare team are very important. Be a good patient by following medical suggestions, watching your weight, eating healthily, taking your prenatal vitamins and attending all your antenatal appointments and tests.

Being able to help make decisions that affect your medical care, including birth positions, pain-relief methods, feeding baby and your partner's level of participation in labour and delivery, helps you feel more in control during labour and delivery. Discuss questions and various situations with your doctor at antenatal appointments.

✣ *Will Working at a Computer Terminal Hurt Your Baby?*

Many women are concerned about working in front of a computer screen. Currently nothing suggests that working at a computer terminal is likely to harm your unborn baby.

If you work at a computer, consider the way you sit and how long you sit. (This is true for any job where you sit most of the time.) Sit in a chair that offers good support for your back and legs. Don't slouch or cross your legs when sitting. Rest your feet on a low stool or box to relieve back strain. Be sure to get up and walk around at least once every 15 minutes—you need to keep good circulation in your legs.

৯ Home Uterine Monitoring

Home uterine monitoring is used to identify women with premature labour. Conditions associated with premature delivery include a previous preterm delivery, infections, premature rupture of membranes, pregnancy-induced hypertension and multiple foetuses.

Home uterine monitoring combines recording uterine contractions with daily telephone contact with the doctor. A recording of contractions is transmitted from the woman's home by telephone to a centre where contractions can be evaluated. Thanks to personal computers, your doctor may be able to view the recordings at his or her surgery or home. In the UK as yet, however, it is rarely available.

Not everyone agrees that home monitoring is beneficial or cost-effective, though some believe the cost can be justified if a premature delivery can be prevented. It may be difficult to identify all the women who need this type of monitoring.

Your Nutrition

৯ Eating Fish during Your Pregnancy

Eating fish is beneficial; it is particularly good for you during pregnancy. Women who eat a variety of fish during pregnancy have longer pregnancies and give birth to babies with higher birth weights, according to some studies. This is important because the longer a baby stays in the uterus, the better its chances are of being strong and healthy at delivery.

Recent studies have shown that women who eat fish during pregnancy may have fewer problems with premature labour. This benefit may be from the omega-3 fatty acids contained in fish that cause a hormonal response to help protect you from premature labour. Omega-3 fatty acids may also help prevent pregnancy-induced hypertension and pre-eclampsia.

Many fish are safe to eat, and you should include them in your diet. Most fish is low in fat and high in vitamin B, iron, zinc, selenium and

copper. Many fish choices are excellent, healthy additions to your diet,
and you can eat them as often as you
like. See the chart on page 266 for a
list of good choices.

Dad Tip About now,
your partner may not feel very
attractive. Take her on a date—
go to dinner and the cinema! Tell
her she's beautiful. Take a full-view
picture of her as a remembrance
of how lovely she is now.

Omega-3 Fatty Acids. Anchovies,
herring, mullet, mackerel, sardines
and trout are some fish with a lot of
omega-3 fatty acids. If you're a vegetarian or you don't like fish, add
rapeseed oil, flaxseed, soya beans, walnuts and wheat germ to your food
plan because these foods contain linolenic oil, which is a type of omega-
3 fatty acid.

Some researchers believe eating fatty fish or ingesting omega-3 fatty
acids in another form (such as fish-oil capsules) may also enhance
your baby's intellectual development. Studies have shown that fish oil
is important to foetal brain development. One study of pregnant
women demonstrated that when a pregnant woman eats fish oil, it
reaches the brain of the developing foetus.

It's important to include omega-3 fatty acids in your eating plan.
However, studies have found it's best not to exceed 2.4 g of omega-3
fatty acids a day.

Methyl-mercury Poisoning. Some fish are contaminated with a
dangerous substance as the result of man-made pollution. People
who eat these fish are at risk of methyl-mercury poisoning. Mercury
is a naturally occurring substance as well as a pollution by-product.
Mercury becomes a problem when it is released into the air as a pol-
lutant. It settles into the oceans and from there winds up in some
types of fish.

The government's Food Standards Agency has determined that a
certain level of methyl mercury in fish is dangerous for humans. We
know methyl mercury can pass from mother to foetus across the placenta. Research has shown that a significant number of children are

Good Fish and Shellfish Choices

Below is a list of fish you can eat as often as you like during pregnancy.

bass	mackerel
catfish	marlin
cod	ocean perch
flounder	pollack
freshwater perch	red snapper
haddock	sole
herring	

You may eat the following shellfish as often as you like if you thoroughly cook them.

clams	oysters
crab	scallops
lobster	prawns

Remember: Don't exceed a total of 340 g (12 oz) of fish a week!

born each year who are at risk of developing neurological problems linked to the consumption of seafood by their mothers during pregnancy. Because of rapid brain development, a foetus may be more vulnerable to methylmercury poisoning.

Studies indicate that pregnant women and those trying to conceive should be cautious—some kinds of fish should not be eaten more than once a month. These fish include shark, swordfish and tuna (fresh or frozen). If you're nursing, limit your consumption of these fish to once a week. Canned tuna is a little safer but don't eat more than one 170 g (6 oz) can a week.

Some freshwater fish may also be risky to eat, such as pike. To be on the safe side, consult local authorities or the Food Standards Agency for up-to-date advice on eating freshwater fish.

Some Additional Cautions about Fish. Other environmental pollutants can appear in fish. Dioxin and PCBs (polychlorinated biphenyls) are found in some fish, such as bluefish (snapper) or lake trout; avoid them.

Parasites, bacteria, viruses and toxins can also contaminate fish. Eating infected fish can make you sick, sometimes severely so. Sushi and ceviche are fish dishes that could contain viruses or parasites. Raw shellfish, if contaminated, could cause hepatitis-A, cholera or gastroenteritis. Avoid *all* raw fish during pregnancy! Other fish to avoid during pregnancy include some found in warm tropical waters. Avoid the following 'local' fish from those areas: amberjack, barracuda, blue-fish, grouper, mahimahi, snapper and fresh tuna.

We advise pregnant women not to eat sushi; however there are a couple of 'sushi' dishes that are OK to eat. Sushi made with *cooked* eel and rolls with *steamed* crab and veggies are acceptable.

If you are unsure about whether you should eat a particular fish or if you would like further information, contact the Food Standards Agency at www.foodstandards.gov.uk or call 0207 276 8000.

You Should Also Know

৵ *Retin-A*

Retin-A (tretinoin), not to be confused with Roaccutane (isotretinoin), is a cream or lotion used to treat acne and to help get rid of fine wrinkles on the face. **If you are pregnant and using Retin-A, stop using it immediately!**

We don't have enough data to know if it's safe to use during pregnancy. We do know any type of medication you use—whether taken internally, inhaled, injected or used topically (spread on the skin)—gets into your bloodstream. Any substance in your bloodstream can be passed to your baby.

Some medications a mother-to-be uses become concentrated in the baby. Your body can handle it, but your baby's body may not be able to. If some substances build up in the baby, they can have significant effects on its development. In the future, we may know more about its effects on a growing baby. At this time, it's best to avoid using Retin-A for the sake of your baby.

৵ *Steroid Creams and Ointments*

Skin conditions may arise during pregnancy that require treatment with creams or ointments. This treatment could include steroid preparations. Before you use anything of this type, consult with your doctor.

⨯ *Seizures*

A history of seizures—before pregnancy, during a previous pregnancy or during this pregnancy—is information you must share with your doctor. Another term for seizure is *convulsion.*

Seizures can and usually do occur without warning. A seizure indicates an abnormal condition related to the nervous system, particularly the brain. During a seizure, a person often loses body control. The serious nature of this problem during pregnancy is compounded because of concern about the baby's safety.

If you have never had a problem with seizures, know that a short episode of dizziness or lightheadedness is *not* usually a seizure. Seizures are usually diagnosed by someone observing the seizure and noting the symptoms previously mentioned. An electroencephalogram (EEG) may be needed to diagnose a seizure.

Medications to Control Seizures. If you take medication for seizure control or prevention, share this important information with your doctor at the beginning of pregnancy. Medication can be taken during pregnancy to control seizures, but some can cause birth defects in a baby, which include facial problems, microcephaly (a small head) and developmental delay. Other medications are used during pregnancy for seizure prevention. One of the more common is phenobarbital, but there is some concern about the safety of this medication.

Seizures during pregnancy or at any other time require serious discussion with your doctor and increased monitoring during pregnancy. If you have questions or concerns about a history of possible seizures, talk to your doctor about them.

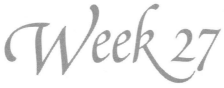

Week 27

Age of Foetus—25 Weeks

How Big Is Your Baby?

This week marks the beginning of the 3rd trimester. In addition to weight and crown-to-rump length, we're adding total length of your baby's body from head to toe. This will give you an even better idea of how big your baby is during this last part of your pregnancy.

Your baby now weighs about 1 kg (2¼ lb), and crown-to-rump length is about 24 cm (9⅔ in) by this week. Total length is about 34 cm (15¼ in). See the illustration on page 271.

How Big Are You?

Your uterus is about 7 cm (2¾ in) above your belly-button. If measured from the pubic symphysis, it is more than 27 cm (10½ in) from the pubic symphysis to the top of the uterus.

Tip for Week 27 Childbirth-education classes are not just for couples. Classes are often offered for single mothers or for pregnant women whose partners cannot come to classes. Ask your doctor about classes for you.

How Your Baby Is
Growing and Developing

᠕ *Eye Development*

Eyes first appear around day 22 of development in the embryo (about 5 weeks gestation). In the beginning, they look like a pair of shallow grooves on each side of the developing brain. These grooves continue to develop and eventually turn into pockets called *optical vesicles*. The lens of each eye develops from the ectoderm. (We discuss ectoderm in Week 4.)

Early in development, eyes are on the side of the head. They move towards the middle of the face between 7 and 10 weeks of gestation.

At about 8 weeks gestation, blood vessels form that lead to the eye. During the 9th week of gestation, the pupil forms, which is the round opening in the eye. At that time, the nerve connection from the eyes to the brain begins to form, called the *optic nerve*.

Eyelids that cover the eyes are fused (connected together) at around 11 to 12 weeks. They remain fused until about 27 to 28 weeks of pregnancy, when they open.

The retina, at the back of the eye, is light-sensitive. It is the part of the eye where light images come into focus. It develops its normal layers by about 27 weeks of pregnancy. These layers receive light and light information, and transmit it to the brain for interpretation—what we know as 'sight.'

Congenital Cataracts. A congenital cataract is an eye problem that may be present at birth. Most people believe cataracts occur only in old age, but that's a misconception. They can appear in a newborn baby!

Instead of being transparent or clear, the lens that focuses light onto the back of the eye is opaque or cloudy. This problem is usually caused by a genetic predisposition (it is inherited). However, it has been found in children born to mothers who had German measles (rubella) around the 6th or 7th week of pregnancy.

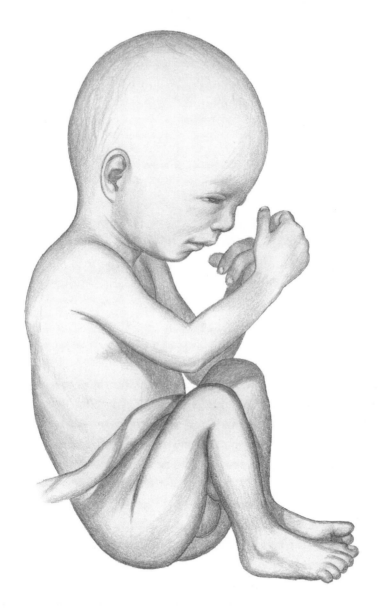

Around this time, your baby's eyelids open. Your baby begins opening and closing its eyes while still inside your uterus.

Microphthalmia. Another congenital eye problem is microphthalmia, in which the overall size of the eye is too small. The eyeball may be only two-thirds its normal size. This abnormality often occurs with other abnormalities of the eyes. It frequently results from maternal infections, such as cytomegalovirus (CMV) or toxoplasmosis, while the baby is developing inside the uterus.

Changes in You

✍ *Feeling Baby Move*

Feeling your baby move (quickening) is one of the more precious parts of pregnancy. This action can be the beginning of your bonding with your baby. Many women feel they begin to relate to the baby and its personality before delivery by feeling the baby's movements. This movement is usually reassuring and a sensation most pregnant women enjoy. Your partner can experience and enjoy the baby's movements by feeling your abdomen when the baby is active.

✍ **Your Baby's Movements.** Movement of your baby can vary in intensity. It can range from a faint flutter, sometimes described as a feeling of a butterfly or a gas bubble in early pregnancy, to brisk motions or even painful kicks and pressure as your baby gets larger.

Women often ask how often a baby should move. They want to know if they should be concerned if the baby moves too much or doesn't move enough. These are hard questions to answer because your sensation is different from that of another woman. The movement of each baby you carry may be different. It is usually more reassuring to have a baby move frequently. But it isn't unusual for a baby to have quiet times when there is not as much activity.

If you've been on the go, you may not have noticed the baby move because you've been active and busy. It may help to lie on your side to notice if the baby is moving or still. Many women report their baby is much more active at night, keeping them awake and making it hard to sleep.

If your baby is quiet and not as active as what seems normal or what you expected, discuss it with your doctor. You can always go to the doctor's surgery to hear the baby's heartbeat if the baby hasn't been moving in its usual pattern. In most instances, there is nothing to worry about.

Kick Count. Towards the end of pregnancy, you may be asked to record how often you feel the baby move. This test is done at home and is called a *kick count*. It provides reassurance about foetal well-being; this information is similar to that learned by a non-stress test. See the discussion in Week 41.

Your doctor/midwife may use one of two common methods. The first is to count how many times the baby moves in an hour. The other is to note how long it takes for baby to move 10 times. Usually you can choose when you want to do the test. After eating a meal is a good time because baby is often more active then. This test is usually done at home.

Pain Under Your Ribs When Baby Moves. Some women complain of pain under their ribs and in their lower abdomen when their baby moves. This type of pain isn't an unusual problem, but it may cause enough discomfort to concern you. The baby's movement has increased to a point where you will probably feel it every day, and movements are getting stronger and harder. At the same time, your uterus is getting larger and putting more pressure on all your organs. Your growing, expanding uterus presses on the small bowel, bladder and rectum.

If the pressure really is pain, don't ignore it. You need to discuss it with your doctor. In most cases, it isn't a serious problem.

↣ *Discovering a Breast Lump*

Discovering a breast lump is important, during pregnancy or any other time. It's important for you to learn at an early age how to do a breast exam on yourself and to perform this on a regular basis (usually after every menstrual period). Nine out of 10 breast lumps are found by women examining themselves.

Your doctor may perform breast exams at regular intervals, often when you have your Pap smear. If you have an exam every year and are lump-free, it helps assure you no lumps are present before you begin pregnancy.

Finding a breast lump may be delayed during pregnancy because of changes in your breasts. It may be more difficult to feel a lump. Enlargement of the breasts during pregnancy and nursing tends to hide lumps or masses in the tissue of the breast.

Examine your breasts during pregnancy as you do when you are not pregnant. Do it every 4 or 5 weeks—the first day of every month is a good time to do it.

Tests for Breast Lumps. The routine test for breast lumps is examination by yourself or your doctor. Other tests include X-ray examination, called a *mammogram*, and ultrasound examination of the breast.

If a lump is found, it may be necessary to have a mammogram or an ultrasound exam performed on the breast. Because a mammogram utilizes X-rays, your pregnancy must be protected during the procedure, usually by shielding your abdomen with a lead apron.

It has not been shown that pregnancy accelerates the course or growth of a breast lump. But we do know it is sometimes more difficult to find a breast lump because of breast changes during pregnancy.

Treatment during Pregnancy. Often a lump in the breast can be drained or aspirated. Fluid removed from the cyst is sent to the lab for evaluation to ensure there are no abnormal cells. If a lump or cyst cannot be drained by a needle, a biopsy of the cyst or lump may be necessary. If fluid is clear, it's a good sign. Bloody fluid is of more concern and must be studied under a microscope in the laboratory.

If examination of a lump indicates breast cancer, treatment may begin during pregnancy. Treatment complications during pregnancy include risks to the foetus related to chemotherapy, radiation or medication, such as anaesthesia or pain medicine for a biopsy. If a lump is cancerous, the need for radiation therapy and chemotherapy must be considered, along with the needs of the pregnancy.

How Your Actions Affect Your Baby's Development

∼ *Antenatal Classes*

When should you think about signing up for antenatal classes? Even though it's just the beginning of the third trimester, now's the time to register for these classes. It's a good idea to get signed up for classes so you can finish them before you get to the end of your pregnancy. By doing this, you'll have time to practise what you learn. You won't be just beginning your classes when you deliver!

Should You and Your Partner Take Antenatal Classes?   During pregnancy, you have probably been learning what's going to happen at delivery by talking with your doctor/midwife and by asking questions. You have also learned what lies ahead from reading materials given to you at antenatal visits, from our other books, such as *Your Pregnancy Questions and Answers, Your Pregnancy after 35, Your Pregnancy for the Father-to-Be* or *Your Pregnancy—Every Woman's Guide* or from other sources. Childbirth classes offer yet another way to learn about this important part of pregnancy. They help you prepare for labour and delivery.

By meeting in class on a regular basis, usually once a week for 4 to 6 weeks, you can learn about many things that concern you. Classes often cover a wide range of subjects, including the following areas.

- What are the different childbirth methods?
- What is 'natural childbirth'?
- What is a Caesarean delivery?
- What pain-relief methods are available?
- What you need to know (and practise) for the childbirth method you choose.
- Will you need an episiotomy?
- Will you need an enema?
- When is a foetal monitor necessary?
- What's going to happen when you reach the hospital?
- Is an epidural or some other type of anaesthesia right for you?

These are important questions. Discuss them with your doctor, if they are not answered in your childbirth-education classes.

Who Goes to Antenatal Classes? Classes are usually held for small groups of pregnant women and their partners or labour coaches. This is an excellent way to learn. You can interact with other couples and ask questions. You'll discover other women are concerned about many of the same things you are, such as labour and pain management. It's good to know you aren't the only one thinking about what lies ahead.

Antenatal classes are not only for first-time pregnant women. If you have a new partner, if it has been a few years since you've had a baby, if you have questions or if you would like a review of what lies ahead, an antenatal class can help you.

These classes may help reduce any worry or concern you and your partner feel about labour and delivery. And they'll help you enjoy the birth of your baby even more.

Where Do You Take Classes? Childbirth classes are offered in various settings. Most hospitals that deliver babies offer antenatal classes, often taught by a midwife. Other types of classes have different degrees of involvement.

This means the time commitment or depth of the subject covered is different for each of the various classes that may be available. Ask at the doctor's surgery about classes they recommend. They can help you decide which type of class would be best for you.

What Will You Learn? Classes are intended to inform you and your partner or labour coach about pregnancy, what happens at the hospital and what happens during labour and delivery. Some couples find classes are a good opportunity to get a partner more involved and to help make him feel more comfortable with the pregnancy. This may give him the opportunity to take a more active part at the time of labour and delivery, as well as during the rest of the pregnancy. See also the discussion in Week 31 of different childbirth methods.

Can You Take Antenatal Classes if You Have Problems? If you have problems getting to an antenatal class because of cost or time or because you're on bed rest, it may be possible to take classes at home. Some instructors will come to your home for private sessions with you and your partner.

~ Infant-Restraint Seats
It isn't too early to think about infant- and child-restraint systems. Some people believe they can hold their baby safely in an accident. Others say their child won't sit still in a restraint.

Dad Tip Offer to do chores that may be more difficult for your partner now. Cleaning the bathtub or the toilet can be a big help. You can add to her safety by putting away anything that belongs in a high or difficult-to-reach location.

Babies should always be in a suitable seat or carry cot restrained by straps. In an accident, an unrestrained child becomes a missile. The force of a crash can literally pull a child out of an adult's arms! One study in America showed *more than 30 deaths a year* occur to unrestrained infants going home from the hospital after birth. In nearly all cases, if the baby had been in an approved infant-restraint system, he or she would have survived the accident.

Start early to teach your child safety. If you always place your child in a restraint system in the car, it will become a natural thing to do. You can increase your child's acceptance of a restraint if you wear seat belts, too!

Your Nutrition

Some important vitamins you may need during pregnancy include vitamin A, vitamin B and vitamin E. Let's examine each vitamin and how it helps you during pregnancy.

Vitamin A—This vitamin is essential to human reproduction. Fortunately, deficiency in the United Kingdom is not common. What is of more concern today is the *excessive use* of the vitamin before conception and in early pregnancy. (This discussion concerns only the retinol forms of vitamin A, usually derived from fish oils. The beta-carotene form, of plant origin, is believed to be safe.)

The RDA (recommended dietary allowance) is 2700 IU (international units) for a woman of childbearing age. The maximum dosage is 5000 IU. Pregnancy does not change these requirements. You probably get vitamin A from the foods you eat, so supplementation during pregnancy is not recommended. Read food labels to check your vitamin-A intake.

Vitamin B—B vitamins important to you in pregnancy include B_6, B_9 (folic acid) and B_{12}. They influence the development of your baby's nerves and the formation of blood cells. If you don't take in enough B_{12} during pregnancy, you could develop anaemia. Good food sources of B vitamins include milk, eggs, bananas, potatoes, kale, avocados and brown rice.

Vitamin E—This is an important vitamin during pregnancy because it helps metabolize fats and helps build muscles and red-blood cells. You can usually get enough vitamin E if you eat meat. Vegetarians and pregnant women who can't eat meat may have a harder time getting enough vitamin E. Foods rich in the vitamin include olive oil, wheat germ, spinach and dried fruit. You may want to check with your doctor or read the label on your prenatal vitamin to see if it supplies 100 per cent of the RDA.

Be cautious with *every* substance you take during pregnancy. If you have questions, discuss them with your doctor/midwife.

You Should Also Know

∽ Systemic Lupus Erythematosus (SLE)

Some women have conditions before pregnancy that require them to take medication for the rest of their lives. They are often concerned about the effects medication may have on their developing babies. One such condition is *systemic lupus erythematosus* (SLE).

Many young women have lupus and take steroids to control the problem. They want to know if medication they take can harm their baby. Should they continue to take steroids during pregnancy?

Lupus is an autoimmune disorder of unknown cause that occurs most often in young or middle-aged women. (Women have lupus much more frequently than men—about nine women to every man.) Those who have lupus have a large number of antibodies in their bloodstream. These antibodies are directed towards the woman's own tissues, which causes problems.

The diagnosis of SLE is made through blood tests, which look for the suspect antibodies. Blood tests done for lupus are a lupus antibody test and an antinuclear antibody test.

Antibodies can be directed to various organs in the body and may actually damage an organ. Affected organs include joints, skin, kidneys, muscles, lungs, the brain and the central nervous system. The most common symptom of lupus is joint pain, which is often mistaken for arthritis. Other symptoms include lesions, rashes or sores on the skin, fever and hypertension.

We don't have a cure for lupus. Systemic lupus erythematosus is generally unaffected by pregnancy. However, miscarriage, premature delivery and complications around the time of delivery are slightly increased in a woman with lupus. If kidneys were involved and there was kidney damage during flareups, you must be on the lookout for kidney problems during pregnancy.

Steroids, short for corticosteroids, are generally prescribed to treat lupus. The primary medication used is prednisone. It is usually prescribed on a daily basis. It may be unnecessary to take prednisone every day, unless complications from lupus occur during pregnancy.

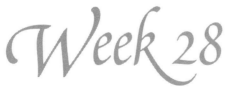

Week 28

Age of Foetus—26 Weeks

How Big Is Your Baby?

Your baby weighs nearly 1.1 kg (2½ lb). Crown-to-rump length is close to 25 cm (10 in). Total length is 35 cm (15¾ in).

How Big Are You?

Your uterus is now well above your umbilicus. Sometimes this growth seems gradual. At other times, it may seem as though changes happen rapidly, as if overnight.

Your uterus is about 8 cm (3¾ in) above your belly-button. If you measure from the pubic symphysis, it is about 28 cm (11 in) to the top of the uterus. Your weight gain by this time should be between 7.7 and 10.8 kg (17 and 24 lb).

Tip for Week 28 Even though delivery is several weeks away, it is not too early to begin making plans for the trip to the hospital. This includes knowing how to reach your partner (keep all of his phone numbers with you). Also consider what you will do if he isn't near enough to take you. Who are potential drivers? How do you get hold of them? Make plans now!

How Your Baby Is
Growing and Developing

Until this time, the surface of the baby's developing brain has appeared smooth. At around 28 weeks of pregnancy, the brain forms characteristic grooves and indentations on the surface. The amount of brain tissue also increases.

Your baby's eyebrows and eyelashes may be present. Hair on the baby's head is growing longer. The baby's body is becoming plumper and rounder. It's beginning to fill out a little because of increased fat underneath the skin. Before this time, the baby had a thin appearance.

Your baby now weighs almost 1.1 kg (2½ lb). This is an amazing growth compared to just 11 weeks ago, when it weighed only about 100 g (3½ oz) at 17 weeks of pregnancy. Your baby has increased its weight more than 10 times in 11 weeks! In the last 4 weeks, from the 24th week of your pregnancy to this week, its weight has doubled. Your baby is growing rapidly!

Changes in You

✌ *The Placenta*
The placenta plays a critical role in the growth, development and survival of the baby. The illustration on page 283 shows the foetus attached to the umbilical cord, which attaches to the placenta.

Two important cell layers, the amnion and the chorion, are involved in the development of the placenta and the amniotic sac. Development and function of the cell layers is complicated, and their description is beyond the scope of this book. However, the amnion is the layer around the amniotic fluid in which the foetus floats.

The placenta begins to form with trophoblastic cells. These cells grow through the walls of maternal blood vessels and establish contact with your bloodstream without your blood and foetal blood mixing. (Foetal circulation is separate from your circulation.) These cells grow

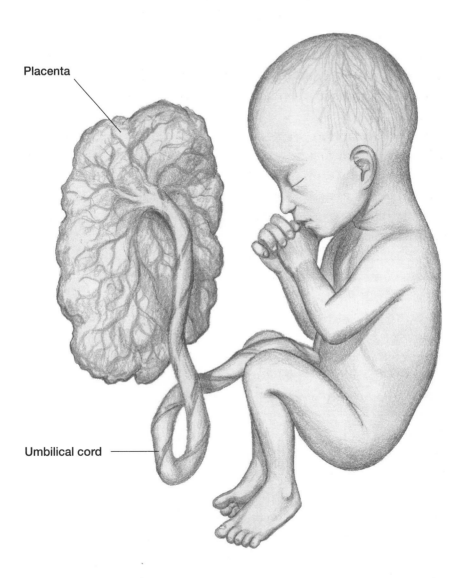

Placenta

Umbilical cord

The placenta, shown here with the foetus, carries oxygen and nutrients to the growing baby. It is an important part of pregnancy.

into the blood vessels without making a vascular connection (or opening) between the blood vessels. But foetal blood flow in the placenta is close to your blood flow in the placenta.

We have closely followed your baby's weight gain in this book. The placenta is also growing at a rapid rate. At 10 weeks gestation, the placenta weighed about 20 g (¾ oz). Ten weeks later, at 20 weeks gestation, it weighs almost 170 g (6 oz). In another 10 weeks, the placenta will have increased to 430 g (15 oz). At full term, 40 weeks, it can weigh almost 650 g (1½ lb)!

Foetal blood vessels and the developing placenta begin connecting as early as the 2nd or 3rd week of development. Around the 3rd week of gestation, projections (villi) at the base of the placenta become firmly attached to the underlying layer of the uterus.

Villi are important during pregnancy. The space around the villi (intervillus space) becomes honeycombed with maternal blood vessels. The villi absorb nutrients and oxygen from the maternal blood; these are transported to the growing baby through the umbilical vein in the umbilical cord. Waste products from the baby are brought through the umbilical arteries to the intervillus space and are transferred to the maternal bloodstream. In this way, the baby gets rid of waste products.

What Does the Placenta Do? The placenta is involved in moving oxygen and carbon dioxide to and from the baby. It is also involved in nutrition and the excretion of waste products from the baby.

In addition to these functions, the placenta has an important hormonal role. It produces human chorionic gonadotropin (HCG) (discussed in Week 5). This hormone is found in your bloodstream in measurable amounts within 10 days after fertilization. Pregnancy tests check HCG levels to determine if a woman is pregnant. The placenta also begins making the hormones oestrogen and progesterone by the 7th or 8th week of pregnancy.

What Does the Placenta Look Like? At full term, a normal placenta is flat, has a cake-like appearance and is round or oval. It is about 15 to

20 cm (6 to 8 in) in diameter and 2 to 3 cm (¾ and 1¼ in) thick at its thickest part. It weighs between 500 to 650 g (17½ and 24 oz) on average.

Placentas vary widely in size and shape. A placenta that is too large (placentamegaly) can be found when a woman is infected with syphilis or when a baby has erythroblastosis (Rh-sensitization of the baby). Sometimes it occurs without any obvious explanation. A small placenta may be found in normal pregnancies but may also be found with intrauterine-growth restriction.

The part of the placenta that attaches to the wall of the uterus has a beefy or spongy appearance. The foetal side of the placenta, the side closest to the baby inside the amniotic sac, is smooth. It is covered with amniotic and chorionic membranes.

The placenta is a red or reddish-brown colour. Around the time of birth, the placenta may have white patches on it, which are calcium deposits.

In multiple pregnancies, there may be more than one placenta, or there may be one placenta with more than one umbilical cord coming from it. Usually with twins, there are two amniotic sacs, with two umbilical cords running to the foetuses from one placenta.

The umbilical cord, which is the attachment from the placenta to the baby, contains two umbilical arteries and one umbilical vein, which carry blood to and from the baby. The cord is about 55 cm (22 in) long and is usually white.

A few women experience problems involving the placenta during pregnancy. These include placental abruption (see Week 33) and placenta previa (see Week 35). After delivery, a retained placenta is sometimes a problem (see Week 38).

How Your Actions Affect Your Baby's Development

✑ Dealing with Maternal Asthma

Asthma is a respiratory illness characterized by an increased responsiveness or sensitivity to stimulation of the trachea and the bronchi, both important to breathing. Problems with asthma are manifested by difficulty breathing, shortness of breath, coughing and wheezing. (Wheezing is a noise like a whistling or a hissing made as air moves through narrowed airways.)

Asthma comes and goes, with acute worsening of symptoms interspersed with symptom-free periods. It affects an estimated 8 million people in the UK. It is equally common in other countries.

Ðad Tip Your partner has been feeling the baby move for 2 or 3 months. Around this time, you may be able to feel it, too! Gently place your hand on her abdomen, and leave it there for a while. Your partner can tell you when the baby is moving.

It may occur at any age, but about 50 per cent of all asthma cases occur before age 10. Another 33 per cent of the cases occur by age 40. Pregnancy does not seem to cause any consistent, predictable problem with asthma. Some pregnant women appear to get better during pregnancy, while others remain about the same. A few get worse.

Asthma in Pregnancy. Uncontrolled asthma can be serious during pregnancy. It can contribute to high blood pressure in the mother and to premature birth, low-birthweight babies or smaller babies. Medications currently in use to treat asthma appear to be safe. Research has shown that inhalers have less of an effect on baby because less medication enters the mother's bloodstream.

ᴥ Treating Asthma Attacks

Most pregnant women with asthma can have a safe pregnancy, labour and delivery. If a woman has severe asthma attacks when she isn't pregnant, she may also have severe attacks during pregnancy.

During pregnancy, your oxygen consumption increases by about 25 per cent. That's why asthma treatment is so important during pregnancy—so baby can get the oxygen it needs to grow and to develop.

The treatment plan used before pregnancy will probably continue to be helpful. This includes medications prescribed for asthma before or during pregnancy.

Asthma medication, such as terbutaline, and steroids, such as hydrocortisone or methylprednisolone, can be used during pregnancy. Aminophylline or theophyline may also be used. Also safe to use while you're pregnant are orciprenaline (Alupent) and salbutamol (Ventolin).

If your asthma is severe, your doctor may prescribe an anti-inflammatory nasal spray or an inhaled steroid, such as beclometasone (Becotide). Discuss the situation at one of your early antenatal visits.

Your Nutrition

You may be wondering what kinds of foods to eat and what to delete from your diet during this stage of your pregnancy. Look at the chart below; it offers you some guidance.

What Kinds of Foods Do I Eat?

Foods to Eat	Servings per Day
Dark-green or dark-yellow fruits and vegetables	1
Fruits and vegetables with vitamin C (tomatoes, citrus)	2
Other fruits and vegetables	2
Whole-grain breads and cereals	4
Dairy products, including milk	4
Protein sources (meat, poultry, eggs, fish)	2
Dried beans and peas, seeds and nuts	2

Foods to Eat in Moderation		Foods to Avoid
Caffeine	200 mg	Anything containing alcohol
Fat	limited amounts	Food additives, when possible
Sugar	limited amounts	

You Should Also Know

৵ *Additional Testing and Procedures*

Twenty-eight weeks of gestation is a time when many doctors initiate or repeat certain blood tests or procedures. Glucose-tolerance testing for diabetes may also be done at this time.

If you are Rh-negative, you will probably receive an injection of Anti-D at this point in your pregnancy. This injection keeps you from becoming sensitized if your baby's blood mixes with yours. Anti-D protects against sensitization until the time of delivery.

Home Birth

In the recent past, there has been a growing interest in giving birth at home, in part because some women feel giving birth at home is 'more natural.' Indeed, there are many clear advantages to having your baby at home, such as the security of knowing you are in familiar surroundings with all the privacy you require. There is sufficient evidence that births in hospital are no more or less safe for women with uncomplicated pregnancies than those that take place at home. The Expert Maternity Group in 1993 concluded that the evidence for the relative safety of home compared with hospital did not justify a general recommendation for hospital delivery. Evidence suggests that given the opportunity, support, and informed choice, more women would consider home birth as an option (Changing Childbirth 1993). For more detailed information on home birth, see www.homebirth.org.uk or www.midirs.org.

Some women who start their labour at home may require transfer to hospital. This is by ambulance with your midwife accompanying you. Reasons for transfer include lack of progress in labour, foetal distress, exhausted mother, bleeding, or retained placenta. It is a good idea to have a bag packed with the essentials should a transfer be required. If you have any concerns regarding your place of birthing, discuss them with your doctor/midwife.

৵ *How Is the Baby Lying?*

It is common at this point in pregnancy to ask your doctor how the baby is lying. Is the baby head first? Is it bottom first (breech)? Is the baby lying sideways?

It's difficult—usually impossible—at this point in pregnancy to tell just by feeling your abdomen how the baby is lying and if it is coming bottom first, feet first or head first. The baby changes position throughout pregnancy.

It doesn't hurt to try to feel the abdomen to see where the head or other parts are located. In another 3 to 4 weeks, the baby's head will be harder; it will be easier at that time for your doctor/midwife to determine how the baby is lying (called *presentation of the foetus*).

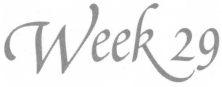

Week 29

Age of Foetus—27 Weeks

How Big Is Your Baby?

By this time, your baby weighs about 1.25 kg (2¾ lb). Crown-to-rump length is almost 26 cm (10½ in). Total foetal length is 37 cm (16¾ in).

How Big Are You?

Measuring from your bellybutton, your uterus is about 7.6 to 10.2 cm (3½ to 4 in) above it. Your uterus is about 29 cm (11½ in) above the pubic symphysis. If you saw your doctor 4 weeks ago, around the 25th week of pregnancy, you probably measured about 25 cm (10 in) at that time. You've grown about 4 cm (1½ in) in 4 weeks. Your total weight gain by this week should be between 8.55 and 11.25 kg (19 and 25 lb).

Tip for Week 29 **If your** doctor advises bed rest, follow his or her instructions. It may be difficult for you to stop your activities and sit idly by when you have lots of things to do, but remember, it's for the good health of you and your baby!

How Your Baby Is Growing and Developing

ᴥ *Foetal Growth*

Week by week, we've noted the change in your baby's size as pregnancy progresses. We use average weights to give you an idea of about how large your baby is at a particular time. However, these are only averages; babies vary greatly in size and weight.

Because growth is rapid during pregnancy, infants born prematurely may be tiny. Even a few weeks less time in the uterus can have a dramatic effect on the size of your baby. The baby continues to grow after 36 weeks of gestation but at a slower rate.

A couple of interesting factors about birthweight have been identified.

- Boys weigh more than girls.
- Birthweight of an infant increases with the increasing number of pregnancies you have or the number of babies you deliver.

Ðad Tip Are you also having pregnancy symptoms? Studies show that as many as 50 per cent of all fathers-to-be experience physical symptoms of pregnancy when their partner is pregnant. *Couvade,* a French term meaning 'to hatch,' is used to describe the condition in a man. Symptoms for an expectant father may include nausea, weight gain and cravings for certain foods.

These are general statements and don't apply to everyone, but they appear to apply in many cases. The average baby's birthweight at full term is 3.28 kg to 3.4 kg (7 to 7½ lb).

How Mature Is Your Baby? A baby born between the 37th and 42nd weeks of pregnancy is a *term baby* or *full-term infant.* Before the 37th week, the term *preterm* can be applied to the baby. After 42 weeks of pregnancy, your baby is overdue and the term *postdate* is used.

When a baby is born before the end of pregnancy, many people use the terms *premature* and *preterm* interchangeably. There is a difference. An infant that is 32 weeks gestational age but has mature pulmonary or lung function at the time of birth is more appropriately called a 'preterm infant' than a premature infant. 'Premature' best describes an infant that has immature lungs at the time of birth.

✣ Premature Babies

Premature birth increases the risk of problems in the baby. It also increases the risk of foetal death. Babies born prematurely usually weigh less than 2.5 kg (5½ lb).

The illustration on page 297 shows a premature baby with several leads attached to its body to monitor its heart rate. Many other attachments are used, such as IVs, tubes and masks that provide oxygen.

In 1976, the neonatal death rate was 9.7 per 1000 live births. In 2002, the rate was 3.6. More than twice the number of preterm infants survive today than 25 years ago.

The decreasing death rate applies primarily to infants delivered during the 3rd trimester (27 weeks or more of gestation) who weigh at least 1 kg (2¾ lb) and are without birth defects. When gestational age and birthweight are below these levels, the death rate increases.

Better methods of caring for premature babies have contributed to higher survival statistics. Today, infants born as early as 25 weeks of pregnancy may survive. However, the long-term survival and quality of life for these babies remains to be seen as they grow older.

What is the survival rate for premature babies? Recent information indicates for infants who weighed about 500 to 700 g (1 to 1½ lb), the survival rate is about 43 per cent. For babies weighing between 700 g to 1.25 kg (1½ and 2¾ lb), the survival rate is about 72 per cent. These rates vary from hospital to hospital.

The average hospital stay for premature babies ranges from 125 days for infants weighing between 600 and 700 g (1⅓ and 1½ lb) to 76 days for babies in the 900-g to 1.25-kg (2- to 2¾-lb) birthweight range.

Any discussion of survival rates must include the frequency rate of disabilities these premature babies suffer. In the lower-birthweight range, many babies who survived had disabilities. Higher-weight babies also had disabilities, but statistics for this group were much lower.

It's usually best for the baby to remain in the uterus as long as possible, so it can grow and develop fully. Occasionally it is best for the baby to be delivered early, such as when the foetus is not receiving adequate nutrition.

Causes of Premature Labour and Premature Birth. In most cases, the causes of premature labour and premature birth are unknown. Causes we do understand include a uterus with an abnormal shape, multiple foetuses, polyhydramnios or hydramnios, placental abruption or placenta previa, premature rupture of membranes, an incompetent cervix, abnormalities of the foetus, foetal death, a retained IUD, serious maternal illness or incorrect estimate of gestational age.

Finding the cause of premature labour and delivery may be difficult. An attempt is always made to determine what causes preterm labour before active labour begins. In this way, treatment may be more effective.

Tests Your Doctor May Do. One test, called *SalEst,* can help determine if a woman might go into labour too early. The test measures levels of the hormone oestriol in a pregnant woman's saliva. Research has shown that there is often a surge in this chemical several weeks before early labour. A positive result means a woman has a 7 times greater chance of delivering her baby before the 37th week of pregnancy. Another test is foetal fibronectin (fFN); see Week 22. This test is not available in all maternity care units in the U.K.

Some difficult questions that must be answered when premature labour begins include those below.

• Is it better for the infant to be inside the uterus or to be delivered?
• Are the dates of the pregnancy correct?
• Is this really labour?

Changes in You

༺ Treatment of Premature Labour

Can anything be done about premature labour? Yes. We now treat premature labour in several different ways.

The treatment most often used for premature labour is bed rest. A woman is advised to stay in bed and lie on her side. (Either side is OK.) Not everyone agrees on this treatment, but bed rest is often successful in stopping contractions and premature labour. If this happens to you and you are advised to rest in bed, it may mean you can't go to work or to continue many activities. It's worth it to agree to bed rest if you can avoid premature delivery of your baby.

If you are confined to bed during your pregnancy, take it easy getting back into the swing of things after baby is born. Lying down for quite a while may result in loss of muscle tone, which can lead to you being out of shape. It can take some time to return to your normal level of activity. Take it easy, and don't rush into any physical activities until you feel up to them. Ease into your post-bed rest life slowly!

Medications to Help Stop Premature Labour. Beta-adrenergic agents, also called *tocolytic agents,* such as ritodrine (Yutopart), may be used to suppress labour. Beta-adrenergics are muscle relaxants. They relax the uterus and decrease contractions. (The uterus is mainly muscle, which pushes the baby out through the cervix during labour.)

The muscle relaxant is given in three different forms—intravenously, as an intramuscular injection and as a pill. It is usually initially given intravenously and may require a hospital stay of a couple of days or more. Maternal side effects include rapid heartbeat, hypotension, the feeling of apprehension or fear, chest tightness or chest pain, changes in the heart's electrical activity, fluid in the lungs, maternal metabolic problems, including increased blood sugar, low blood potassium and even acidosis of the blood (similar

Bed-Rest Boredom Relievers

You may be advised to rest in bed if you experience any number of pregnancy complications. Lying in bed takes the pressure of the baby's weight off your cervix, which can help if you experience premature labour. Resting on your side maximizes the blood flow to your uterus, which brings more oxygen and nutrients to baby.

Bed rest can mean anything from staying in bed part of the day to staying in bed 24/7. It can be pretty boring being confined to bed. Below are some suggestions to help beat bed-rest boredom.

- Spend the day in a room other than your bedroom. Use the living-room or family-room sofa for daytime activities.
- Use foam mattress pads and extra pillows for comfort.
- Keep a telephone close at hand.
- Keep reading material, the television remote control, a radio and other essentials nearby.
- Establish a daily routine. When you get up, change into daytime clothes. Shower or bathe every day. Comb your hair, and put on lipstick. Nap if you need it. Go to bed when you normally do.
- Keep food and drinks close at hand. Use a cooler to keep food and drinks cold. Use an insulated container for hot soup or coffee.
- Start a diary. Our book, *Your Pregnancy Journal Week by Week*, is easy to use and lets you record your thoughts and feelings to share with your partner now and your child later.
- Do some crafts that aren't messy, such as cross stitch, knitting, crocheting, drawing or hand sewing. Make something for baby!
- Use the time to read and to prepare for baby's arrival.
- Spend some time planning baby's room (someone else will have to carry through on it), deciding what you'll need for a layette and making a list of all the necessary items you'll need after baby comes home.
- Sort! Use the time to sort through recipes, to put pictures in albums or make a scrapbook of information for after baby's arrival.
- Call your favourite local charity or political organization, and volunteer to make phone calls, stuff envelopes or write letters.
- For support, contact other women who have been on bed rest. Your doctor or midwife may be able to put you in touch with other women who have had the same experience. If not, start your own support group!

to a diabetic reaction), headaches, vomiting, shaking, fever and/or hallucinations.

When premature contractions stop, you can be switched to oral medications, which you take every 2 to 4 hours. Ritodrine is used in pregnancies over 20 weeks and under 36 weeks gestation. In some cases, the medication is used without giving an IV first. This is done most often in women with a history of premature labour or for a woman with multiple pregnancies.

Similar problems as those described above probably occur in the baby. Low blood-sugar levels have been seen in babies after birth in some mothers who took ritodrine before delivery. Rapid heartbeat is also commonly seen in these babies.

Terbutaline may also be used as a muscle relaxant to halt premature labour. Its safety in early pregnancy is not established, although it is used in late pregnancy. Side effects of terbutaline are similar to those of ritodrine.

> A study was recently conducted to investigate ways to help stop premature labour. Researchers found that use of a hormone in some women may reduce their risk of giving birth to a premature baby. The hormone is called *progesterone (17 alpha-hydroxyprogesterone caproate)*.
>
> In the study, women who had had problems with premature labour in previous pregnancies were given a weekly injection of progesterone. This course of treatment substantially reduced the rate of premature deliveries. More studies are needed, but there is hope that this treatment will lead to a decrease in premature birth, which can be a very serious problem.

Magnesium sulfate is used to treat pre-eclampsia (see Week 31 for information on pre-eclampsia). We have known for quite a while that magnesium sulfate may also help stop labour. This medication is most often given through an IV and requires hospitalization. However, it is occasionally given as an oral preparation, without hospitalization. You must be monitored frequently if you take magnesium sulphate.

Sedatives or narcotics may also be used in early attempts to stop labour. This may consist of an injection of morphine or meperidine. This is not a long-term solution but may be effective in initially stopping labour.

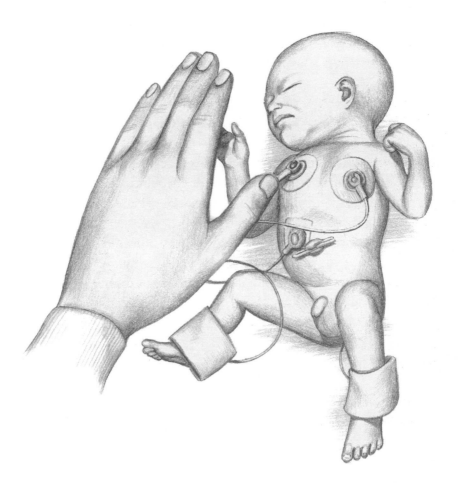

Premature baby (born at 29 weeks of pregnancy) shown with foetal monitors attached to it. Note size of adult hand in comparison.

Benefits of Stopping Premature Labour. Benefits of stopping premature labour include reducing the risks of foetal problems and problems related to premature delivery. If you experience premature labour, you may need to see your doctor frequently. Your doctor will probably monitor your pregnancy with ultrasound or non-stress tests. (See the discussion of the non-stress test in Week 41.)

How Your Actions
Affect Your Baby's Development

Most of our discussion this week has been devoted to the premature infant and treatment of premature labour. If you are diagnosed as having premature labour and your doctor prescribes bed rest and medications to stop it, follow his or her advice!

If you're concerned about your doctor's or midwife's instructions, discuss them. If you're told not to work or advised to reduce your activities and you ignore the advice, you're taking chances with your well-being and your unborn baby's. It isn't worth taking risks.

Your Nutrition

We hope you have been listening to your body during your pregnancy. You rest when you're tired. You go to the bathroom when you first feel the urge. You pay attention to any new discomforts. You may also listen to your body when it comes to food and drink. When you feel hungry or thirsty, you eat or drink something. Eating smaller, more frequent meals provides a constant supply of nutrients to your growing baby.

Keep nourishing snacks near at hand. Raisins, dried fruit and nuts are good choices when you're on the go. Know what time of day or night hunger strikes you the hardest. Be prepared.

Be different, if you want to be. Eat spaghetti for breakfast and cereal for lunch, if that's what appeals to you. Don't force yourself to eat something that turns you off or makes you sick. There's always an alternative. As long as you eat nourishing food and pay attention to the types of foods you eat, you are helping yourself and your growing baby.

You Should Also Know

ஃ *Group-B Streptococcus Infection*
Group-B streptococcus *(GBS)* infection rarely causes problems in adults but can cause life-threatening infections in newborns. GBS is often transmitted from person to person by sexual contact.

In women, GBS is most often found in the vagina or rectum. It is possible to have GBS in your system and not be sick or have any symptoms.

One recommendation aimed at preventing this infection in newborns is that all women who have risk factors be treated for GBS. Risk factors include the following:

- a previous infant with GBS infection
- preterm labour
- ruptured membranes for more than 18 hours
- a temperature of 38°C (100.4°F) immediately before or during childbirth

The second recommendation is that a GBS culture be taken from the rectal and vaginal areas of all pregnant women at 35 to 37 weeks gestation. Antibiotics, such as penicillin or ampicillin, are given during labour to women with a positive culture.

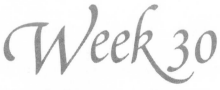

Week 30

Age of Foetus—28 Weeks

How Big Is Your Baby?

At this point in your pregnancy, your baby weighs about 1.35 kg (3 lb). Its crown-to-rump length is a little over 27 cm (10¾ in), and total length is 38 cm (17 in).

How Big Are You?

Measuring from your bellybutton, your uterus is about 10 cm (4 in) above it. From the pubic symphysis, the top of your uterus measures about 30 cm (12 in).

It may be hard to believe you still have 10 weeks to go! You may feel like you're running out of room as your uterus grows up under your ribs. However, your foetus, placenta and uterus, along with the amniotic fluid, will continue to get larger.

The average total healthy weight gain during pregnancy is 11.4 to 15.9 kg (25 to 35 lb). About half of this weight is concentrated in the growth of the uterus, the baby and the placenta, and in the volume of amniotic fluid. This growth is mostly in the front of your abdomen and in your pelvis, where it is noticeable to you. You may experience increasing discomfort in your pelvis and abdomen as pregnancy progresses. At this point, you should be gaining about 450 g (1 lb) a week.

How Your Baby Is Growing and Developing

✑ *Umbilical-Cord Knots*

The illustration this week, page 302, shows a foetus and its umbilical cord. Can you see the knot in the cord? You may wonder how a knot like this can occur. We do not believe the cord grows in a knot.

A baby is usually quite active during pregnancy. We believe these knots occur as the baby moves around in early pregnancy. A loop forms in the umbilical cord; the baby moves through the loop, and a knot results. Your actions do not cause or prevent this kind of complication, which can be serious. A knot in the umbilical cord does not occur often.

Dad Tip Now is the time to think about changing your work schedule so you can be around home more during the last part of the pregnancy and after baby is born. Nearly all parents wish they were able to spend more time at home. If you travel a great deal, you may need to alter your schedule so you can be home towards the end of the pregnancy. Babies come on their own schedule. If you want to be present for the delivery, plan ahead!

Changes in You

✑ *Rupture of Membranes*

The membranes around the baby that contain the amniotic fluid are called the *bag of waters*. They usually do not break until just before labour begins, when labour begins or during labour. But that isn't always the case; sometimes they break earlier in pregnancy.

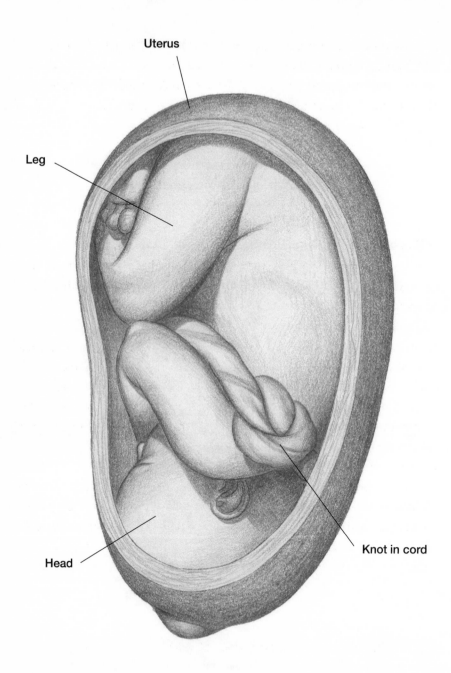

Uterus

Leg

Knot in cord

Head

This foetus has a knot in its umbilical cord.

After your waters break, you need to take certain precautions. The membranes of pregnancy help protect your baby from infection. When your waters break and you leak fluid, your risk of infection increases. An infection could be harmful to your baby. Call your doctor immediately when your waters break.

How Your Actions Affect Your Baby's Development

✑ *Bathing during Pregnancy*

Many women wonder if bathing in the latter part of pregnancy will in some way harm their baby. Most doctors believe it's safe to bathe throughout pregnancy. They may caution you to be careful as you get in or out of the bathtub. And be sure bath water is not too hot. Most will not tell you to avoid bathing while you're pregnant. However, if you think your waters have broken, avoid having a bath.

Tip for Week 30 Good posture can help relieve lower-back stress and eliminate some backache discomfort. Maintaining good posture may take some effort, but it's worth it if it relieves your pain.

Women also want to know how they'll know if their waters break while they are in the bath or shower. When your waters break, you'll usually notice a gush of water followed by slow leakage. If your waters break while you're bathing, you may not notice the initial gush of fluid. However, you'll probably notice the leakage of fluid, which can last for quite a while.

Your Nutrition

Some women ask if herbal teas are safe to drink during pregnancy. They have heard that some herbal teas can be beneficial to a pregnant

Benefits of Drinking Some Herbal Teas

camomile	aids digestion
dandelion	helps with swelling and can soothe an upset stomach
ginger root	helps with nausea and nasal congestion
nettle leaf	rich in iron, calcium and other vitamins and minerals
peppermint	relieves gas pains and calms the stomach
red raspberry	helps with nausea and stabilizes hormones

woman. Many herbal teas are safe to use; some are not. Herbal teas you can use safely include camomile, dandelion, ginger root, nettle leaf, peppermint and red raspberry.

You should *not* use some herbal teas while you're pregnant. Studies indicate herbal teas to avoid include blue cohosh, black cohosh, penny-royal leaf, yarrow, goldenseal, fever-few, psyllium seed, mugwort, comfrey, coltsfoot, juniper, rue, tansy, cottonroot bark, large amounts of sage, senna, cascara sagrada, buckthorn, fern, slippery elm and squaw vine.

You Should Also Know

✑ Child-Care Decisions

You may think this is an odd place to put a discussion of child care for a baby that won't even be born for another 10 weeks, but it's important to start thinking about this now if you plan to return to work. Quality care is in high demand and short supply! Experts advise you to begin looking for a child-care situation *at least 6 months* before you need it. For some women, that may be the end of the second trimester!

If you find a situation you like, sign up as soon as possible; there may be a waiting list. If you find something more suitable later, you can always change your mind.

Deciding what type of child care is best for your baby can be a challenging task. You and your partner must make many decisions in selecting the type of care you want for baby. The best way to do that is to know your options before you begin.

Before you can determine which care situation is the best for your family, you must examine your needs and the needs of your child. Your options for child care include:

- in-your-home care by a family member or by a non-relative
- care in a caregiver's home
- a child-care centre

In-home Care. You may choose in-home care, either by a relative or non-relative. It's fairly easy when someone comes to your home to take care of your child. You don't have to get baby ready before you go in the morning, and you never have to take your child out in bad weather. It also takes less time in the morning and evening if you don't have to drop off or to pick up baby.

When the caregiver is a non-relative, it can be very expensive to have someone come to your home. You are also hiring someone you do not know to come into your home and tend your child. You must be diligent in asking for references and checking them out thoroughly as there is no formal registration of nannies and no plans by the government to introduce such a scheme.

Care in a Caregiver's Home. You may decide to take your child to someone else's home. A home-like setting may make a child feel more comfortable. The Children Act 1989 provides for local authorities to operate a registration and inspection service for childminders—as well as day nurseries, playgroups, private nursery schools and crèches—and all registered providers are expected to meet national standards. However, this does not absolve you from the responsibility of checking each situation very carefully.

Child-Care Centres. A child-care centre is an environment in which many children are cared for in a larger setting. Centres vary widely in the facilities and activities they provide, the amount of attention they give each child, group sizes and child-care philosophy.

Some child-care centres do not accept infants. Babies have special needs; be sure the place you choose for your infant can meet those needs.

The Cost of Child Care. It can cost you a lot to provide child care for your baby. We're not talking about a situation that is out of the ordinary—we're talking about a regular care situation in your home, someone else's home or in a day-care centre.

Whether a person comes to your home or you take baby to theirs, you will probably have to pay your care provider's income tax and national insurance. Contact the Inland Revenue for further information. If the person works in your home, be sure you have homeowner's or renter's insurance to cover them while they are at your home.

Be prepared in advance; child-care costs can be pretty high in many areas of the country.

♻ *Cancer and Pregnancy*
Pregnancy is a happy time for most women, filled with anticipation and excitement. Occasionally, however, serious problems can occur. Cancer in pregnancy is one serious complication that occurs rarely.

This discussion is included not to scare you but to provide you with information. It is not a pleasant subject to discuss, especially at this time. However, every woman should have this information available. Its inclusion in this book is twofold:

• to increase your awareness of a serious problem
• to provide you with a resource to help you formulate questions for a dialogue with your doctor if you wish to discuss it

Cancer before Pregnancy. If you are now pregnant and you have had cancer in the past, tell your doctor as soon as you discover you are pregnant. He or she may need to make decisions about individualized care for you during pregnancy.

Cancer in Pregnancy. The occurrence of cancer at any time is stressful. When cancer occurs during pregnancy, it is even more stressful. The doctor must consider how to treat the cancer, but he or she is also concerned about the developing baby.

The way in which these issues are handled depends on when cancer is discovered. A woman's concerns may include the following.

- Will the pregnancy have to be terminated so the cancer can be treated?
- Will treatment or medications used harm the baby?
- Will the malignancy affect the baby or be passed to the baby?
- Should therapy be delayed until after delivery or after termination of the pregnancy?

Fortunately, many cancers in women occur after the reproductive years, which lowers the likelihood of cancer during pregnancy. Cancer during pregnancy is a rare occurrence and must be treated on an individual basis.

Some cancers found during pregnancy include breast tumours, leukaemia and lymphomas, melanomas, gynaecologic cancers (cancer of the female organs, such as the cervix, uterus and ovaries) and bone tumours.

Tremendous changes affect your body during pregnancy. Researchers suggest ways these changes can affect the possible discovery of cancer during pregnancy.

- Some believe cancers influenced by the increased hormone levels during pregnancy may increase in frequency during pregnancy.
- Increased blood flow, with accompanying changes in the lymphatic system, may contribute to the transfer of cancer to other parts of the body.
- Anatomical and physiological changes of pregnancy (growth of the abdomen and changes in the breasts) can make it difficult to find or to diagnose an early cancer.

These three beliefs about cancer during pregnancy appear to have some validity but vary widely depending on the cancer and the organ involved.

Breast Cancer. Breast cancer is rare in women younger than 35. Fortunately, it is an uncommon complication of pregnancy.

During pregnancy, it may be harder to find breast cancer because of changes in the breasts, such as tenderness, increased size and even lumpiness. Of all women who have breast cancer, about 2 per cent are pregnant at the time of diagnosis. Most evidence indicates pregnancy does not increase the rate of growth or spread of a breast cancer.

Treatment of breast cancer during pregnancy varies and must be individualized. It may require surgery, chemotherapy or radiation; a combination of all these treatments may be used.

A form of breast cancer you should be aware of is *inflammatory breast cancer (IBC)*. Although it is very rare, it can occur during and after pregnancy and may be mistaken for mastitis, which is inflammation of the breast. Symptoms of inflammatory breast cancer include swelling or pain in the breast, redness, nipple discharge or swollen lymph nodes above the collarbone or under the arm. You may feel a lump, although one is not always present.

If you experience any of these symptoms, *do not panic!* Nearly all of the time it will be a breast infection related to breastfeeding. However, if you are concerned, contact your doctor. A biopsy is used to diagnose the disease. To learn more about IBC, visit www.ibcsupport.org.

Cervical Cancers and Pelvic Cancers. Cervical cancer is believed to occur about once in every 10,000 pregnancies. However, about 1 per cent of the women who have cancer of the cervix are pregnant when it is diagnosed. Cancer of the cervix is curable, particularly if it is found and treated in its early stages.

Malignancies of the vulva, the tissue surrounding the opening to the vagina, have also been reported during pregnancy. It is a rare complication; only a few cases have occurred.

Other Cancers in Pregnancy. *Hodgkin's disease* (a form of cancer) commonly affects young people. It is now being controlled for long periods with radiation and chemotherapy. The disease occurs in about 1 of every 6000 pregnancies. Pregnancy does not appear to have a negative effect on the course of Hodgkin's disease.

Pregnant women who have *leukaemia* have demonstrated an increased chance of premature labour. They may also experience an increase in bleeding after pregnancy. Leukaemia is usually treated with chemotherapy or radiation therapy.

Melanoma may occur during pregnancy. A melanoma is a cancer derived from skin cells that produce *melanin* (pigment). A malignant melanoma can spread through the body. Pregnancy may cause symptoms or problems to worsen. A melanoma can spread to the placenta and to the baby.

Bone tumours are rare during pregnancy. However, two types of benign (non-cancerous) bone tumours can affect pregnancy and delivery. These tumours, *endochondromas* and *benign exostosis*, can involve the pelvis; tumours may interfere with labour. The possibility of having a Caesarean delivery is more likely with these tumours.

Week 31

Age of Foetus—29 Weeks

How Big Is Your Baby?

Your baby continues to grow. It weighs about 1.6 kg (3½ lb), and crown-to-rump length is 28 cm (11¾ in). Its total length is nearly 40 cm (18 in).

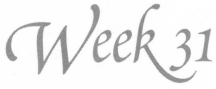

Dad Tip Now's the time to begin discussing baby equipment, such as cots, car seats and layette items, with your partner. You'll need to make some of these purchases before baby's birth. Most hospitals or birthing centres won't let you take baby home without a car seat.

How Big Are You?

Measuring from the pubic symphysis, it is now a little more than 31 cm (12 in) to the top of the uterus. From your bellybutton, it is almost 11 cm (4½ in).

At 12 weeks gestation, the uterus was just filling your pelvis. As you can see in the illustration on page 313, by this week the uterus fills a large part of your abdomen.

Your total pregnancy weight gain by this time should be between 9.45 and 12.15 kg (21 and 27 lb).

How Your Baby Is
Growing and Developing

✤ *Intrauterine-Growth Restriction (IUGR)*

Intrauterine-growth restriction (IUGR) indicates a newborn infant is small for its gestational age. By definition, its birthweight is below the 10th percentile (in the lowest 10 per cent) for the baby's gestational age. This means 9 out of 10 babies of normal growth are larger.

When gestational age is appropriate—meaning dates are correct and the pregnancy is as far along as expected—and weight falls below the 10th percentile, there is reason for concern. Growth-restricted infants have a higher rate of death and injury than infants in the normal-weight range.

Diagnosing and Treating IUGR. Diagnosing IUGR can be difficult. One reason your doctor measures you at each visit is to see how your uterus and baby are growing. A problem is usually found by measuring the uterus over a period of time and finding no change. If you measured 27 cm (10¾ in) at 27 weeks gestation and at 31 weeks you measure only 28 cm (11 in), your doctor might become concerned about IUGR and tests may be ordered.

Diagnosis of this type of problem is one important reason to keep all your antenatal appointments. You may not like being weighed at every appointment, but it helps your doctor see that your pregnancy is growing and the baby is getting bigger.

Intrauterine-growth restriction can be diagnosed or confirmed by ultrasound. Ultrasound may also be used to assure that the baby is healthy and no malformations exist that must be taken care of at birth.

When IUGR is diagnosed, avoid doing anything that could make it worse. Stop smoking. Improve your nutrition. Stop using drugs and alcohol.

Bed rest is another treatment. Resting on your side enables the baby to receive the best blood flow, and better blood flow is the best chance it has to improve growth. If maternal disease causes IUGR, treatment involves improving the mother's general health.

An infant with intrauterine-growth restriction is at risk of dying before delivery. Avoiding this may involve delivering the baby before it is full term. Infants with IUGR may not tolerate labour well; a C-section is more likely because of foetal distress. The baby may be safer outside the uterus than inside of it, in some cases.

Causes of IUGR. What causes intrauterine-growth restriction? Below are some conditions that increase the chance of intrauterine-growth restriction or a small foetus.

Smoking and other tobacco use can inhibit a baby's growth. The more cigarettes smoked, the greater the impairment and the smaller the baby.

A woman of average size or smaller who doesn't gain enough weight may have a growth-restricted baby. This is one of the reasons that good nutrition and a healthy diet are so important during pregnancy. Do not attempt to restrict normal weight gain during pregnancy. Research indicates that when calories are restricted to under 1500 a day for an extended time, IUGR may result.

Pre-eclampsia and high blood pressure (hypertension) can have a marked effect on foetal growth. Cytomegalovirus, rubella and other infections may also restrict foetal growth.

Maternal anaemia may be a cause of intrauterine-growth restriction. (Anaemia is discussed in Week 22.) Abnormalities may cause inhibited growth because the baby receives less nutrition during pregnancy. A woman who has delivered a growth-restricted infant may be more likely to do so again in subsequent pregnancies.

Women who live at high altitudes are more likely to have babies who weigh less than those born to women who live at lower altitudes. Alcoholism and drug use, kidney disease and carrying more than one baby may also be causes of a smaller-than-normal baby.

Other reasons for a small baby, unrelated to IUGR, include the fact that a woman who is small might have a small baby. In addition, prolonged pregnancy can lead to an undernourished, smaller baby. A malformed or abnormal foetus may also be smaller, especially when chromosomal abnormalities are present.

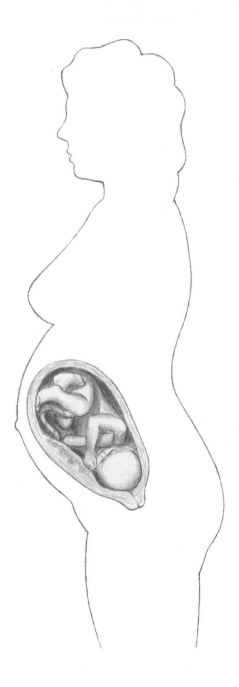

Comparative size of the uterus at 31 weeks of pregnancy (foetal age—
29 weeks). The uterus can be felt about 11 cm (4½ in) above the bellybutton.

Changes in You

↭ *Swelling in Your Legs and Feet during Pregnancy*

You may notice, especially as you near the end of pregnancy, that if you take your shoes off and leave them off for a while, you may not be able to put them back on. This problem is related to swelling.

You may also notice that wearing nylon stockings that are tight at the knee (or tight socks) leaves an indentation in your legs. It may look like you still have clothing on. Avoid tight, restrictive clothing if you experience swelling.

Your body produces as much as 50 per cent more blood and body fluids during pregnancy to meet baby's needs. Some of this extra fluid leaks into your body tissues. When your enlarging uterus pushes on pelvic veins, blood flow in the lower part of your body is partially blocked. This pushes fluid into your legs and feet, causing swelling.

The way you sit can also affect circulation of these body fluids. Crossing your legs, either at the knee or at the ankle, restricts blood flow to your legs. To improve circulation, don't cross your legs.

Carpal Tunnel Syndrome During Pregnancy

Carpal tunnel syndrome is characterized by pain in the hand and wrist, which can extend into the forearm and shoulder. The cause of the pain is compression of the median nerve in the wrist. Symptoms can be numbness, tingling or burning of the inner half of one or both hands. At the same time, the fingers feel numb and useless. More than half of the time, both hands are involved.

The problem may occur during pregnancy, due to water retention and swelling in the wrist and arm area. Up to 25 per cent of all women experience mild symptoms during pregnancy, but no treatment is necessary. The full syndrome, in which treatment may be needed, is less frequent; it occurs in only 1 to 2 per cent of all pregnant women.

Treatment depends on symptoms. Carpal tunnel syndrome may be treated with surgery; however, this is rarely performed during pregnancy. In pregnant women, splints are often used during sleep and rest, in an attempt to keep the wrist straight. Most often, symptoms disappear after delivery.

Occurrence of carpal tunnel syndrome during pregnancy does *not* mean you will suffer from this problem after baby's birth. In rare instances, symptoms may recur long after pregnancy. In these cases, surgery may be necessary.

How Your Actions
Affect Your Baby's Development

✂ *Sleeping Positions*
We've already described the importance of resting on a regular basis and lying on your side when you sleep. (See Week 15.) Now is when it will pay off. You may notice you begin to retain water if you don't lie on your side when sleeping or resting. Lying on your side could help you feel better quickly.

✂ *Visiting Your Doctor/Midwife*
It's important to keep all antenatal appointments with your doctor/ midwife. It may seem to you that not much happens at these visits, especially when everything is normal and going well. But the information your doctor/midwife collects tells him or her a lot about your condition and your baby's.

Your doctor/midwife is watching for signs that indicate you might have a problem, such as changes in your blood pressure, changes in your weight or the inadequate growth of the baby. If these problems are not discovered early, they may have serious consequences for you and your baby.

✂ *Childbirth Methods*
It's time to start thinking about how you want to deliver your baby. You may think it's too early to do this, but now is the time to start thinking about it. Why? Because many of the methods that are commonly practised need a lot of time to prepare you and your partner to use them.

If you decide you want a particular method or class, such as those offered by the National Childbirth Trust (NCT), you will probably have to sign up fairly early to get a place. In addition, you will want the time to practise what you learn so you will be able to use it during labour and delivery.

What Is Natural Childbirth? Some women decide before the birth of their baby that they are going to labour and deliver with *natural* *childbirth.* What does this mean? The description or definition of natural childbirth varies from one couple to another.

Many people equate natural childbirth with a drug-free labour and delivery. Others equate natural childbirth with the use of mild pain medications or local pain medications, such as numbing medications in the area of the vagina for delivery or for an episiotomy and repair of episiotomy. Most agree that natural childbirth is birth with as few artificial procedures as possible. A woman who chooses natural childbirth usually needs some advance instruction to prepare for it.

Childbirth Philosophers. A number of people have influenced the way women approach childbirth today. Most seek to enable the woman to follow the lead in her body, in a loving and intimate environment. The following are some of the most well known in this country.

- *Grantley Dick-Read* pioneered a method that attempted to break the fear-tension-pain cycle of labour and delivery. His classes were the first to include fathers in the birth experience, and his teachings were so basic that they are now taken for granted by all centres.
- *Lamaze* conditions mothers, through training, to replace unproductive labouring efforts with fruitful ones and emphasizes relaxation and breathing as ways to relax during labour and delivery. It forms the basis of the teaching of the National Childbirth Trust in Britain.
- *Frederick Leboyer* was influenced by the psychiatrists Reich, Rank and Janov, who shared the belief that later problems in life stem from birth's trauma. His concern was therefore primarily for the baby rather than the mother. In order to minimize the trauma of birth, he suggested that the birthing room have soft lighting and that noise and movement be kept to a minimum. Leboyer also believed that the baby should be placed on the mother's stomach as soon as possi-

ble, as immediate skin-to-skin contact was essential to calm the baby.

- *Sheila Kitzinger* believes that birth is a very personal experience, and that the labouring mother should be an active 'birth-giver' rather than a passive patient. The challenge, she believes, facing the maternity services today is to enable parents to have a real choice in how their babies are born. Birth, according to Kitzinger, is not an illness, and a labouring mother and her partner should not be treated as patients, but as intelligent adults whose right it is to have the final say in the decisions surrounding the birth of their baby.

Should You Consider Natural Childbirth? Natural childbirth isn't for every woman. If you arrive at the hospital dilated 1 cm, with strong contractions and in pain, natural childbirth may be hard for you. In this situation, an epidural might be appropriate.

On the other hand, if you arrive at the hospital dilated 4 or 5 cm and contractions are OK, natural childbirth might be a reasonable choice. It's impossible to know what will happen ahead of time, but it helps to be aware of, and ready for, everything.

It's important to keep an open mind during the unpredictable process of labour and delivery. Don't feel guilty or disappointed if you can't do all the things you planned before labour. You may need an epidural. Or the birth may not be accomplished without an episiotomy. Don't let anyone make you feel guilty or make you feel as though you've accomplished less if you end up needing a C-section, an epidural or an episiotomy.

Beware of instructors in childbirth-education classes who tell you labour is free of pain, no one really needs a C-section, IVs are unnecessary or an episiotomy is foolish. This can create unrealistic expectations for you. If you do need any of the above procedures, you may feel as though you failed during your labour.

The goal in labour and delivery is a healthy baby and a healthy mum. If this means you end up with a C-section, you haven't failed. Be grateful a Caesarean delivery can be performed safely. Babies that would not have survived birth in the past can now be delivered safely. This is a wonderful accomplishment!

Your Nutrition

Pregnancy precautions can often be applied to everyday life, such as avoiding *salmonella* poisoning. Salmonella bacteria can cause a range of problems, from mild gastric discomfort to severe, sometimes fatal, food poisoning. Any of these could be serious for you.

Salmonella bacteria has many sources—there are over 1400 different strains! They are found in raw eggs and raw poultry. The bacteria is destroyed when a food is cooked, but it's wise to take additional precautions. Keep in mind the following measures to ensure your safety.

- When preparing poultry or products made with raw eggs, clean your counters, utensils, dishes and pans with hot water and soap or a disinfecting agent when you are finished.
- Cook poultry thoroughly.
- Don't eat products made with raw eggs, such as Caesar salad, hollandaise sauce, homemade or restaurant mayonnaise, homemade ice cream, mousse and so on. Don't taste cake batter, biscuit dough or anything else that contains raw eggs before it is cooked.
- When you eat eggs, be sure they are cooked thoroughly. Boil eggs for at least 7 minutes. Poach eggs for 5 minutes. Fry them on each side for 3 minutes. Don't eat eggs that are cooked 'sunnyside up' or are still 'runny'.

You Should Also Know

৵ *Pregnancy-Induced Hypertension*
Pregnancy-induced hypertension (high blood pressure) occurs only during pregnancy. With hypertension of pregnancy, the systolic pres-

sure (the first number) increases to higher than 140 ml of mercury or a rise of 30 ml of mercury over your beginning blood pressure. A diastolic reading (the second number) of over 90 or a rise of 15 ml of mercury also indicates a problem. An example is a woman whose blood pressure at the beginning of pregnancy is 100/60. Later in pregnancy, it is 130/90. This indicates she may be developing high blood pressure or pre-eclampsia.

> *Tip for Week 31* Wearing rings and watches can cause circulation problems. Sometimes a ring becomes so tight on a pregnant woman's finger that the ring must be cut off by a jeweller. You might not want to wear rings if swelling occurs. Some pregnant women purchase inexpensive rings in larger sizes to wear during pregnancy. Or you could put your rings on a pretty chain, and wear them around your neck or on a bracelet.

Your doctor/midwife will be able to determine if your blood pressure is rising to a serious level by checking it at every antenatal appointment. That's one of the reasons it is so important to keep all of your antenatal appointments.

✑ What Is Pre-eclampsia?

Pre-eclampsia describes a variety of symptoms that occur only during pregnancy or shortly after delivery. Pre-eclampsia problems are characterized by a collection of symptoms:

- swelling (oedema)
- protein in the urine (proteinuria)
- high blood pressure (hypertension)
- a change in reflexes (hyperreflexia)

Other non-specific, important symptoms of pre-eclampsia include pain under the ribs on the right side, headache, seeing spots or other changes in vision. These are all warning signs. Report them to your doctor immediately, particularly if you've had blood-pressure problems during pregnancy!

Pre-eclampsia can progress to *eclampsia*. Eclampsia refers to seizures or convulsions in a woman with pre-eclampsia. Seizures are not caused by a previous history of epilepsy or a seizure disorder.

Most pregnant women have some swelling during pregnancy; swelling in the legs does not mean you have pre-eclampsia. It is also possible to have hypertension during pregnancy without having pre-eclampsia.

What Causes Pre-eclampsia? No one knows what causes pre-eclampsia or eclampsia. It occurs most often during a woman's first pregnancy. Women over 35 years old who are having their first baby are more likely to develop high blood pressure and pre-eclampsia. (See Week 16 for more information on pregnancy after 35.)

Some researchers believe that working women are more likely to develop pre-eclampsia than women who do not work. They attribute this increase to *job stress;* if you are in a stressful job situation, discuss it with your doctor.

Treating Pre-eclampsia. The goal in treating pre-eclampsia is to avoid eclampsia (seizures). That means keeping a close watch on you throughout pregnancy and checking your blood pressure and weight at every antenatal visit.

Weight gain can be a sign of pre-eclampsia or worsening pre-eclampsia. Pre-eclampsia affects weight gain because it increases water retention. If you notice any symptoms, call your doctor's surgery.

Treatment of pre-eclampsia begins with bed rest at home. You may not be able to work or to spend much time on your feet. Bed rest allows for the most efficient functioning of your kidneys and the greatest blood flow to the uterus. You might want to read the section on *Bed-Rest Boredom Relievers* in Week 29 if you are advised to rest in bed.

Lie on your side, not on your back. Drink lots of water. Avoid salt, salty foods and foods that contain sodium, which make you retain fluid. Diuretics, which were used in the past, are not prescribed to treat pre-eclampsia today and are not recommended.

If you can't rest at home in bed or if symptoms do not improve, your doctor/midwife may have to admit you to the hospital or deliver your baby. A baby is delivered for the baby's well-being and to avoid seizures in you.

During labour, pre-eclampsia may be treated with magnesium sulphate. It is given by IV to prevent seizures during and after delivery. High blood pressure may be treated with antihypertensive medication.

If you think you've had a seizure, call your doctor/midwife immediately! Diagnosis may be difficult. If possible, someone who observed the possible seizure should describe it to your doctor/midwife. Eclampsia is treated with medications similar to those prescribed for seizure disorders (see Week 26).

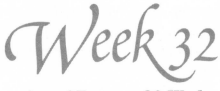

Week 32

Age of Foetus—30 Weeks

How Big Is Your Baby?

By this week, your baby weighs almost 1.8 kg (4 lb). Crown-to-rump length is over 29 cm (11½ in), and total length is nearly 42 cm (19 in).

How Big Are You?

Measurement to the top of the uterus from the pubic symphysis is about 32 cm (12¾ in). Measuring from your bellybutton to the top of the uterus now measures almost 12 cm (5 in).

How Your Baby Is Growing and Developing

Twins? Triplets? More?
When talking about pregnancies of more than one baby, in most cases we refer to twins. The chance of a twin pregnancy is more likely than pregnancy with triplets, quadruplets or quintuplets (or even more!).

You and your partner may be in shock if you learn you have more than one baby on the way. It's a normal reaction. Eventually the joy of expecting more than one baby may help offset the apprehension and responsibility you may feel. If you are expecting two or more babies, you will visit your doctor more often. You will need to plan carefully for delivery and for the care of the babies after you go home. Read the following pages for information on the many different issues surrounding multiples.

Identical Twins and Fraternal Twins. Twin foetuses usually result (over 65 per cent of the time) from the fertilization of two separate eggs. These are called *dizygotic twins* or *fraternal twins*. With fraternal twins, you can have a boy and a girl.

About 33 per cent of the time, twins come from a single egg that divides into two similar structures. Each has the potential of developing into a separate individual. These are known as *monozygotic twins* or *identical twins*. Identical twins are not always identical. It is possible for fraternal twins to appear more alike than identical twins!

Either or both processes may be involved when more than two foetuses are formed. For example, quadruplets may result from fertilization of one, two, three or four eggs.

Division of the fertilized egg occurs between the first few days and about day 8. In this book, we refer to it as the 3rd week of pregnancy. If division of the egg occurs after 8 days, the result can be twins that are connected, called *conjoined twins*. (Conjoined twins used to be called *Siamese twins*.) These babies may share important internal organs, such as the heart, lungs or liver. Fortunately this is a rare occurrence.

Frequency of Multiple Births. The frequency of twins depends on the type of twins. Identical twins occur about once in every 250 births around the world. This type of twin formation appears to be uninfluenced by age, race, heredity, number of pregnancies or medications taken for infertility (fertility drugs). The incidence of fraternal twins, however, is influenced by race, heredity, maternal age, the number of previous pregnancies and the use of fertility drugs.

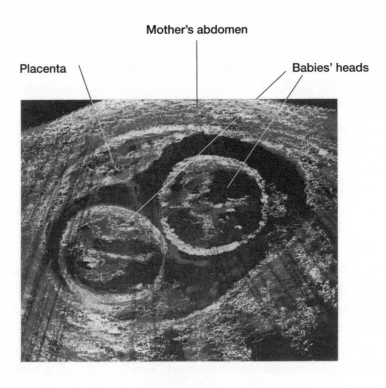

Mother's abdomen

Placenta

Babies' heads

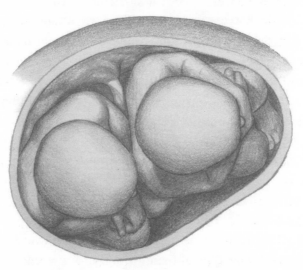

Ultrasound of twins shows two babies in the uterus. If you look closely, you can see the two heads. The interpretive illustration shows how the babies are lying.

The frequency of multiple foetuses varies significantly among different races. Twins occur in 1 out of every 100 pregnancies in white women compared to 1 out of every 79 pregnancies in black women. Certain areas of Africa have an incredibly high frequency of twins. In some places, twins occur once in every 20 births! Hispanic women also have a higher number of twin births than white women. The occurrence of twins among Asians is less common—about 1 in every 150 births.

Heredity also plays a part in the occurrence of twins. In one study of fraternal twins, the chance of a female twin giving birth to a set of twins herself was about 1 in 58 births.

The occurrence of twins is probably more common than we know. Early ultrasound exams often reveal two sacs or two pregnancies. Later ultrasounds of the same woman may show that one sac (or one pregnancy) has disappeared, while the other pregnancy continues to grow and to develop normally. Some researchers believe these ultrasound results should not be disclosed in the first 8 to 10 weeks of pregnancy. Parents who are informed of twins at this point may be distraught to learn later that one of the babies will not be born.

Triplets occur once in every 8,000 deliveries. Many doctors never deliver or participate in the delivery of triplets in their medical careers. (Dr Curtis has been fortunate to deliver two sets of triplets.)

Some families are more blessed than others. In one case we know of personally, a woman had three single births. Her 4th pregnancy was twins, and her 5th pregnancy (a year later) was triplets! She and her husband decided on another pregnancy—they were surprised (and probably relieved) when the 6th pregnancy resulted in only one baby.

Fertility Medication, In-Vitro Fertilization and Multiple Pregnancies. We have known for a long time that fertility drugs increase the chance of multiple pregnancies. Several different medications are used to treat infertility. Each one affects, to a different degree, a woman's chances of conceiving more than one foetus. One of the more common medications is clomiphene (Clomid). It increases the chance of multiple foetuses somewhat less than other medications. But an increased chance is still there.

Twins are more common in pregnancies that result from the use of fertility drugs or with the implantation of more than one embryo with in-vitro fertilization. The percentage of male foetuses decreases as the number of foetuses per pregnancy increases. This means more females are born in these multiple pregnancies.

Discovering You're Carrying More than One Baby. Diagnosis of twins was more difficult before ultrasound was available. The illustration on page 324 shows an ultrasound of twins. You can see parts of both foetuses.

It is uncommon to discover twin pregnancies just by hearing two heartbeats. Many people believe when only one heartbeat is heard, there could be no possibility of twins. This may not be the case. Two rapid heartbeats may have a similar or almost identical rate. That could make it difficult to determine that there are two babies.

Measuring and examining your abdomen during pregnancy is important. Usually a twin pregnancy is noted during the second trimester because you are too big and growth seems too fast for a single pregnancy.

Ultrasound examination is the best way to tell if you are carrying more than one baby. Diagnosis can also be made by X-ray after 16 to 18 weeks of pregnancy, when foetal skeletons are visible. However, this method is used infrequently today.

Do Multiple Pregnancies Have More Problems?   With a multiple pregnancy, the possibility of problems goes up. Possible problems include the following:

- increased risk of miscarriage
- foetal death or mortality
- foetal malformations
- low birthweight or growth restriction
- pre-eclampsia
- problems with the placenta, including placental abruption and placenta previa
- maternal anaemia

• maternal bleeding or haemorrhage
• problems with the umbilical cord, including entwinement or tangling of the babies' umbilical cords
• hydramnios or polyhydramnios
• labour complicated by abnormal foetal presentation, such as breech or transverse lie
• premature labour

One of the biggest problems with multiple pregnancies is premature delivery. As the number of foetuses increases, the length of gestation and the birthweight of each baby decreases, although this is not true in every case.

The average length of pregnancy for twins is about 37 weeks. For triplets it is about 35 weeks. For every week the babies remain in the uterus, their birthweights increase, along with the maturity of organs and systems.

Major malformations in multiple pregnancies are more common than they are in single pregnancies. The incidence of minor malformation is twice as high as it is in a single pregnancy. Malformations are more common among identical twins than fraternal twins.

One of the main goals in dealing with multiple foetuses is to continue the pregnancy as long as possible to avoid premature delivery. This may best be accomplished by bed rest. You may not be able to carry on with regular activities during your entire pregnancy. If your doctor recommends bed rest, follow his or her advice.

Weight gain is important with a multiple pregnancy. You will gain more than the normal 11.4 to 15.9 kg (25 to 35 lb), depending on the number of foetuses you are carrying. Supplementation with iron is essential.

Some researchers believe use of a *tocolytic agent* (medication to stop labour), such as ritodrine, is critical in preventing premature delivery. (See Week 29.) These agents are used to relax the uterus to keep you from going into premature labour.

Follow your doctor's instruction closely. Every day and every week you're able to keep the babies inside you are days or weeks you won't have to visit them in an intensive-care nursery while they grow, develop and finish maturing.

Delivering More Than One Baby. How multiple foetuses are delivered often depends on how the babies are lying in your uterus. Possible complications of labour and delivery, in addition to prematurity, include the following:

• abnormal presentations (breech or transverse)
• prolapse of the umbilical cord (the umbilical cord comes out ahead of the babies)
• placental abruption
• foetal distress
• bleeding after delivery

Because there is higher risk during labour and delivery, precautions are taken before delivery and during labour. These include the need for an IV, the presence of an anaesthesiologist and the availability and possible presence of paediatricians or other medical personnel to take care of the babies.

With twins, all possible combinations of foetal positions can occur. Both babies may come head first (vertex). They may come *breech*, meaning bottom or feet first. They may come sideways or *oblique*, meaning at an angle that is neither breech nor vertex. Or they may come in any combination of the above. (See the discussion of birth presentation in Week 38.)

When both twins are head first, a vaginal delivery may be attempted and may be accomplished safely. It may be possible for one baby to deliver vaginally. The second one could require a C-section if it turns, the cord comes out ahead of the baby or the baby is distressed following delivery of the first foetus. Some doctors believe delivery of two or more babies requires a C-section.

After delivery of two or more babies, doctors pay close attention to maternal bleeding because of the rapid change in the size of the uterus. It is greatly overdistended with more than one baby. Medication, usually oxytocin (Pitocin), is given by IV to contract the uterus to stop bleeding so the mother doesn't lose too much blood. A heavy blood loss could produce anaemia and make a blood transfusion or long-term treatment with iron supplementation necessary.

Changes in You

Until this week, your visits to the doctor/midwife have probably been on a monthly basis, unless you've had complications or problems. At week 32, most doctors/midwives begin seeing a pregnant woman every 2 weeks. This will continue until you reach your last month of pregnancy; at that time, you'll probably switch to weekly visits.

By this time, you probably know your doctor/midwife fairly well and feel comfortable talking about your concerns. Now is a good time to ask questions and to discuss concerns about labour and delivery. If there are complications or problems later in pregnancy or at delivery, you'll be able to communicate

Dad Tip Together with your partner, make a list of important telephone numbers and keep it with you. Include numbers of your work, your partner's work, the hospital, the doctor's surgery, a back-up driver, baby-sitter or others. You may also want to make a list of numbers of people you want to call after the delivery of your baby. Take this list to the hospital with you.

better with your doctor/midwife and know what is going on. You'll feel comfortable with the care you're receiving.

Your doctor/midwife may plan on talking to you about many things in the weeks to come, but you can't always assume this. You may be taking antenatal classes and hearing different things about labour and delivery, such as stories about enemas, IVs and complications. Don't be afraid to ask any questions you have. Most doctors and nurses are receptive to your queries. They want you to discuss things you're concerned about instead of worrying about them unnecessarily.

How Your Actions
Affect Your Baby's Development

∽ Keep Taking Your Prenatal Vitamins

The vitamins and iron in prenatal vitamins are still essential to your well-being and the well-being of your baby or babies. If you're anaemic at the time of delivery, a low blood count could have a negative effect on both or all of you. Your chance of needing a blood transfusion could be higher. Keep taking your prenatal vitamins every day!

Your Nutrition

If you're expecting more than one baby, your nutrition and weight gain are extremely important during pregnancy. Food is your best source of nutrients and calories, but it's also important for you to take your prenatal vitamin every day. If you don't gain weight early in pregnancy, you have a greater chance of developing pre-eclampsia. Your babies may be tiny, too.

> *Tip for Week 32* Your requirements for calories, protein, vitamins and minerals increase if you carry more than one baby. You'll need to eat about 300 calories a day more *per baby* than for a normal pregnancy. For ideas on how to add those 300 calories, see Week 15.

If you're expecting twins, target weight gain (for a normal-weight woman) is about 20.4 kg (45 lb). Don't be alarmed when your doctor/midwife discusses the amount of weight he or she wants you to gain. Studies show that if a woman gains the targeted amount of weight with a multiple pregnancy, her babies are often healthier.

How can you gain the amount of weight you need to gain? Just adding extra calories won't benefit you or your developing babies. Junk food, full of empty calories, doesn't add much. Get your calories from specific sources. For example, it's important to eat an extra serving of a dairy product and an extra serving of a protein each day. These two servings provide you with the extra calcium, protein and iron you require to meet the needs of your growing babies. Discuss the situation with your doctor/midwife; he or she may suggest you see a nutritionist.

You Should Also Know

ᏊᎨᏊ *Postpartum Bleeding and Haemorrhage*

It is normal to lose blood during labour and delivery. However, a heavy postpartum haemorrhage is different and significant. Postpartum haemorrhage is a loss of blood in excess of 500 ml (17 fl oz) in the first 24 hours after your baby's birth.

There can be many reasons for postpartum haemorrhage. The most common causes include a uterus that will not contract and lacerations or tearing of the vagina or cervix during the birth process.

Other causes include trauma to the genital tract, such as a large or bleeding episiotomy, or a rupture, hole or tear in the uterus. Blood loss may be related to the failure of blood vessels to compress to stop bleeding inside the uterus (where the placenta was attached). This may occur if the uterus fails to contract because of rapid labour, a long labour, several previous deliveries, a uterine infection, an overdistended uterus (with multiple foetuses) or with certain agents used for general anaesthesia.

Heavy bleeding may also result from retained placental tissue. In this situation, most of the placenta delivers, but part of it remains inside the uterus. Retained placental tissue may cause bleeding immediately, or bleeding may occur weeks or even months later.

Problems with blood clotting can cause haemorrhaging. This may be related to pregnancy, or it may be a congenital medical problem. Bleeding following delivery requires constant attention from your doctor and the midwives caring for you.

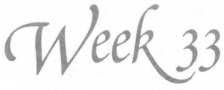

Week 33

Age of Foetus—31 Weeks

How Big Is Your Baby?

Your baby weighs about 2 kg (4½ lb) by this week. Its crown-to-rump length is about 30 cm (12 in), and total length is nearly 43 cm (19½ in).

How Big Are You?

Measuring from the pubic symphysis, it is now about 33 cm (13¼ in) to the top of the uterus. Measurement from your bellybutton to the top of your uterus is about 13 cm (5¼ in). Your total weight gain should be between 9.9 and 12.6 kg (22 and 28 lb).

How Your Baby Is Growing and Developing

Placental Abruption
The illustration on the opposite page shows placental abruption, which is premature separation of the placenta from the wall of the uterus.

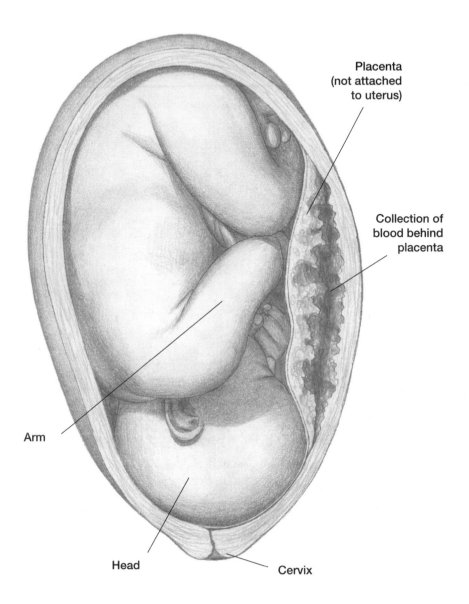

Placenta (not attached to uterus)

Collection of blood behind placenta

Arm

Head

Cervix

This illustration of placental abruption shows that the placenta has separated from the wall of the uterus.

Normally, the placenta does not separate from the uterus until after the baby is delivered. Separation before delivery (placental abruption) can be very serious.

The frequency of placental abruption is estimated to be about 1 in every 80 deliveries. We do not have a more exact statistic because time of separation varies, altering the risk to the foetus. If the placenta separates at the time of delivery and the infant is delivered without incident, it is not as significant as a placenta separating during pregnancy.

The cause of placental abruption is unknown. Certain conditions may increase its chance of occurrence, including:

- physical injury to the mother, as from a car accident or a bad fall
- a short umbilical cord
- sudden change in the size of the uterus (from rupture of membranes)
- hypertension
- dietary deficiency
- a uterine abnormality, such as a band of tissue or a scar in the uterus where the placenta cannot attach properly
- previous surgery on the uterus (removal of fibroids) or D&C for abortion or miscarriage

Studies indicate that folic-acid deficiency can play a role in causing placental abruption. Others suggest maternal smoking and alcohol consumption may make a woman more likely to have placental abruption.

A woman who has had placental abruption in the past is at increased risk of having it recur. Rate of recurrence has been estimated to be as high as 10 per cent. This can make a pregnancy following placental abruption a high-risk pregnancy.

Separation of the placenta may involve partial or total separation from the uterine wall. The situation is most severe when the placenta totally separates from the uterine wall. The foetus relies entirely on circulation from the placenta. With separation, it cannot receive blood from the umbilical cord, which is attached to the placenta.

Symptoms of Placental Abruption. Symptoms of placental abruption can vary a great deal. There may be heavy bleeding from the vagina, or you may experience no bleeding at all. The illustration on page 333 shows bleeding behind the placenta with complete separation.

Ultrasound may be helpful in diagnosing this problem, although it does not always provide an exact diagnosis. This is particularly true if the placenta is located on the back surface of the uterus where it cannot be seen easily with ultrasound examination.

Other symptoms can include lower-back pain, tenderness of the uterus or abdomen, and contractions or tightening of the uterus. Of the various symptoms associated with placental abruption, the following are the most common.

- Vaginal bleeding occurs in about 75 per cent of all cases.
- Tenderness of the uterus occurs about 60 per cent of the time.
- Foetal distress or problems with the foetal heart rate occur about 60 per cent of the time.
- Tightening or contraction of the uterus occurs about 34 per cent of the time.
- Premature labour occurs in about 20 per cent of the cases.

Serious problems, such as shock, may occur with separation of the placenta. Shock occurs because of the rapid loss of large quantities of blood. Intravascular coagulation, in which a large blood clot develops, can also be a problem. Factors that clot the blood may be used up, which can make bleeding a problem.

Can Placental Abruption Be Treated? Treatment of placental abruption varies, based on the ability to diagnose the problem and the status of the mother and baby. With heavy bleeding, delivery of the baby may be necessary.

When bleeding is not heavy, the problem may be treated with a more conservative approach. This depends on whether the foetus is in distress and if it appears to be in immediate danger.

Placental abruption is one of the most serious problems related to the second and third trimesters of pregnancy. If you have any symptoms, call your doctor immediately!

Changes in You

↣ *How Will You Know Your Membranes Have Ruptured?*

How will you know when your waters break? It isn't usually just one gush of water, with no further leakage. There is often a gush of amniotic fluid, usually followed by a leaking of small amounts of fluid. Women describe it as a constant wetness or water running down their leg when they stand. *Continuous* leakage of water is a good clue that your waters have broken.

Amniotic fluid is usually clear and watery. Occasionally it may have a bloody appearance, or it may be yellow or green.

It isn't uncommon to have an increase in vaginal discharge or to lose urine in small amounts as your baby puts pressure on your bladder. But there are ways for your doctor to tell if your waters have broken. Two tests can be done on the amniotic fluid.

One is a *nitrazine test,* though this is not routinely used in the U.K. When amniotic fluid is placed on a small strip of paper, it changes the colour of the paper. This test is based on the acidity or pH of the amniotic fluid. However, blood can also change the colour of nitrazine paper, even if your waters haven't broken.

Another test that may be done is a *ferning test*. Amniotic fluid or fluid from the back of the vagina is taken with a swab and placed on a slide for examination under a microscope. Dried amniotic fluid has the appearance of a fern or branches of a pine tree. Ferning is often more helpful in diagnosing ruptured membranes than looking at colour changes on nitrazine paper.

What Do You Do When Your Waters Break? Your membranes may rupture at any point in pregnancy. Don't assume it will happen only around the time of labour.

If you think your waters have broken, call your community midwife or maternity unit if you're having a hospital delivery. Avoid sexual intercourse at this time. Intercourse increases the possibility of introducing an infection into your uterus and thus to your baby.

How Your Actions Affect Your Baby's Development

⁓ *Weight Gain Continues*

You are continuing to gain weight as your pregnancy progresses. You may be gaining weight faster than at any other time during pregnancy. However, *you* are not putting on most of this weight—the baby is! Your baby is going through a period of increased growth and may be gaining as much as 225 g (8 oz) or more every week!

Continue to eat the right foods for you. Heartburn may be more of a problem now because your growing baby may not allow your stomach much room. You may find eating several small meals a day, rather than three large meals, makes you feel more comfortable.

Your Nutrition

You know the importance of eating a well-balanced diet during pregnancy. Eating fresh fruit and vegetables, dairy products, whole-grain products and protein all contribute to the healthy development of your baby. You may be concerned about what foods to avoid. Some foods may be OK to eat when you're not pregnant but should be avoided now.

Tip for Week 33 Don't stop eating or start skipping meals as your weight increases. Both you and your baby need all the calories and nutrition you receive from a healthy diet.

When possible, avoid food additives. We aren't certain how they can affect a developing baby, but if you can avoid them, do so. Be careful about pesticides, too. Thoroughly wash and wipe dry all fruits and vegetables before you eat or prepare them, even if you don't normally eat the peel. Contaminants could get on your hands if you don't wash them. Peel a fruit or vegetable *after* you wash it, if that's the way you normally eat it. It helps to remove even more of the fruit that might be contaminated.

Avoid fish that might be contaminated with PCBs. (See Week 26 for further information.) Buy fish only from a reputable market, or eat those caught only in areas free from contamination. Be vigilant about the foods you consume to protect your growing baby.

You Should Also Know

ᴣ Will You Have an Episiotomy?

An *episiotomy* is an incision made from the vagina towards the rectum during delivery to avoid undue tearing of the area as the baby's head passes through the birth canal. It may be a cut directly in the midline toward the rectum, or it may be a cut to the side. After the baby is delivered, layers are closed separately with absorbable sutures that do not require removal after they heal.

There is little you can do if you need an episiotomy. Some people practice, teach and believe in stretching the birth canal during labour and at the time of delivery to try to avoid an episiotomy. It may work for some, but it doesn't work for every woman. Others suggest an episiotomy to avoid stretching the vagina, bladder and rectum. Stretching the vagina can result in loss of control of your urine or bowels and can change sensations experienced during sexual intercourse.

Ðad Tip Is your home safe for your new baby? Things to consider when thinking about safety include pets, furniture, secondhand smoke, window coverings or anything else in your home that could pose a danger to your little one. Start now to check for problems so you'll have time to take care of them before baby's birth.

The reason for an episiotomy usually becomes clear at delivery when the baby's head is in the vagina. An episiotomy is a controlled, straight, clean cut. That's better than a tear or rip that could go in many directions, including tearing or ripping into the bladder, large blood vessels or rectum. An episiotomy also heals better than a ragged tear.

Ask your doctor/midwife if he or she thinks you may need an episiotomy. Discuss why an episiotomy is necessary. Find out whether it might be a cut in the middle or to the side of the vagina. You might also ask if there is anything you can do to prepare for the possibility of an episiotomy, such as having an enema or stretching the vagina. If a vacuum extractor (ventouse) or forceps are used for delivery, an episiotomy may be done before the device is placed on the baby's head.

Description of an episiotomy also includes a description of the depth of the incision.

- A *first-degree* episiotomy cuts only the skin.
- A *second-degree* episiotomy cuts the skin and underlying tissue.
- A *third-degree* episiotomy cuts the skin, underlying tissue and rectal sphincter, which is the muscle that goes around the anus.
- A *fourth-degree* episiotomy goes through the three layers and through the rectal mucosa.

The most painful part of the entire birth experience might be an episiotomy. It may continue to cause some discomfort as it heals. Don't be afraid to ask for medication to ease any pain. There are many medications that are safe to take, even if you breastfeed your baby, including paracetamol. Paracetamol with codeine or other medications may also be prescribed for pain.

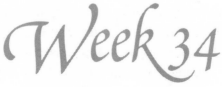

Week 34

Age of Foetus—32 Weeks

How Big Is Your Baby?

Your baby weighs almost 2.28 kg (5 lb) by this week. Its crown-to-rump length is about 32 cm (12¾ in). Total length is 44 cm (19¾ in).

How Big Are You?

Measuring up from your bellybutton, it's about 14 cm (5½ in) to the top of your uterus. From the pubic symphysis, you will measure about 34 cm (13½ in).

It's not important that your measurements match any of your friends' at similar points in their pregnancies. What's important is that you're growing appropriately and that your uterus grows and gets larger at an appropriate rate. These are the signs of normal growth of your baby inside your uterus.

Tip for Week 34 A strip of paper, tape or a bandage can help cover a bellybutton that is sensitive or unsightly (poking through your clothing).

How Your Baby Is Growing and Developing

⁓ *Testing Your Baby before Birth*

An ideal test done before delivery would determine if the foetus is healthy. It would be able to detect major foetal malformations or foetal stress, which could indicate an impending problem.

Ultrasound accomplishes some of these goals by enabling doctors to observe the baby inside the uterus, as well as to evaluate the brain, heart and other organs of the foetal body. Along with ultrasound examinations, foetal monitoring in the form of a non-stress test and a contraction stress test can indicate foetal well-being or problems. (See Week 41 for discussions of the non-stress test and the contraction stress test.)

Changes in You

⁓ *Will Your Baby Drop?*

A few weeks before labour begins or at the beginning of labour, you may notice a change in your abdomen. When examined by your doctor, measurement from your bellybutton or the pubic symphysis to the top of the uterus may be smaller than what you noticed on a previous visit. This phenomenon occurs as the head of the baby enters the birth canal. This change is often called *lightening*.

Don't be concerned if you don't notice lightening or a drop of the foetus. This doesn't occur with every woman or with every pregnancy. It's also common for your baby to drop just before labour begins or during labour.

With lightening, you may experience benefits and problems. One benefit may be more room in your upper abdomen. This gives you more room to breathe because there's more room for your lungs to expand. However, with the descent of the baby, you may notice more pressure in your pelvis, bladder and rectum, which can make you more uncomfortable.

In some instances, your doctor/midwife may examine you and tell you your baby is 'not in the pelvis' or 'is high up.' He or she is saying the baby has not yet descended into the birth canal. However, this situation can change quickly.

If your doctor/midwife says your baby is 'floating' or 'ballotable' it means part of the baby is felt high in the birth canal. But the baby is not engaged (fixed) in the birth canal at this point. The baby may even move away from your doctor's/midwife's fingers when you are examined.

↝ *Uncomfortable Feelings You May Experience*

At this point in their pregnancies, some women have the uncomfortable feeling the baby is going to 'fall out.' This feeling is related to pressure the baby exerts because it has moved lower in the birth canal. Some women describe the feeling as an increase in pressure.

If you're concerned or worried about it, consult your doctor. It may be a reason to perform a pelvic exam to see how low the baby's head is. In almost all cases, the baby will not be coming out. But because it is at a lower position than what you're used to, the baby will exert more pressure than you have noticed during recent weeks.

Another feeling associated with increased pressure may occur around this week. Some pregnant women have described it as a 'pins-and-needles' sensation. The feeling is tingling, pressure or numbness in the pelvis or pelvic region from the pressure of the baby. It is a common symptom and shouldn't concern you.

These feelings may not be relieved until delivery occurs. You can lie on your side to help decrease pressure in your pelvis and on the nerves, vessels and arteries in the pelvic area. If the problem is severe, talk to your doctor/midwife about it.

↝ *Braxton-Hicks Contractions and False Labour*

Ask your doctor/midwife what the signs of labour contractions are; they are usually regular. They increase in duration and strength over time. You'll notice a regular rhythm to real labour contractions. You'll want to time them so you know how frequently they occur and how long they last. When you go to the hospital depends in part on your contractions.

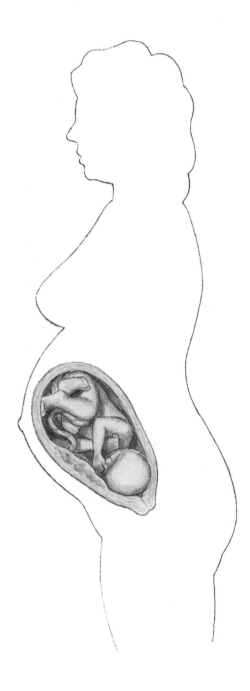

Comparative size of the uterus at 34 weeks of pregnancy (foetal age—
32 weeks). The uterus can be felt about 14 cm (5½ in) above your bellybutton.

Braxton-Hicks contractions are painless, non-rhythmical contractions you may be able to feel when you place your hand on your abdomen. These contractions often begin early in pregnancy and are felt at irregular intervals. They may increase in number and strength when the uterus is massaged. Like false labour, they are not positive signs of true labour.

False labour often occurs before true labour begins. False-labour contractions can be painful and may appear to be real labour to you. See the box below.

In most instances, false-labour contractions are irregular. They are usually of short duration (less than 45 seconds). The discomfort of the contraction may occur in various parts of your body, such as the groin, lower abdomen or back. With true labour, uterine contractions produce pain that starts at the top of the uterus and radiates over the entire uterus, through the lower back into the pelvis.

False labour is usually seen in late pregnancy. It seems to occur more often in women who have been pregnant before and delivered more babies. It usually stops as quickly as it begins. There doesn't appear to be any danger to your baby.

True Labour or False Labour?

Considerations	True Labour	False Labour
Contractions	Regular	Irregular
Time between contractions	Come closer together	Do not get closer together
Contraction intensity	Increases	Doesn't change
Location of contractions	Entire abdomen	Various locations or back
Effect of anaesthetic or pain relievers	Will not stop labour	Sedation may stop or alter frequency of contractions
Cervical change	Progressive cervical change (effacement and dilatation)	No cervical change

How Your Actions Affect Your Baby's Development

The end of your pregnancy begins with labour. Some women are concerned (or hope!) that their actions can cause labour to begin. The old wives' tales about going for a ride over a bumpy road or taking a long walk to start labour aren't true.

We do know intercourse and stimulation of the nipples may cause labour to start in some cases, but this isn't true for every woman. Going about your daily activities (unless your doctor/midwife has advised bed rest) will not cause labour to start before your baby is ready to be born. In the following weekly discussions, we continue to discuss what labour involves and the many issues surrounding this climactic event.

Your Nutrition

ᔓ *Cholesterol Check*

It's a waste of time and effort to have your cholesterol level checked during pregnancy. The level of cholesterol in your blood rises during pregnancy due to hormonal changes. Wait until after you have your baby or stop breastfeeding to check your cholesterol.

ᔓ *A Vitamin-Rich Snack*

When you're looking for something to snack on, you might not think of a baked potato, but it's an excellent snack! You get protein, fibre, calcium, iron, B vitamins and vitamin C when you eat a potato. Bake up a few, and store them in the refrigerator. Heat one up when you're hungry. Broccoli is another food filled with vitamins. Add it to your baked potato, and top both with some natural yoghurt, cottage cheese or non-fat soured cream for a delicious treat!

> **Dad Tip** Your partner may begin to feel nervous and apprehensive as her delivery date draws near. A reassuring cuddle may be all she needs to dispell her anxiety.

You Should Also Know

ᴣ *What Is a 'Bloody Show'?*

Often following a vaginal examination or with the beginning of early labour and early contractions, you may bleed a small amount. This is called a *bloody show;* it can occur as the cervix stretches and dilates. You should not lose a lot of blood. If it causes you concern or appears to be a large amount of blood, call your doctor immediately.

Along with a bloody show, you may pass a mucus plug at the beginning of labour. This is different from your bag of waters breaking (ruptured membranes). Passing this mucus plug doesn't necessarily mean you'll have your baby soon or even that you'll go into labour in the next few hours. It poses no danger to you or your baby.

ᴣ *Timing Contractions*

Most women are instructed in antenatal classes or by their doctor about how to time contractions during labour. To time how long a contraction lasts, begin timing when the contraction starts and end timing when the contraction lets up and goes away.

It's also important to know how often contractions occur. There is much confusion about this. You can choose from two methods. Ask your doctor/midwife which method he or she prefers.

- Note the time period from when a contraction starts to the time the next contraction starts. This is the most commonly used method and the most reliable.
- Note the time period from when a contraction ends to the time the next contraction starts.

It's helpful for you or your partner to time your contractions before calling your midwife or the hospital. Your midwife will probably want to know how often contractions occur and how long each contraction lasts. With this information, your midwife can decide when you should go to the hospital.

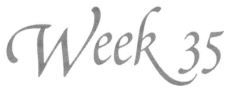

Week 35

Age of Foetus—33 Weeks

How Big Is Your Baby?

Your baby now weighs over 2.5 kg (5½ lb). Crown-to-rump length by this week of pregnancy is about 33 cm (13¼ in). Its total length is 45 cm (20¼ in).

How Big Are You?

Measuring from your bellybutton, it is now about 15 cm (6 in) to the top of your uterus. Measuring from the pubic symphysis, the distance is about 35 cm (14 in). By this week, your total weight gain should be between 10.8 and 13 kg (24 and 29 lb).

Dad Tip At an antenatal visit, ask the midwife about your part in the delivery. There may be some things you'd like to do, such as cutting the cord or videotaping your baby's birth. It's easier to talk about these things ahead of time. Not every new father wants an active role in the delivery. That's OK, too.

How Your Baby Is Growing and Developing?

✧ *How Much Does Your Baby Weigh?*

You have probably asked your doctor/midwife several times how big your baby is or how much your baby will weigh when it's born. Next to asking about the sex of a baby, this is the most frequently asked question.

You're getting larger. Your increasing size is due to the growth of baby and placenta as well as the increased amount of amniotic fluid. All these factors make estimating foetal weight more difficult.

Using Ultrasound to Estimate Foetal Weight. Ultrasound can be used to estimate foetal weight, but errors in weight estimates can and do occur. The accuracy of predicting foetal weight using ultrasound has improved. Making an accurate estimate can be valuable.

Several measurements are used in a formula or computer programme to estimate a baby's weight. These include diameter of the baby's head, circumference of the baby's head, circumference of the baby's abdomen, length of the femur of the baby's leg and, in some instances, other foetal measurements.

Many feel that ultrasound is the method of choice to estimate foetal weight. But even with ultrasound, estimates may vary as much as 225 g (8 oz) or more in either direction.

Will Your Baby Fit through the Birth Canal? Even with a foetal-weight estimate, whether by your doctor or by ultrasound, we can't tell if the baby is too big for you or whether you'll need a C-section. Usually, it's necessary for you to labour to be able to see how the baby fits into your pelvis and if there is room for it to pass through the birth canal.

In some women who appear to be average or better-than-average size, a 2.7- to 2.9-kg (6- or 6½-lb) baby won't fit through the pelvis. Experience has also shown that women who may appear petite are sometimes able to deliver 3.4-kg (7½-lb) or larger babies without much

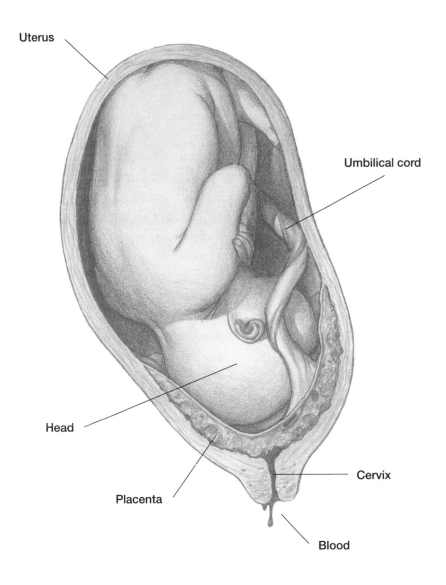

Uterus

Umbilical cord

Head

Cervix

Placenta

Blood

In this illustration of placenta previa, note how the placenta completely covers the cervical opening to the uterus. (See page 352 for more information.)

difficulty. The best test or method of evaluating whether your baby will deliver through your pelvis is labour.

Changes in You

✑ *Emotional Changes in Late Pregnancy*

As you come closer to delivery, you and your partner may become more anxious about the events to come. You may even have more mood swings, which seem to occur for no reason. You may become more irritable, which can place a significant strain on your relationship. You may be concerned about insignificant or unimportant things. Your concern about the health and well-being of the baby may also increase during the last weeks of your pregnancy. This can include concern about how well you will tolerate labour and how you will get through delivery. You may be concerned about whether you'll be a good mother or be able to raise a baby properly.

While these emotions rage inside you, you'll notice you're getting bigger and aren't able to do things you used to do. You may feel more uncomfortable, and you may not be sleeping well. These things can all work together to make your emotions swing wildly from highs to lows.

How Can You Deal with These Changes? Emotional changes are normal; don't feel as though you're alone. Other pregnant women and their partners have the same concerns.

Talk with your partner about your concerns. Tell him how you feel and what's going on. You may be surprised to discover the concerns your partner has about you, the baby and his role during labour and delivery. By talking about these things, your partner may find it easier to understand what you're experiencing, including mood swings and crying spells.

Discuss emotional problems with your doctor. He or she may be able to reassure you that what you're going through is normal. Take advantage of antenatal classes and information available about pregnancy and delivery.

Emotional changes often occur, so be ready for them. Ask your partner, the nurse in the doctor's surgery and your doctor to help you understand what is normal and what can be done about mood swings.

How Your Actions Affect Your Baby's Development

ᴥ Preparing for Baby's Birth

At this point, you may be feeling a little nervous about the birth. You might be afraid you won't know when it's time to call your community midwife or go to the hospital. Don't hesitate to talk to your doctor about it at one of your visits. He or she will tell you what signs to watch for. In antenatal classes, you should also learn to recognize the signs of labour and when you should call your doctor or go to the hospital.

Your bag of waters may rupture before you go into labour. In most cases, you'll notice this as a gush of water followed by a steady leaking. (See Week 33.)

During the last few weeks of pregnancy, have your suitcase packed and ready to go. See the list in Week 36 for some helpful suggestions, so you'll have the things you want when you get to the hospital.

If you can, tour the hospital facilities a few weeks ahead of your scheduled due date. Find out where to go and what to do when you get there.

Talk with your partner about the best ways to reach him if you think you are in labour. If either of you has a mobile phone, it's probably the easiest way to stay in touch. You might have him check with you periodically. It's also common for a partner to wear a pager if he is often away from a phone, especially during the last few weeks of pregnancy.

Ask your doctor what you should do if you think you're in labour. Is it best to call the surgery? Should you go directly to the hospital? By knowing what to do, and when, you'll be able to relax a little and not worry about the beginning of labour and delivery.

Your Nutrition

Your body continues to need lots of vitamins and minerals for your developing baby. And you'll need even more of them if you choose to breastfeed! On the opposite page is a chart showing your daily vitamin and mineral requirements during pregnancy and breastfeeding. It's important to realize how necessary your continued good nutrition is for you and your baby.

Nutrient Requirements during Pregnancy and Breastfeeding

Vitamins & Minerals	During Pregnancy	During Breastfeeding
A	800 mcg	1300 mcg
B_1 (thiamine)	1.5 mg	1.6 mg
B_2 (riboflavin)	1.6 mg	1.8 mg
B_3 (niacin)	17 mg	20 mg
B_6	2.2 mg	2.2 mg
B_{12}	2.2 mcg	2.6 mcg
C	70 mg	95 mg
Calcium	1200 mg	1200 mg
D	10 mcg	10 mcg
E	10 mg	12 mg
Folic acid (B_9)	400 mcg	280 mcg
Iron	30 mg	15 mg
Magnesium	320 mg	355 mg
Phosphorous	1200 mg	1200 mg
Zinc	15 mg	19 mg

You Should Also Know

✣ What Is Placenta Previa?
With *placenta previa*, the placenta lies close to the cervix or covers the cervix. This problem is not common; it happens about once in every 170 pregnancies. The illustration on page 349 shows placenta previa.

Placenta previa is serious because of the chance of heavy bleeding. Bleeding may occur during pregnancy or during labour.

The cause of placenta previa is not completely understood. Risk factors for an increased chance of placenta previa include previous Caesarean delivery, many previous pregnancies and increased maternal age.

Symptoms of Placenta Previa. The most characteristic symptom of placenta previa is painless bleeding without any contractions of the uterus. This doesn't usually occur until close to the end of your second trimester or later when the cervix thins out, stretches and tears the placenta loose.

Bleeding with placenta previa may occur without warning and may be extremely heavy. It occurs when the cervix begins to dilate with early labour, and blood escapes.

Placenta previa should be suspected when a woman experiences vaginal bleeding during the latter half of pregnancy. The problem cannot be diagnosed with a physical exam because a pelvic examination may cause heavier bleeding. Doctors use ultrasound to identify placenta previa. Ultrasound is particularly accurate in the second half of pregnancy because the uterus and placenta get bigger, and things are easier to see.

Your doctor may advise you not to have a pelvic exam if you have placenta previa. This is important to remember if you see another doctor or when you go to the hospital.

The baby is more likely to be in a breech position with placenta previa. For this reason, and to control bleeding, a Caesarean delivery is usually performed. Caesarean delivery with placenta previa offers the advantage of delivering the baby, then removing the placenta so the uterus can contract. Bleeding can be kept to a minimum.

Tip for Week 35 Maternity bras are designed to provide extra support to your growing breasts. You may feel more comfortable wearing one during the day and at night while you sleep.

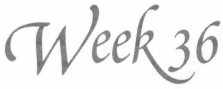

Week 36

Age of Foetus—34 Weeks

How Big Is Your Baby?

By this week, your baby weighs about 2.75 kg (6 lb). Its crown-to-rump length is over 34 cm (13½ in), and total length is 46 cm (20¾ in).

How Big Are You?

Measuring from the pubic symphysis, it's about 36 cm (14½ in) to the top of your uterus. If you measure from your bellybutton, it's more than 14 cm (5½ in) to the top of your uterus.

You may feel as though you've run out of room! Your uterus has grown bigger in the past few weeks as the baby has grown inside of it. Now your uterus is probably up under your ribs.

Tip for Week 36 Take time to relax. Remember to put your feet up; this will prevent water retention and varicose veins.

How Your Baby Is Growing and Developing

↷ *Maturity of Your Baby's Lungs and Respiratory System*

An important part of your baby's development is maturation of the lungs and respiratory system. When a baby is born prematurely, a common problem is development of *respiratory-distress syndrome* in the newborn. This problem is also called *hyaline membrane disease*. In this situation, lungs are not completely mature, and the baby can't breathe on its own without help. Oxygen is necessary. The baby may require a machine, such as a ventilator, to breathe for it.

In the early 1970s, scientists developed two methods for evaluating foetal-lung maturity. An amniocentesis test must be done for both tests. The first method, the *L/S ratio*, enables doctors to determine in advance if a baby can breathe on its own after delivery.

The L/S-ratio test doesn't usually indicate a baby's lungs are mature until at least 34 weeks of pregnancy. At that time, the relationship between two factors in the amniotic fluid changes. Levels of lecithin go up, while levels of sphingomyelin stay the same. The ratio between these two levels indicates if a baby's lungs are mature.

The *phosphatidyl glycerol (PG)* test is another way doctors can evaluate the maturity of the baby's lungs. This test is either positive or negative. If phosphatidyl glycerol is present in the amniotic fluid (positive result), the infant will probably not suffer respiratory distress upon delivery.

Specific cells in the lungs produce chemicals that are essential for respiration immediately after birth. An important part of a newborn baby's breathing is determined by the chemical *surfactant*. A baby born prematurely may not have surfactant in its lungs. Surfactant can be introduced directly into the lungs of the newborn to prevent respiratory-distress syndrome. The chemical is available for immediate use by the baby. Many premature babies who receive surfactant do not have to be put on respirators—they can breathe on their own!

Changes in You

You have only 4 to 5 weeks to go until your due date. It's easy to get anxious for your baby to be delivered. However, don't ask your doctor/midwife to induce labour at this point.

You may have gained 11.25 to 13.5 kg (25 to 30 lb), and you still have a month to go. It isn't unusual for your weight to stay the same at each of your weekly visits after this point.

The maximum amount of amniotic fluid surrounds the baby now. In the weeks to come, the baby continues to grow. However, some amniotic fluid is reabsorbed by your body, which decreases the amount of fluid around the baby and decreases the amount of room in which the baby has to move. You may notice a difference in sensation of foetal movements. For some women, it feels as if the baby is not moving as much as it had been.

↪ *What Is Labour?*

It is important to understand a little about the labour process. Then you'll be more informed when labour occurs, and you'll know what to do when it begins. What causes labour? Why does it happen?

Unfortunately, we don't have good answers to these questions. The factors that cause labour to begin are still unknown. There are many theories as to why labour happens when it does. One theory is that hormones made by the mother and foetus together trigger labour. Or it could be that the foetus produces some hormone that causes the uterus to contract.

Labour is defined as the dilatation (stretching and thinning) of your cervix. This occurs because the uterus, which is a muscle, contracts (tightens) and relaxes to squeeze out its contents (the baby). As the baby is pushed out, the cervix stretches.

At various times, you may feel tightening, contractions or cramps, but it isn't actually labour until there is a *change in the cervix*. As you can see from the discussion that begins on the next page, there are many aspects to labour. You'll go through them all as you deliver your baby.

Three Stages of Labour. There are three distinct stages of labour.

Stage one—The first stage of labour begins with uterine contractions of great enough intensity, duration and frequency to cause thinning (effacement) and opening (dilatation) of the cervix. The first stage of labour ends when the cervix is fully dilated (usually 10 cm) and sufficiently open to allow the baby's head to come through it.

Stage two—The second stage of labour begins when the cervix is completely dilated at 10 cm. This stage ends with the delivery of the baby.

Stage three—The third stage of labour begins after delivery of the baby. It ends with delivery of the placenta and the membranes that have surrounded the foetus.

Some doctors have even described a 4th stage of labour, referring to a time period after delivery of the placenta during which the uterus contracts. Contraction of the uterus is important in controlling bleeding that can occur after delivery of the baby and the placenta.

How Long Will Labour Last? The length of the first and second stages of labour, from the beginning of cervical dilatation to delivery of the baby, can last 14 to 15 hours or more in a first pregnancy. Women have had faster labours than this, but don't count on it.

A woman who has already had one or two children will probably have a shorter labour, but don't count on that either! The average time for labour is usually decreased by a few hours for a second or third delivery.

Everyone's heard of women who barely make it to the hospital or had a 1-hour labour. For every one of those patients, there are many women who have laboured 18, 20, 24 hours or longer.

It's almost impossible to predict the amount of time that will be required for labour. You may ask your doctor about it, but his or her answer is only a guess.

Dad Tip Pack for yourself, too! Some essential items you might need include magazines, phone numbers, a change of clothes and something to sleep in, a camera, film, new battery, snacks, a phone card or lots of change, a comfortable pillow and extra cash.

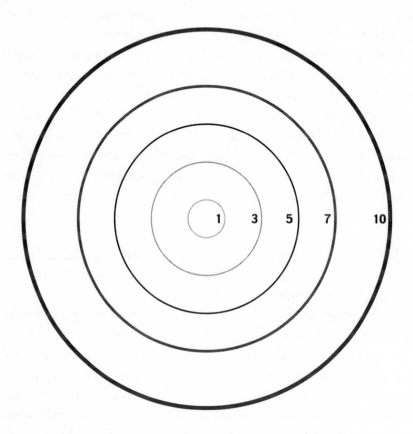

Cervical dilatation in centimetres (shown actual size).

Your Nutrition

You're getting close to the end of your pregnancy. You may be having a harder time with your food plan than you had earlier in your pregnancy. You may be bored with the foods you've been eating. Your baby is getting larger, and you don't seem to have as much room for food. Heartburn or indigestion may also be problems now.

Don't give up on good nutrition! It's important to continue to pay attention to what you eat. Be vigilant so you continue to provide your baby the best nutrition it needs before its birth.

Every day, try to eat one serving of a dark-green leafy vegetable, a serving of food or juice rich in vitamin C, and one serving of a food rich in vitamin A (many foods that are yellow, such as yams, carrots and cantaloupes, are good sources of vitamin A). Remember to keep up your fluid intake.

You Should Also Know

∾ *How Is Your Baby Presenting?*

At what point in your pregnancy can your doctor/midwife tell how baby is presenting for delivery—for example, if the baby's head is down or if the baby is breech? At what point will the baby stay in the position it is in?

Usually between 32 and 34 weeks of pregnancy, you can feel the baby's head in the lower abdomen below your umbilicus. Some women can feel different parts of the baby earlier than this. But the baby's head may not be hard enough yet to identify as the head.

The head gradually becomes harder as calcium is deposited in the foetal skull. Your baby's head has a distinct feeling. It is different from the feeling your doctor gets with a breech. A breech position has a soft, round feeling.

Beginning at 32 to 34 weeks, your doctor/midwife will probably feel your abdomen to determine how the baby is lying inside you. This position may have changed many times during pregnancy.

At 34 to 36 weeks of pregnancy, the baby usually gets into the position it's going to stay in. If you have a breech at 37 weeks, it's possible

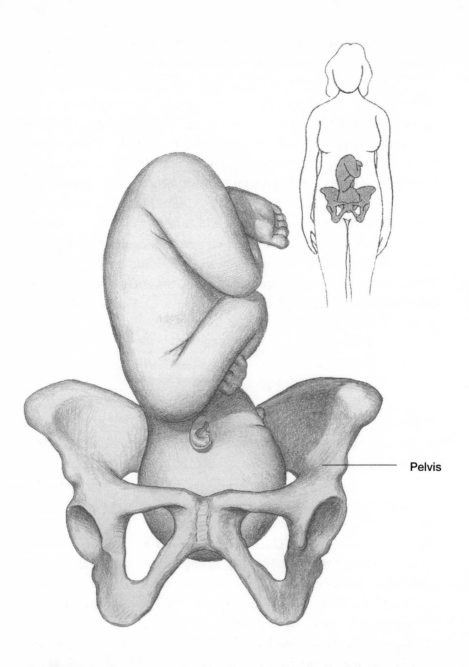

Pelvis

Alignment of baby with head in pelvis before delivery. This is the preferable presentation.

the baby can still turn to be head-down. But it becomes less likely the closer you get to the end of your pregnancy.

∿ Packing for the Hospital

Packing for the hospital can be unnerving. You don't want to pack too early and have your suitcase staring at you. But you don't want to wait till the last minute, throw your things together and take the chance of forgetting something important.

It's probably a good idea to pack about 3 or 4 weeks before your due date. Pack things you'll need during labour for you and your partner, items you and the baby will need after delivery and personal articles for your hospital stay.

There are a lot of things to consider, but the list below should cover nearly all of what you might need:

- hospital notes
- heavy socks to wear in the delivery room
- an item to use as a focal point
- 1 cotton nightgown or T-shirt for labour
- lip balm, lollipops or fruit drops, to use during labour
- light diversion, such as books or magazines, to use during labour
- breath spray
- 1 or 2 nightgowns for after labour (bring a nursing gown if you're going to breastfeed)
- slippers with rubber soles
- 1 long robe for walking in the halls
- 2 bras (nursing bras and pads if you breastfeed)
- 3 pairs of panties
- toiletries you use, including brush, comb, toothbrush, toothpaste, soap, shampoo, conditioner
- hairband or ponytail holder, if you have long hair
- loose-fitting clothes for going home
- sanitary pads, if the hospital doesn't supply them
- glasses, if you wear contacts (you can't wear contacts during labour)

You may also want to bring one or two pieces of fruit to eat after the delivery. Don't pack them too early!

It's also a good idea to include some things in your hospital kit for your partner to help you both during the birth. You might bring the following:

- a watch with a second hand
- talc or cornflour for massaging you during labour
- a paint roller or tennis ball for giving you a low-back massage during labour
- tapes or CDs and a player, or a radio to play during labour
- camera and film
- list of telephone numbers and phone card
- change for telephones and vending machines
- snacks for your partner

The hospital will probably supply most of what you need for your baby, but you should have a few things:

- clothes for the trip home, including a vest, stretch suit, outer clothes (a hat if it's cold outside)
- a couple of baby blankets
- nappies, if your hospital doesn't supply them

Be sure you have an approved infant car seat in which to take your baby home. It's important to start your baby in a car seat the very first time he or she rides in a car! Many hospitals will not let you take your baby home without one.

Week 37

Age of Foetus—35 Weeks

How Big Is Your Baby?

Your baby weighs almost 2.95 kg (6½ lb). Crown-to-rump length is 35 cm (14 in). Its total length is around 47 cm (21 in).

How Big Are You?

Your uterus may stay the same size as measured in the last week or two. Measuring from the pubic symphysis, the top of the uterus is about 37 cm (14¾ in). From the bellybutton, it is 16 to 17 cm (6½ to 6¾ in). Your total weight gain by this time should be about as high as it will go at 11.3 to 15.9 kg (25 to 35 lb).

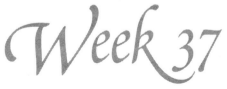 *Dad Tip* Let your partner know how she can reach you at work or when you're out. You may not understand how nervous she can be about getting in touch with you when she needs you. Carry a mobile phone or a pager with you all the time. This can comfort her and provide her with peace of mind.

How Your Baby Is
Growing and Developing

Is Your Baby's Head Down in Your Pelvis?

Your baby is continuing to grow and to gain weight, even during these last few weeks of pregnancy. As discussed in Week 36, the baby's head is usually directed down into the pelvis around this time. However, in about 3 per cent of all pregnancies, the baby's bottom or legs come into the pelvis first. This is called a *breech presentation*, which we discuss in Week 38.

Changes in You

ᴄᴦ *Pelvic Exam in Late Pregnancy*

About this time in your pregnancy, your doctor/midwife may do a pelvic exam. This pelvic exam helps your doctor/midwife evaluate the progress of your pregnancy. One of the first things he or she will observe is whether you are leaking amniotic fluid. If you think you are, it's important to tell your doctor.

Your doctor will examine your cervix during the pelvic exam. During labour, the cervix usually becomes softer and thins out. This process is called *effacement*. Your doctor/midwife will evaluate the cervix for its softness or firmness and the amount of thinning.

Before labour begins, the cervix is thick and is '0 per cent effaced.' When you're in active labour, the cervix thins out; when it is half-thinned, it is '50 per cent effaced.' Immediately before delivery, the cervix is '100 per cent effaced' or 'completely thinned out.'

The dilatation (amount of opening) of the cervix is also important. This is usually measured in centimetres. The cervix is fully open when the diameter of the cervical opening measures 10 cm. The goal is to be a 10! Before labour begins, the cervix may be closed. Or it may be open a little way, such as 1 cm (nearly ½ in). Labour is the stretching and opening of the cervix so the baby fits through it and can pass out of the uterus.

Your doctor also evaluates whether the baby's head, bottom or legs are coming first. (He or she may refer to a 'presenting part.') The shape of your pelvic bones is also noted.

The station is then determined. Station describes the degree to which the presenting part of the baby has descended into the birth canal. If the baby's head is at a -2 station, it means the head is higher inside you than if it were at a +2 station. The 0 point is a bony landmark in the pelvis, the starting place of the birth canal.

Think of the birth canal as a tube going from the pelvic girdle down through the pelvis and out the vagina. The baby travels through this tube from the uterus. It's possible that you may dilate during labour but the baby doesn't move down through the pelvis. In this case, a C-section may be needed because the baby's head doesn't fit through the pelvic girdle.

Information Your Doctor/Midwife Learns. When your doctor/midwife examines you, he or she may describe your situation in medical terms. You might hear you are '2 cm, 50 per cent and a -2 station.' This means the cervix is open 2 cm (about 1 in), it is halfway thinned out (50 per cent effaced) and the presenting part (baby's head, feet or buttocks) is at a -2 station.

Try to remember this information. It's helpful when you go to the hospital and are checked there. You can tell the medical personnel in labour and delivery what your dilatation and effacement were at your last checkup so they can know if your situation has changed.

How Your Actions Affect Your Baby's Development

✄ *Caesarean Delivery*

Most women plan on a normal vaginal birth, but a Caesarean delivery is always a possibility. With a Caesarean, the baby is delivered through an incision made in the mother's abdominal wall and uterus. The illustration on page 367 shows a Caesarean delivery. Common names for this type of surgery are *C-section, Caesarean section* and *Caesarean delivery*.

Reasons for a C-Section. C-sections are done for many reasons. The most common reason for having a C-section is a previous Caesarean delivery. However, some women who have had C-sections can have a vaginal delivery with later pregnancies; this is called *vaginal birth after Caesarean (VBAC)*. See the discussion that begins on page 370. Discuss the matter with your doctor/midwife if you've had a C-section and believe you would like to attempt a vaginal delivery this time.

A Caesarean delivery may be necessary if your baby is too big to fit through the birth canal. This condition is called *cephalo-pelvic disproportion (CPD)*. CPD may be suspected during pregnancy, but usually labour must begin before it can be confirmed. A C-section may be recommended if an ultrasound shows your baby is very large—4.5 kg (9 lb 14 oz) or larger—and may not be easily delivered vaginally.

Foetal distress is another reason for a Caesarean section. Doctors use foetal monitors during labour to watch the foetal heartbeat and its response to labour. If the heartbeat indicates the baby is having trouble with labour contractions, a C-section may be necessary for the baby's well-being.

If the umbilical cord is compressed, a C-section may be necessary. The cord may come into the vagina ahead of the baby's head or the baby can press on part of the cord. This is a dangerous situation because a compressed umbilical cord can cut off the blood supply to the baby.

A C-section is usually necessary if the baby is in a breech presentation, which means the baby's feet or buttocks enter the birth canal first. Delivering the shoulders and the head after the baby's body may damage the baby's head or neck, especially with a first baby.

Placental abruption or placenta previa are also reasons for a Caesarean delivery. If the placenta separates from the uterus before delivery (placental abruption), the baby loses its supply of oxygen and nutrients. This is usually diagnosed when a woman has heavy vaginal bleeding. If the placenta blocks the birth canal (placenta previa), the baby cannot be delivered any other way.

Rising Rate of Caesarean Deliveries. In the 1950s, only 5 per cent of all deliveries were by C-section. In 1970, the rate had risen to 11 per cent.

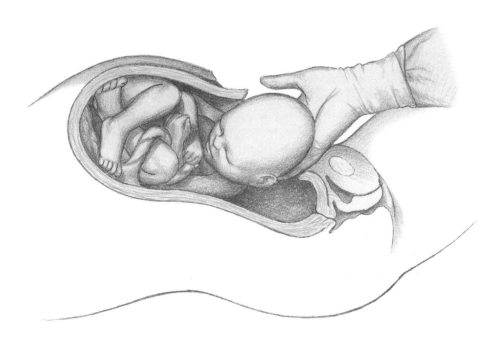

Delivery of a baby by Caesarean section.

Today, in the UK, Caesarean deliveries account for about 22 per cent of all deliveries. This increase is related in part to more stringent monitoring during labour and safer procedures for C-sections. Another reason for more Caesarean deliveries is bigger babies. With bigger babies, a C-section is sometimes the only way to deliver. Researchers believe this increase in the size of babies is due to pregnant women eating a better diet, not smoking during pregnancy and being older when they deliver.

How Is a C-Section Performed? You are often awake when a C-section is done. An anaesthesiologist usually gives you an epidural or spinal anaesthetic. (Types of anaesthesia are discussed in Week 39.) If you're awake for the procedure, you may be able to see your baby immediately after delivery!

With a C-section, an incision is made through the skin of the abdominal wall to the uterus. The wall of the uterus is cut, then the amniotic sac containing the baby and placenta is cut. The baby is removed through the incision. Next, the placenta is removed. The uterus is closed in layers with sutures that absorb and do not have to be removed. The remainder of the abdomen is sewn together with absorbable sutures.

Most Caesarean deliveries done today are *low-cervical* Caesareans or *low-transverse* Caesareans. This means the incision is made low in the uterus.

In the past, a Caesarean was often done with a classical incision, in which the uterus is cut down the midline. This incision doesn't heal as well as a low-cervical incision. Because the incision is made in the muscular part of the uterus, it is more likely to pull apart with contractions (as in a vaginal birth after Caesarean). This can cause heavy bleeding and injure the baby. If you have had a classical Caesarean section in the past, you *must* have a C-section every time you have a baby.

A T-incision is another type of C-section incision. This incision goes across and up the uterus in the shape of an inverted T. It provides more room to get the baby out. If you have had this type of incision, you will need to have a Caesarean delivery with all subsequent pregnancies. It too is more likely to rupture than other types of incisions.

Advantages and Disadvantages of Having a C-Section. There are advantages to having a C-section. The most important advantage is delivery of a healthy infant. The baby you are carrying may be too large to fit through your pelvis. The only safe method of delivery might be a C-section. Usually a woman needs to experience labour before her doctor will know if the baby will fit. It may be impossible to predict ahead of time.

The disadvantage is that a Caesarean section is a major operation and carries with it all the risks of surgery. Risks include infection, bleeding, shock due to blood loss and the possibility of blood clots and injury to other organs, such as the bladder or rectum.

Will You Need a Caesarean? It would be nice to know you're going to need a C-section before delivery so you wouldn't have to go through labour. Unfortunately, it's usually necessary to wait for labour contractions for a couple of reasons. You won't know ahead of time if your baby will be stressed by labour contractions. And it is often hard to predict if the baby will fit through your birth canal.

Some women believe that if they have a Caesarean, 'it won't be like having a baby.' They falsely believe they won't experience the entire birth process. That's not true. If you deliver by C-section, try not to feel this way. You haven't failed in any way!

Remember, having a baby has taken 9 long months. Even with a Caesarean delivery, you have accomplished an amazing feat.

After Your Caesarean Delivery. After a C-section, you can hold the baby and perhaps even nurse. You may need pain relief for the incision. A new drug-pump system to deliver pain relief is available that may help you feel better without side effects for baby. Called the *ON-Q*, it sends a local painkiller to the *incision* area to help relieve pain. This system delivers medication to the pain site instead of sending it through your body, so very little, if any, medication can get to your baby through your breast milk. Ask your doctor about it at one of your antenatal visits. As this is a new method of analgesia, it may not be available in your hospital.

You will probably stay in the hospital a couple of days longer than if you had a vaginal delivery, usually about 5 days. In the past, doctors usually recommended a woman have no solid food until 2 days after delivery. Recent research shows that this time can be cut from a few days to a *few hours* after the procedure. Why? In the past, many Caesarean deliveries required general anaesthesia; food is not recommended after general anaesthesia. However, today most C-sections require only regional anaesthesia, so the same rules may not apply.

Recovery at home from a Caesarean section takes longer than recovery from a vaginal delivery. The normal time for full recovery from a C-section is usually 4 to 6 weeks.

↬ Vaginal Birth after Caesarean (VBAC)

Should you attempt a vaginal delivery after having had a C-section? Vaginal birth after Caesarean (VBAC) is becoming more common. Medically speaking, the method of delivery is not as important as the well-being of you and your baby.

Before you and your doctor make a final decision, you need to weigh the risks and the benefits to you and your baby with both types of delivery. In some cases, there may not be any choice in the matter. In other cases, you and your doctor may decide to let you labour for a while to see if you can deliver vaginally.

Some women like having a repeat Caesarean section. They request one because they don't want to go through labour only to end up with a Caesarean delivery anyway.

If you've had a previous C-section and want to try VBAC, you may need another C-section if you have gestational diabetes or other problems. Discuss it with your doctor if you have questions.

Advantages and Risks of VBAC. Advantages of a vaginal delivery include a decreased risk of problems associated with major surgery, which Caesarean birth is. Recovery after a vaginal delivery is shorter. You can be up and about in the hospital and at home in a much shorter amount of time.

If you are small and the baby is large, you may need another C-section. Multiple foetuses may make vaginal delivery difficult or impossible without danger to the babies. Problems, such as high blood pressure or diabetes, may require a repeat C-section.

There is some risk that the internal surgical scar from an earlier C-section could stretch and pull apart, called *uterine rupture,* during subsequent labour and delivery, with serious consequences. Research has shown this is especially true if hormones are used to ripen the cervix and/or induce labour. In one study, it was shown that a woman's risk of uterine rupture increased *15 times* if topical hormones are applied to the cervix to ripen it. Researchers believe the contractions that are produced using this method are too strong for a uterus that is scarred by previous surgery. If an intravenous hormone is used to induced labour, such as oxytocin, the risk of rupture increases *5 times*.

In this case, a repeat C-section may be advised to avoid rupture of the uterus. However, if pregnancy and labour are closely monitored, a woman may be able to have a vaginal delivery.

Risk also increases for a woman who gets pregnant within 9 months of having a previous C-section. In this case, the uterus is *3 times* more likely to rupture during a Caesarean delivery. Researchers believe this might occur because it can take from 6 to 9 months for the uterine scar to heal (this is the scar on the uterus—not your abdomen). Until enough healing time has elapsed, the uterus may not be strong enough to stand up to the stress of a vaginal delivery. VBACs are safest when at least 18 months has passed between the previous C-section and the attempted vaginal delivery.

If you want to attempt VBAC, discuss it with your doctor in advance so plans can be made. During labour, you will probably be monitored more closely with foetal monitors. You may be attached to IVs, in case a Caesarean section becomes necessary.

Consider the benefits and risks in deciding whether to attempt a vaginal delivery after a previous Caesarean section. Discuss advantages and disadvantages at length with your doctor and your partner before making a final decision. Don't be afraid to ask your doctor his or her opinion of your chances for a successful vaginal delivery. He or she knows your health and pregnancy history.

Your Nutrition

You and your partner have been invited to a big party. You've been diligent about your nutrition, and your pregnancy is almost over. Should you let yourself go, and eat and drink whatever you want? It's probably a good idea to maintain your good eating habits. You *can* party healthily. Below are some suggestions to help you have a good time.

Eat food when it's fresh or hot—at the beginning of the party. As the party goes on, the food may not be chilled or heated enough to prevent bacteria from growing. So eat early or when dishes are refilled.

Eat something before you go to take the edge off your appetite. Or drink a large glass of water. It may be easier to avoid high-fat, high-calorie foods if you're not ravenous.

Avoid alcohol. Drink fruit juice 'spiked' with ginger ale or lemon-and-lime soda.

Raw fruits and vegetables can be satisfying. Avoid raw seafood, raw meat and soft cheeses, such as Brie, Camembert and feta. They may contain listeriosis.

Stay away from the refreshment table if you can't resist the goodies. It may feel better to sit down (away from food), relax and talk with friends.

You Should Also Know

✨ *Will You Have an Enema?*
Will you be required to have an enema when you arrive at labour and delivery? An *enema* is a procedure in which fluid is injected into the rectum for the purpose of clearing out the bowel.

Many hospitals offer an enema at the beginning of labour, but it is not always mandatory. However, there are certain advantages to having an enema early in labour. You may not want to have a bowel movement soon after your baby's delivery because of discomfort with an episiotomy. Having an enema before labour can prevent this discomfort.

An enema before labour can also make the birth of your baby a more pleasant experience. When the baby's head comes out through the birth canal, anything in the rectum comes out, too. An

Tip for Week 37 Be prepared for delivery with bags packed, hospital notes ready and available, and other important details taken care of.

enema decreases the amount of contamination by bowel movement during labour and at the time of delivery. This can also help prevent possible infection.

Ask your doctor/midwife if an enema is routine or considered helpful. Tell him or her you'd like to know about the benefits of an enema and the reason for giving one. It isn't required by all hospitals.

✂ *What Is Back Labour?*

Some women experience back labour. Back labour refers to a baby that is coming through the birth canal looking straight up. With this type of labour, you will probably experience lower-back pain.

The mechanics of labour work better if the baby is looking down at the ground so it can extend its head as it comes out through the birth canal. If the baby can't extend its head, its chin points towards its chest. This can cause pain in your lower back during labour.

This type of labour can also last longer. Your doctor may need to rotate the baby so it comes out looking down at the ground rather than up at the sky.

It may be difficult at times to tell the exact location of different parts of the baby. You may have a good idea according to where you feel kicks and punches. Ask your doctor to show you on your tummy how the baby is lying. Some doctors will take a marking pen and draw on your stomach to show you how the baby is lying. You can leave it so you can show your partner how your baby was lying when you were seen in the surgery that day.

✁ *Will Your Doctor Use Forceps or a Vacuum Extractor?*

The use of forceps—metal instruments used in the delivery of babies—has decreased in recent years for a couple of reasons. One reason is the more frequent use of Caesarean delivery to deliver a baby that might be high up in the pelvis. A C-section may be much safer than a forceps delivery for the baby if it's not close to delivering on its own.

Another reason for the decrease in the use of forceps is the use of a *vacuum extractor (ventouse)*. There are two types of vacuum extractors. One has a plastic cup that fits on the baby's head by suction. The other has a metal cup that fits on baby's head. The doctor is able to pull on the vacuum cup to deliver baby's head and body.

The goal with every birth is to deliver the baby as safely as possible. If a large amount of traction with forceps is needed to deliver the baby, a Caesarean section might be a better choice.

If the possible use of a vacuum extractor or forceps causes you concern, discuss it with your doctor/midwife. It's important to establish good communication with your doctor/midwife so you can communicate before and during labour about these concerns.

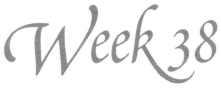

Week 38

Age of Foetus—36 Weeks

How Big Is Your Baby?

At this time, your baby weighs about 3.1 kg (6¾ lb). Crown-to-rump length hasn't changed much; it's still about 35 cm (14 in). Total length is around 47 cm (21 in).

How Big Are You?

Many women don't grow larger during the last several weeks of pregnancy, but they feel very uncomfortable. The distance between your uterus and the pubic symphysis is about 36 to 38 cm (14½ to 15¼ in). From your bellybutton to the top of your uterus is about 16 to 18 cm (6½ to 7¼ in).

How Your Baby Is Growing and Developing

✕ Foetal Monitoring during Labour

You may wonder how your doctor/midwife can tell your baby is all right, especially during labour. In many hospitals, the baby's heart rate is monitored throughout labour. Being able to detect problems early is important so they can be resolved.

Every time the uterus contracts during labour, less oxygenated blood flows from you to the placenta. Most babies are able to handle this stress without any problem. However, some babies are affected; this is called *foetal stress* or *foetal distress*.

There are two ways to monitor the baby's heartbeat during labour. *External foetal monitoring* can be used before your membranes rupture. A belt with a receiver is strapped to your abdomen. It uses a principle similar to ultrasound to detect the baby's heartbeat.

An *internal foetal monitor* monitors the baby's heartbeat more precisely. An electrode is placed on the baby's scalp and is connected by wires to a machine that records the foetal heart rate. Only women whose membranes are broken and who are dilated at least 1 cm can be attached to an internal foetal monitor.

Foetal Blood Sampling. Doctors can also test your baby's blood pH to see how well baby is tolerating the stress of labour. Before this test can be done, your membranes must be ruptured, and you must be dilated at least 2 cm .

An instrument is applied to the scalp of the baby to make a small nick in the skin. The baby's blood is collected in a small tube or pipette, and the pH (acidity) is checked. If the baby is having trouble with labour and is under stress, the pH level can help determine this. This test may be useful in making a decision as to whether labour can continue or if a C-section needs to be done.

Changes in You

↭ *Postnatal Depression*

After your baby is born, you may feel very emotional. You may even wonder if having a baby was a good idea. This is called the 'baby blues.' Most women experience some degree of postnatal emotional problems, and many experts consider some degree of baby blues to be normal.

Up to 80 per cent of all women have 'baby blues.' See the discussion below. It usually appears between 2 days and 2 weeks after the baby is born. Baby blues are temporary and usually leave as quickly as they come.

However, symptoms of *postnatal depression (PND),* which affects about 10 per cent of all mothers, may not appear until several months *after* delivery. They may occur when the woman starts getting her period again and experiences hormonal changes.

Postnatal depression can resolve on its own, but it can often take as long as a year. With more severe problems, treatment may relieve symptoms in a matter of weeks, and improvement should be significant within 6 to 8 months. Often medication is necessary for complete recovery.

Different Degrees of Depression. The mildest form of postnatal distress is *baby blues.* This situation lasts only a couple of weeks, and symptoms do not worsen. See ways to handle baby blues on page 378.

A more serious version of postnatal distress is called *postnatal depression (PND).* The difference between baby blues and postnatal depression lies in the frequency, intensity and duration of the symptoms. PND can occur from 2 weeks to 1 year after the birth. A mother may have feelings of anger, confusion, panic and hopelessness. She may experience changes in her eating and sleeping patterns. She may fear she will hurt her baby or feel as if she is going crazy. Anxiety is one of the major symptoms of PND.

The most serious form of postnatal depression is *puerperal psychosis* and affects about 1 in 1,000 mothers. The woman may have hallucinations, think about suicide or try to harm the baby. Many women who develop puerperal psychosis also exhibit signs of bipolar mood disorder, which is unrelated to childbirth. Discuss this situation with your doctor if you are concerned.

After you give birth, if you believe you are suffering from some form of postnatal depression, contact your doctor. Every postnatal reaction, whether mild or severe, is usually temporary and treatable.

In addition, if after 2 weeks of motherhood you are just as exhausted as you were shortly after you delivered, you may be at risk of developing postnatal depression. It's normal to feel extremely tired, especially after the hard work of labour and delivery and adjusting to the demands of being a new mum. However, if your exhaustion doesn't get better within 2 weeks, contact your GP/health visitor.

Causes of Postnatal Depression. A new mother must make many adjustments, and many demands are placed on her. Either or both of these situations may cause distress. We aren't sure what causes postnatal depression; not every woman experiences it. We believe a woman's individual sensitivity to hormonal changes may be part of the cause; the drop in oestrogen and progesterone after delivery may contribute to postnatal depression.

Other possible factors include a family history of depression, lack of familial support after the birth, isolation and chronic fatigue. You may also be at higher risk of suffering from postnatal depression (PND) if:

- your mother or sister suffered from the problem—it seems to run in families
- you suffered from PND with a previous pregnancy—chances are you'll have the problem again
- you had fertility treatments to achieve this pregnancy—hormone fluctuations may be more severe, which may cause PND
- you suffered extreme PMS before the pregnancy—hormonal imbalances may be greater after the birth
- you have a personal history of depression
- you have experienced any major life changes recently—you may experience a hormonal drop as a result

Handling the Baby Blues. One of the most important ways you can help yourself handle baby blues is to have a good support system near at hand. Ask family members and friends to help. Ask your mother or mother-in-law to stay for a while. Ask your partner to take some work leave, or hire someone to come in and help each day.

There are other things you can do to help relieve the symptoms. You might want to try any or all of the following.

- Rest when your baby sleeps.
- Find other mothers who are in the same situation; it helps to share your feelings and experiences.
- Don't try to be perfect.
- Pamper yourself.
- Do some form of moderate exercise every day.
- Eat nutritiously, and drink plenty of fluids.
- Go out every day.

Talk to your doctor about using antidepressants if the above steps don't work for you. Over a period of time, these will bring about a gentle and gradual improvement, so it's important to keep taking your medication even after you start feeling better.

Dealing with the More Serious Forms of PND. Beyond the relatively minor symptoms of baby blues, postnatal depression can be evidenced in two ways. Some women experience acute depression that can last for weeks or months; they cannot sleep or eat, they feel worthless and isolated, they are sad and they cry a great deal. For other women, they are extremely anxious, restless and agitated. Their heart rate increases. Some unfortunate women experience both sets of symptoms at the same time.

If you experience any of these symptoms, call your doctor/health visitor immediately. He or she will probably prescribe a course of treatment for you. Do it for you and your family.

How Your Actions Affect Your Baby's Development

ᔑ *Breech Presentation*

As we've mentioned already, it's common for your baby to be in the breech presentation early in pregnancy. However, when labour starts, only 3 to 5 per cent of all babies, not including multiple pregnancies, present as a breech. Do your actions determine how your baby presents?

Certain factors make a breech presentation more likely. One of the main causes is the baby's prematurity. Near the end of the second trimester, a baby may be in a breech presentation. By taking care of yourself, you may avoid going into premature labour. That gives your baby the best opportunity to change its position naturally.

Although we don't always know why a baby is in the breech position, we know breech births occur more often when:

- you have had more than one pregnancy
- you are carrying twins, triplets or more
- there is too much or too little amniotic fluid
- the uterus is shaped abnormally
- you have abnormal uterine growths, such as fibroids
- you have placenta previa
- your baby has hydrocephalus

There are different kinds of breech presentations. A *frank breech* occurs when the legs are flexed at the hips and extended at the knees. This is the most common type of breech found at term or the end of pregnancy; feet are up by the face or head.

Tip for Week 38 If your doctor suspects your baby is in a breech position, he or she may order an ultrasound to confirm it. It helps identify how the baby is lying in your uterus.

With a *complete breech presentation,* one or both knees are flexed, not extended. See the illustration on page 381.

Delivering a Breech Baby. There is some controversy in obstetrics over the best method of delivering a breech baby. For many years, breech deliveries were performed vaginally. Then it was believed the safest method was to deliver the baby by C-section, especially if it was a first baby. Today, most doctors believe a baby in the breech position can probably be delivered more safely by a Cesarean section performed during early labour or before labour begins.

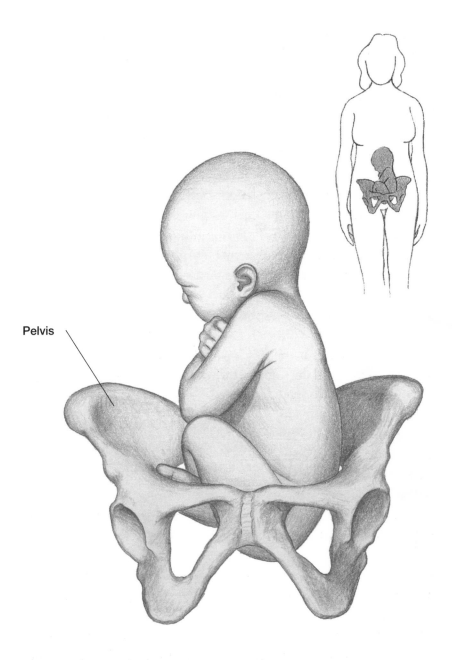

Pelvis

Baby aligned in the pelvis bottom first, with knees flexed, is called a *complete breech presentation*.

Some doctors believe a woman can deliver a breech without difficulty if the situation is right. This usually includes a frank breech in a mature foetus of a woman who has had previous normal deliveries. Most agree a *footling breech presentation* (one leg extended, one knee flexed) should be delivered by Caesarean section.

If your baby is breech, it's important to discuss it with your doctor. When you get to the hospital, tell the midwives and hospital personnel you have a breech presentation. If you call with a question about labour and you have a breech presentation, mention this information to the person you talk with.

Turning Your Baby. Attempts may be made to turn the baby from a breech to a head-down (vertex) presentation before your waters break, before labour begins or in early labour. Using his or her hands, the doctor manually attempts to turn the baby into the head-down birth position. This procedure is called *external cephalic version (ECV)* or just *version*.

Problems can occur with ECV, and it's important to know about them. Talk with your doctor about whether this procedure is an option for you. Possible risks include:

- rupture of membranes
- placental abruption
- affect on baby's heart rate
- onset of labour

More than 50 per cent of the time, a doctor is successful in turning the baby. However, some stubborn babies shift again into a breech presentation. ECV may be tried again, but version is harder to perform as your delivery date draws closer.

Other Types of Abnormal Presentations. Another unusual presentation is a *face presentation*. The baby's head is hyperextended so the face comes into the birth canal first. This type of presentation is most often delivered by C-section if it does not convert to a regular presentation during labour.

In a *shoulder presentation*, the shoulder presents first. In a *transverse lie*, the baby is lying almost as if in a cradle in the pelvis. The baby's head is on one side of your abdomen, and its bottom is on the other side. There is only one way to deliver these types of presentation, and that is by Caesarean section.

Ðad Tip Ask your partner if there are things she would like you to bring to the hospital for her, such as special tapes or CDs and a player for the music. Discuss it ahead of time, and have things ready. If you take a tour of the hospital or birthing centre, you might get other ideas of things you can do to help control the environment your new baby enters.

Your Nutrition

You may not feel much like eating about this time, but it's important to keep eating a healthy diet. Snacks might be the answer. Instead of eating large meals, eat small snacks throughout the day to keep your energy levels up and to help avoid heartburn. You may be tired of the foods you've been eating. The list below offers some smart snacks for your healthy nutrition:

- bananas, raisins, dried fruit and mangoes to satisfy your sweet tooth and to provide you with iron, potassium and magnesium
- fruit shakes made with skimmed milk and yoghurt, ice cream for calcium, vitamins and minerals
- crackers that are high in fibre; spread with a little peanut butter for taste and protein
- cottage cheese and fruit, flavoured with a little sugar and some cinnamon, for tasty milk and fruit servings
- salt-free crisps or tortillas with salsa or bean dip for fibre and good taste
- hummus and pitta slices for fibre and good taste

- fresh tomatoes, flavoured with some olive oil and fresh basil; eat with a few thin slices of Parmesan cheese for a vegetable serving and dairy serving
- chicken or tuna salad (made from fresh chicken or tuna packed in brine) and crackers or tortilla pieces for protein and fibre

You Should Also Know

∽ *What Is a Retained Placenta?*

In most instances, the placenta is delivered within 30 minutes after the birth of your baby and is a routine part of the delivery. In some cases, a piece of placenta remains inside the uterus and does not deliver spontaneously. When this happens, the uterus cannot contract adequately, resulting in vaginal bleeding that can be heavy.

In other cases, the placenta does not separate because it's still attached to the wall of the uterus. This can be a very serious situation. However, this complication is rare.

Bleeding is usually severe after delivery, and surgery may be necessary to stop it. An attempt may be made to remove the placenta by D&C.

Reasons for an abnormally adherent placenta are many. It is believed a placenta may attach over a previous Caesarean-section scar or other previous incisions on the uterus. The placenta may attach over an area that has been scraped, such as with a D&C, or over an area of the uterus that was infected at one time.

Your doctor/midwife will pay attention to the delivery of your placenta while you are paying attention to your baby. Some people ask to see the placenta after delivery; you may wish to have your doctor show it to you.

∽ *Will You Need to Be Shaved?*

Many women want to know if they have to have their pubic hair shaved before the birth of their baby. It is not a requirement any longer. Many women are not shaved these days. However, some women who chose not to have their pubic hair shaved later said they experienced discomfort when their pubic hair became entangled in their underwear due to the normal vaginal discharge after the birth of their baby. So you might want to think about this procedure, and discuss it with your doctor/midwife.

Week 39

Age of Foetus—37 Weeks

How Big Is Your Baby?

Your baby weighs a little more than 3.25 kg (7 lb). By this point in your pregnancy, crown-to-rump length is about 36 cm (14½ in). The baby's total length is close to 48 cm (21½ in).

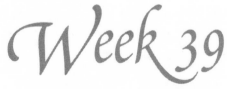

Tip for Week 39 Don't take tags off gifts until after your baby is born. You may need to exchange the gift if its size, colour or 'sex' isn't correct.

How Big Are You?

The illustration on page 388 shows a side view of a woman with a large uterus and her baby inside it. She's about as big as she can get. You probably are, too!

If you measure from the pubic symphysis to the top of the uterus, the distance is 36 to 40 cm (14½ to 16 in). Measuring from the belly-button, the distance is about 16 to 20 cm (6½ to 8 in).

You're almost at the end of your pregnancy. Your weight should not increase much from this point. It should remain between 11.3 and 15.9 kg (25 and 35 lb) until delivery.

How Your Baby Is
Growing and Developing

Your baby continues to gain weight, even up to the last week or two of pregnancy. It doesn't have much room to move inside your uterus. At this point, all the organ systems are developed and in place. The last organ to mature is the lungs.

ᔰ *Can Your Baby Get Tangled in the Cord?*

You may have been told by friends not to raise your arms over your head or reach high to get things because it can cause the cord to wrap around the baby's neck. There doesn't seem to be any truth to this old wives' tale.

Some babies do get tangled in their umbilical cord and can get the cord tied in a knot or wrapped around their neck. However, nothing you do during pregnancy causes or prevents this from happening.

A tangled umbilical cord isn't necessarily a problem during labour. It only becomes a problem if the cord is stretched tight around the baby's neck or is in a knot.

Changes in You

It would be unusual for you *not* to be uncomfortable and feel huge at this time. Your uterus has filled your pelvis and most of your abdomen. It has pushed everything else out of the way.

At this point in pregnancy, you may think you'll never want to be pregnant again because you're so uncomfortable. Or you may be sure your family is complete. At this point, some women consider permanent sterilization, such as tubal ligation.

ᔰ *Tubal Ligation after Delivery?*

Some women choose to have a tubal ligation done while they are in the hospital after having their baby. Now is not the time to make the

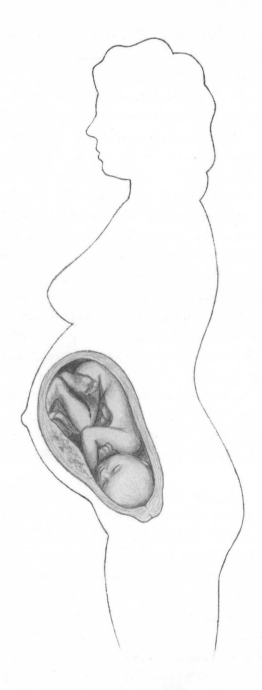

Comparative size of the uterus at 39 weeks of pregnancy (foetal age—
37 weeks) with a baby that is close to full term.

decision about having a tubal ligation if you haven't seriously considered it before.

Being sterilized following delivery of a baby has some advantages. You're in the hospital and won't need another hospitalization. However, there are disadvantages to having a sterilization at this time. Consider the procedure permanent and not reversible. If you have your tubes tied within a few hours or a day after having your baby, then change your mind, you may regret the tubal ligation.

If you have an epidural, it's possible to use the epidural as anaesthesia for a tubal ligation. If you didn't have an epidural, it may be necessary to anesthetize you. This is often done the morning after you've had your baby. This doesn't usually lengthen the time you're in the hospital.

Different kinds of procedures are performed for permanent sterilization. Most common is a small incision underneath your bellybutton. The Fallopian tubes can be seen through this incision.

A piece of the tube can be removed, or a ring or clip can be placed on the tube to block it. This type of surgery usually requires 30 to 45 minutes to perform.

If you have second thoughts or are unsure about having it done, don't have the surgery. Tubal ligations can be reversed, but require a hospital stay of 3 to 4 days. Reversals are about 50 per cent effective, but pregnancy cannot be guaranteed.

How Your Actions Affect Your Baby's Development

↛ *Is Breastfeeding Right for You and Your Baby?*
The discussion on the following pages actually concerns your actions *after* your baby is born—whether you breastfeed your baby. Your decision about breastfeeding is a personal one. One of the more compelling reasons to breastfeed is the bonding that occurs between mother and baby. This close relationship can begin as soon as the baby is born—some women breastfeed on the delivery table. It helps stimulate uterine contractions, which can prevent haemorrhage.

Breastfeeding encourages the natural intimacy of a newborn baby with its mother and the mother with her baby. The opportunity to breastfeed may be a relaxing time for you. It may give you a chance to spend some wonderful time with your new baby. However, if it doesn't work out, it's all right to stop and switch to formula.

Benefits of Breastfeeding. Both you and your baby benefit if you breastfeed. Mother's milk is good for your baby because it contains all the nutrients your baby needs during the first months of life. Commercial formulas have good mixtures of vitamins, protein, sugar, fat and minerals, but none can match your breast milk.

Another advantage of breastfeeding is you pass protection against infection (through antibodies) to your baby in your breast milk. Many people believe a breastfed baby is less likely to get colds and infections than a bottlefed baby.

Breastfeeding is also good for the baby because he or she will probably have to nurse more vigorously than is necessary with some bottle teats. This encourages good tooth and jaw development. Breastfeeding may also help prevent SIDS (sudden infant death syndrome). One study showed that babies breastfed exclusively for 4 months or longer had a lower SIDS rate than babies who were breastfed for less than a month.

Nursing your baby may also protect him or her from high cholesterol levels in adulthood. Although a breastfed baby may have higher cholesterol levels as an infant, studies show that as an adult, cholesterol levels may be lower than those for other adults. In addition, one study reported breastfeeding may have positive effects on adult intelligence—your baby may be smarter as an adult if he or she is breastfed for at least 7 months.

Researchers have found an important reason to breastfeed your baby if he or she is born prematurely. A great deal of a premature baby's protection from infections comes from your breast milk. In America recently, outbreaks of an infection called *E. sakazakii* have been found in neonatal intensive care units and have been associated with milk-based powdered formulas. Based on these findings, it is recommended that powdered infant formulas *not* be used for premature babies.

Another plus for breastfeeding—it's ecologically a better choice for the world! Producing infant formulas uses our resources, and the packaging of formulas adds greatly to our landfills.

Advantages for you include decreased cost as compared to buying formula. It's convenient to breastfeed; you don't have to carry bottles and formula with you for baby. Some women find breastfeeding makes it easier for them to regain their figure.

You may have noticed during pregnancy that your breasts have got larger and were probably tender at times. This happens because increased hormonal activity makes the alveoli in the breasts get larger. Milk in the breast is stored in small sacs of these alveoli.

Colostrum is the first milk that comes from the breasts. Regular breast milk usually arrives 2 or 3 days after delivery. Its arrival is initiated by stimulation from the baby suckling at your breast. The sucking sends a message to your brain to produce prolactin, a hormone that stimulates milk production in the alveoli.

Learning to Breastfeed. You may want to learn how to breastfeed while you're in the hospital. Ask the nurses to show you some of the tricks they've learned to help your baby catch on to it. Ask them any questions you have. What you learn may make the difference in keeping your baby happy with breastfeeding.

Breastfeeding requires a healthful nutrition plan for you, similar to the one you followed during pregnancy. You'll need at least 500 extra calories each day (compared to the extra 300 during pregnancy). Some doctors recommend you continue taking your prenatal vitamins after pregnancy, while you are nursing.

Be careful about what you eat and drink because things you eat can pass into your breast milk. Certain foods may not 'sit' well with you or your baby. Spicy foods and chocolate you eat may cause an upset stomach in your baby! Caffeine can also pass to your baby. Any alcohol you drink passes to your baby through your breast milk, so be careful about your consumption of alcoholic beverages. The longer you breastfeed, the more you'll realize what you can (and cannot) eat and drink.

There may be times when you are away from the baby, but you want to continue to breastfeed. You can do this by using a breast pump and storing your breast milk. You can pump your breasts with battery-operated pumps, electrical pumps or manual pumps. Ask for suggestions before you leave the hospital.

Talk with your doctor/midwife during pregnancy about breastfeeding. Ask friends about their experiences and how much they enjoyed it. You may also want to contact one of the organizations that encourage and promote breastfeeding (see Resources). They offer help to women who may be having trouble getting started with breastfeeding. Give them a call if you need information or support.

Engorgement. A common breastfeeding problem for some women is *breast engorgement.* Breasts become swollen, tender and filled with breast milk. What can you do to relieve this problem?

- The best cure is to drain the breasts, if possible, as you do when breastfeeding. Some women take a hot shower and empty their breasts in the warm water.
- Ice packs may also help.
- Feed your baby from both breasts *each time* you feed. Don't feed on only one side.
- When you're away from your baby, try to express some breast milk to keep your milk flowing and breast ducts open. You'll also feel more comfortable.
- Mild pain medicines, such as paracetamol, are often useful in relieving the pain of engorgement. Paracetamol is safe to use while breastfeeding.
- You might need to use stronger medications, such as paracetamol with codeine.
- Call your doctor/midwife if engorgement is especially painful. He or she will decide on treatment.

Breast Infections. It is possible to get an infection in your breast while breastfeeding. If you think you have an infection, call your doctor. An infection may cause pain in the breast, and the breast may turn red and become swollen. You may have streaks of red discoloration on the breast; you may also feel as though you have the flu.

Sore Nipples. Most nursing mothers have sore nipples at some point, particularly at first. You can take steps to lessen or to relieve the soreness. Try the following.

- Keep your breasts dry and clean.
- Do not air dry—it encourages scab formation and can take quite a while for a sore breast to heal.
- Moist healing is best. Covering the entire nipple area with Vaseline every time baby finishes nursing can help.

Good news! Before too long—a few days to a few weeks—your breasts will become accustomed to breastfeeding, and problems will lessen.

Inverted Nipples. Some women have trouble breastfeeding because of inverted nipples. This happens when the nipple retracts inwards instead of pointing outwards. If you have inverted nipples, it is still possible to breastfeed. Plastic breast shields are available to wear under clothing to help bring out an inverted nipple.

Some midwives also recommend pulling on the nipple and rolling it between the thumb and index finger. Talk about this situation at one of your antenatal appointments.

Support Bras. Some women find wearing a support bra helpful in the last few weeks of pregnancy. A nursing bra is useful while nursing. Many doctors/midwives suggest wearing a nursing bra all the time, even when you sleep, to make you more comfortable. To prepare your breasts for nursing, however, expose them regularly to the air. Not wearing a bra now and then while you are wearing clothes allows your nipples to toughen slightly when they rub against the fabric of your clothes.

Nursing with Silicone Breast Implants. Women have successfully nursed with breast implants; however, implants may make nursing more difficult. Doctors don't agree as to whether it is safe or possibly harmful to nurse with implants. If you are concerned, discuss the matter with your doctor/midwife; ask him or her for the latest information.

The Bottlefeeding Option. It won't harm your baby if you choose to bottlefeed. We don't want any mother to feel guilty if she chooses bottlefeeding over breastfeeding since, with iron-fortified formula, a bottlefed baby receives good nutrition.

Some Reasons You May Not Be Able to Breastfeed. You may be unable to breastfeed if you are extremely underweight or have some medical conditions, such as a prolactin deficiency, heart disease, kidney disease, tuberculosis or HIV/AIDS. Some infants have problems breastfeeding, or they are unable to breastfeed if they have a cleft palate or cleft lip. Lactose intolerance can also cause breastfeeding problems. Sometimes a woman cannot breastfeed because of a physical condition or problem.

Some women want to breastfeed and try to, but it doesn't work out. If breastfeeding doesn't work for you, please don't worry about it. Your baby will be OK.

Advantages to Bottlefeeding. There are advantages to bottlefeeding.

- Some women enjoy the freedom bottlefeeding provides; others can help care for the baby.
- Bottlefeeding is easy to learn; it never causes the mother discomfort if it is done incorrectly.
- Fathers can be more involved in caring for baby.
- Bottlefed babies may go longer between feedings because formula is usually digested more slowly than breast milk.
- A day's supply of formula can be mixed all at once, saving time and effort.
- You don't have to be concerned about feeding your baby in front of other people.

- It's easier to bottlefeed if you plan to return to work soon after your baby is born.
- If you feed your baby iron-fortified formula, he or she won't need iron supplementation.
- If you use fluoridated tap water to mix formula, you may not have to give your baby fluoride supplements.

Your Nutrition

✌ *If You Breastfeed*

If you're going to breastfeed your baby, you need to begin thinking about nutritional needs for the time you will nurse. You will probably be advised to eat about 500 extra calories each day during this time. A breastfeeding mother secretes 425 to 700 calories into her breast milk every day! The extra calories you take in will help you maintain good health. These calories should also be nutritious and healthy, like the ones you've been eating during pregnancy. Choose 9 servings from the bread/cereal/pasta/rice group and 3 servings from the dairy group. Fruit servings should number 4, and vegetable servings should number 5. The amount of protein in your diet should be 225 g (8 oz) during breastfeeding. Be particularly careful with fats, oils and sugars; limit intake to 4 teaspoons.

As previously discussed, you may have to avoid some foods because they can pass into breast milk and cause your baby some stomach distress. Avoid chocolate, foods that produce gas in you, such as Brussels sprouts and cauliflower, highly spiced foods and other foods you have problems with. Discuss the situation with your doctor or health visitor if you have questions and concerns.

In addition to the food you eat, you need to continue to drink lots of fluids. You need to drink at least *2 litres (4 pints)* of fluid every day to make enough milk for your baby and for you to stay hydrated. You'll need more fluid in hot weather. Avoid caffeine-containing foods and drinks because caffeine can act as a diuretic. It can also pass to your baby through your breast milk. Although caffeine is out of your bloodstream in 3 to 5 hours, it can remain in a baby's bloodstream for up to 96 hours!

Keep up your calcium intake. It's important if you breastfeed. You might ask your doctor what kind of vitamin supplement you should take. Some mothers take a prenatal vitamin as long as they breastfeed.

℘ If You Bottlefeed

Even if you bottlefeed, it's important to follow a nutritious eating plan, such as the one you followed during pregnancy. Continue to eat foods high in complex carbohydrates, such as grain products, fruits and vegetables. Lean meats, chicken and fish are good sources of protein. For your dairy products, choose the low-fat or skim types.

If you bottlefeed, you need fewer calories than you would if you were breastfeeding. But don't drastically cut your caloric intake in the hopes of losing weight quickly. You still need to eat nutritiously to maintain good energy levels. Be sure the calories you eat are not from junk foods.

Following is a list of the types and quantities of foods you should try to eat each day: Choose 6 servings from the bread/cereal/pasta/rice group, and 3 servings of fruit. Eat 3 servings of vegetables. From the dairy group, choose 2 servings. Eat about 170 g (6 oz) of protein each day. We still advise caution with fats, oils and sugars; limit intake to 3 teaspoons. And keep up your fluid intake. You can also use the pregnancy nutrition plan as a reference; see Week 6.

You Should Also Know

℘ Pain Relief during Labour

Labour is painful because your uterus has to change shape greatly so your baby can be born. You may request relief from this pain. Pain relief during labour is approached in many ways. When you take pain medication, remember there are two patients to consider—you and your unborn baby. It is best to find out in advance what is available for pain control. Then see how your labour goes for you before making a final decision.

A valuable part of your experience in labour and delivery is your preparation for it. This includes being aware of things that are happening to you, and why, and not being frightened by the pain you feel. You should have confidence in those taking care of you, including your doctor and the staff at the hospital.

An *anaesthetic* is a complete block of all pain sensations and muscle movement. An *analgesic* is full or partial relief of pain sensations. Narcotic analgesics pass to your baby through the placenta and may decrease respiratory function in the newborn infant. They can also affect your baby's Apgar scores (see page 416). These medications should not be given close to the time of delivery.

In many places, anaesthesia for delivery is given by an injection of a particular medication to affect a particular area of the body. This is called a block, such as a *pudendal block*, an *epidural block* or a *cervical block*. Medication is similar to the type used to block pain when you have a tooth filled. The agents are xylocaine or xylocaine-like medications.

Occasionally, it is necessary to use general anaesthesia for delivery of a baby, usually for an emergency Caesarean delivery. A paediatrician attends the birth because it is possible the baby will be asleep following delivery.

What Is an Epidural Block? The epidural block is one of the most popular anaesthetics used today for labour and delivery, and it is used frequently. It provides relief from the pain of uterine contractions and delivery. It should be administered only by someone trained and experienced in this type of anaesthesia. Some obstetricians have this experience, but in most areas an anaesthesiologist or nurse anaesthetist must administer it.

A continuous epidural block is started while you are sitting up or lying on your side. The anaesthesiologist numbs an area of skin over your lower back in the middle of your spinal cord. He or she then introduces a needle through the numbed area of the skin; anaesthetic is placed around the spinal cord but not into the spinal canal. A plastic catheter is left in place.

Epidural pain medication may be given during labour with a pump. The anaesthesiologist uses the pump to inject a small amount of medication at regular intervals or as needed. An epidural provides excellent relief from labour pain.

A combined spinal epidural block/walking epidural uses epidural and spinal techniques to relieve pain. There is often less numbness with this combination, so a woman may be able to walk around more easily. It is sometimes called a *walking epidural.*

You may have heard some confusing information about when you can receive an epidural, if you choose to have one. Most doctors believe an epidural block should be given during labour based on your level of pain. You may *not* be required to be dilated to a specific point before getting an epidural.

A problem with an epidural block is that it can make your blood pressure drop. Low blood pressure may affect blood flow to the baby. Fortunately, IV fluids administered with the epidural help reduce the risk of hypotension (low blood pressure). You may also have problems pushing during delivery. According to recent studies, no link between use of epidurals during labour and the experience of later back pain has been established.

Other Pain Blocks. When contractions are regular and the cervix is beginning to dilate, uterine contractions may be uncomfortable. For pain in this early stage of labour, many hospitals use a mixture of a narcotic analgesic drug, such as meperidine, and a tranquillizer, such as promethazine (Phenergan). This decreases pain and causes some sleepiness or sedation. Medication may be given through an IV or by injection into a muscle.

Spinal anaesthesia may be used for a Caesarean section. With this anaesthesia, pain relief lasts long enough for the Caesarean section to be performed. Today, spinal anaesthesia is not used as often as epidural anaesthesia for labour.

Another type of block used occasionally is a pudendal block. It is given through the vaginal canal and decreases pain in the birth canal itself. You still feel the contraction and tightening with pain in the uterus. Some hospitals use a paracervical block. It provides pain relief for the dilating cervix but doesn't relieve the pain of contractions.

Intrathecal anaesthesia is a single dose of anaesthesia into the area surrounding the spinal cord. It isn't a total block; the woman feels the contraction so she may push.

There is no perfect method for pain relief during labour and delivery. Discuss all the possibilities with your midwife, and mention any concerns. Find out what types of anaesthesia are available and the risks and benefits of each.

Anaesthesia Problems and Complications. There are possible complications from use of anaesthesia. These include increased sedation of the baby with use of narcotics, such as meperidine. The newborn may have lower Apgar scores and depressed breathing. The baby may require resuscitation, or it may need to receive another drug, such as naloxone (Narcan), to reverse the effects of the first drug.

If a mother is given general anaesthesia, increased sedation, slower respiration and a slower heartbeat may also be observed in the baby. The mother is usually 'out' for more than an hour and is unable to see her newborn infant until later.

If you have an epidural or spinal block during delivery, you may experience various side effects after delivery. Some ways to help alleviate these discomforts include the following.

- If you experience itching, put pressure on the area with a towel or blanket. Ease discomfort by applying lots of lotion.
- If you have a headache, drink a beverage that contains caffeine, such as coffee, tea or a caffeinated fizzy drink.
- If you become nauseous, breathing deeply can help. Inhale through your nose, and exhale through your mouth.

It may be impossible to determine before you go into labour which anaesthesia will be best for you. But it's helpful to know what's available and what types of pain relief you might be able to count on during your labour and delivery.

✣ Contraction of the Uterus after Delivery

After you deliver your baby, your uterus shrinks immediately from about the size of a watermelon to the size of a football. When this happens, the placenta detaches from the uterine wall. At this time, there may be a gush of blood from inside the uterus signalling delivery of the placenta.

After the placenta is delivered, you may be given oxytocin. This helps the uterus contract and clamp down so it won't bleed. Extremely heavy bleeding after vaginal delivery is called *postpartum haemorrhage*, which is bleeding more than 500 ml (17 fl oz). It can often be prevented by massaging the uterus and using medications to help the uterus contract.

The main reason a woman experiences heavy bleeding after delivering a baby is her uterus does not contract, called an *atonic* uterus. Your doctor/midwife attending you may massage your uterus after delivery. They may show you how to do it so your uterus will stay firm and contracted. This is important so you won't lose more blood and become anaemic.

✣ Cord-Blood Banking

Are you and your partner thinking about storing blood from your baby's umbilical cord? Researchers have found that stem cells, which are present in cord blood, have proved very successful in treating some diseases. *Cord blood* is blood left in the umbilical cord and placenta after a baby is born. In the past, the placenta and the umbilical cord were usually discarded following delivery.

There is a great deal of interest about saving cord blood after delivery. Umbilical-cord blood can be used to treat cancer and genetic diseases that are now treated by bone-marrow transplants. Cord blood has been used successfully to treat childhood leukaemia, some immune diseases and other blood diseases. At present, research is being conducted in the United States and Europe to use cord blood for gene therapy in a number of diseases, including sickle-cell anaemia, diabetes and AIDS.

Cord blood contains the same valuable cells that are found in bone marrow. These 'stem cells' are the building blocks of the blood and immune systems. These special cells are undeveloped in cord blood. Because they are undeveloped, cord blood does not need to be matched as closely for a transplant as bone-marrow blood does. This feature can be especially important for members of ethnic minority groups or people with rare blood types. These groups traditionally have had more difficulty finding acceptable donor 'matches.'

Since 1996, cord blood banking has been undertaken by NHS facilities within the National Blood Service. Obstetric patients donate cord blood altruistically, in a similar way to bone marrow donors. Recently, however, commercial companies have been targetting women and offering (for a fee) to have the blood stored. This blood can be used by the child from whom it was collected, his siblings or parents.

Blood is collected directly from the umbilical cord immediately after delivery. There is no risk or pain to the mother or baby. The blood is transported to a banking facility where it is frozen and cryogenically stored.

Discuss this situation with your doctor/midwife at an antenatal appointment—especially if your family has a history of certain diseases. Ask about how and where blood is stored and the cost of storing it. If you don't want to waste your baby's cord blood, think about donating it. Ask your doctor for information about cord-blood banking services and cord-blood donation in your area.

Dad Tip Who do you and your partner want in the delivery room? Having a baby is a unique and wonderful experience. Some couples choose the intimacy and privacy of being alone during the birth. Other couples want various family members and friends to share the experience with them. If you talk about it ahead of time, you can decide together what you both want. After all, it's your baby's birth.

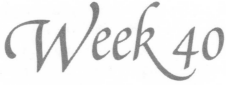

Week 40

Age of Foetus—38 Weeks

How Big Is Your Baby?

Your baby weighs about 3.4 kg (7½ lb). Its crown-to-rump length is about 37 to 38 cm (14¾ to 15¼ in). Total length is 48 cm (21½ in). Your baby fills your uterus and has little room to move. See the illustration on page 404.

How Big Are You?

From the pubic symphysis to the top of the uterus, you probably measure between 36 to 40 cm (14½ and 16 in). From your bellybutton to the top of your uterus is 16 to 20 cm (6½ to 8 in).

By this time, you probably don't care an awful lot about how much you measure. You feel you're as big as you could ever be, and you're ready to have your baby. You may continue to grow and even to get a little bit bigger until you have your baby. But don't be discouraged—you'll have your baby soon.

How Your Baby Is Growing and Developing

Bilirubin is a breakdown product from red blood cells. Before your baby is born, bilirubin is transferred easily across the placenta from the foetus to maternal circulation. Through this process, your body is able to get rid of the bilirubin from the baby. Once your baby is delivered and the umbilical cord is clamped, the baby is on its own to handle the bilirubin produced in its own body.

⌒ *Jaundice in a Newborn*

After birth, if your baby has problems dealing with bilirubin, it may develop high levels of it in the blood. Your baby may develop jaundice—yellowing of the skin and the whites of the eyes. Bilirubin levels typically increase for 3 or 4 days after the baby's delivery, then decrease.

Your neonatologist and midwives check for jaundice by observing your baby's colour. Your baby may have a test to measure his or her bilirubin levels at the hospital or at home.

A baby is treated for jaundice with *phototherapy,* which can be delivered in the hospital or at home with a freestanding device or a fibre-optic blanket. The light from the special device penetrates the skin and destroys the bilirubin. If high levels of bilirubin are present, the baby may undergo an exchange blood transfusion.

Kernicterus in a Newborn. Extremely high levels of bilirubin (hyperbilirubinaemia) in a newborn infant cause doctors concern because a serious condition called *kernicterus* can develop. Kernicterus is seen more frequently in premature infants than in babies delivered at full term. If the baby survives the kernicterus, it may have neurological problems—spasticity, lack of muscle coordination and varying degrees of mental retardation. However, kernicterus in a newborn is rare.

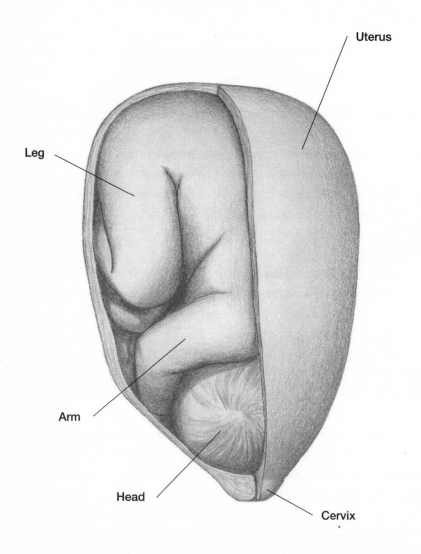

Uterus

Leg

Arm

Head

Cervix

A full-term baby has little room to move. This is one reason foetal movements may slow down in the last few weeks of pregnancy.

Changes in You

✑ *While You Wait to Go to the Hospital*

If you are waiting to go to the hospital and are experiencing pain, there are a few things you can do at home. The following actions may help you manage your pain.

- At the beginning of each contraction, take a deep breath. Exhale slowly. At the end of the contraction, again breathe deeply.
- Get up and move! It helps distract you and may relieve back pain.
- Ask your partner to massage your shoulders, neck, back and feet. It helps ease tension, and it feels good.
- Hot and/or cold compresses can help reduce cramping and various aches and pains. A warm shower or bath can feel very good.
- When a contraction begins, try to distract yourself with mental pictures of pleasant or soothing images.

How Your Actions Affect Your Baby's Development

✑ *Going to the Hospital*

Ask your midwife how you should prepare to go to the hospital; he or she may have specific instructions for you. You might want to ask the following questions.

- When should we go to the hospital once I'm in labour?
- Should we call you before we leave for the hospital?
- How can we reach you after regular surgery hours?
- Are there any particular instructions for me to follow during early labour?
- Where do we go—to A & E or the maternity department?

Many couples are advised to go to the hospital after an hour of contractions that are 5 to 10 minutes apart. However, leave sooner if the hospital is far away or hard to get to, or if the weather is bad.

The delivery of your baby is the event you've been planning for! If this is your first baby, you may be excited and a little apprehensive. Delivery of your baby is something you'll remember for a long time.

You need to decide who you want with you during delivery. Sometimes, family members assume they're invited to the delivery. Some couples choose to bring young children into the delivery room to see the birth of a new brother or sister. Discuss this with your doctor or midwife ahead of time, and get his or her opinion. The delivery of the baby might be exciting and special to you and your partner, but it may be frightening to a young child.

Some places may offer special classes for older siblings to help prepare them for the new baby. This is a good way to help your older children feel they're part of the birth experience.

The Labour Check. When you get to the hospital, you may be sent home! This happens if labour hasn't really started or if it is early labour. When you arrive at the hospital, you will be evaluated for signs of labour. This is sometimes called a *labour check*.

If you are sent home, don't get frustrated, upset or mad. Understand that to determine if a woman is in labour she must often be seen and evaluated at the hospital/home. This is something that can't be determined over the phone!

The people who evaluate you know you want to get on with the birth process and that you don't want to go home. However, if you aren't in true labour, it *is* best to go home. If this happens to you, make the best of it. You'll be back when the time is right!

In the Hospital. When you are admitted to labour and delivery (or a birthing centre), many things happen. You will probably be asked many questions when you check in. They may include the following.

• Have your membranes ruptured? At what time?
• Are you bleeding?
• Are you having contractions? How often do they occur? How long do they last?
• When did you last eat, and what did you eat?

Other important information for you to share includes medical problems you have and any medications you take or have taken during pregnancy. If you've had complications, such as placenta previa, tell medical personnel when you first come to labour and delivery.

Your Initial Exam. A pelvic exam is performed to help determine what stage of labour you are in and to use as a reference point for future exams during labour. This exam and the vital signs are performed by a midwife (who can be male or female). Only in unusual situations, such as in an emergency, will your doctor do this initial exam.

A brief pregnancy history is taken. Vital signs, including blood pressure, pulse, temperature and baby's heart rate, are noted.

Once You Are Admitted. If you are in labour and remain at the hospital, other things will happen. Each hospital has its own set of routine procedures.

You may receive an enema (though not unless you request it), or an IV may be started. You will be asked to give a urine sample, to test for the presence of protein and sugar. Your midwife may want to discuss your birth plan and pain relief, or you may have an epidural put in place, if you have requested one.

If you have decided to have an epidural or if it looks as if labour will last quite awhile, an IV will be started. You may still be able to walk around. You may not be encouraged to eat, but you will be allowed to have more than ice chips and water. During this time, you and your partner may be alone together, with midwives coming into the room to perform various tasks, then leaving. In most instances, a monitoring belt is placed on your abdomen to record your contractions and the baby's heartbeat. The monitoring record can be seen in the room and also by midwives at the nursing station.

Blood pressure is taken at regular intervals, and pelvic exams are performed to follow labour's progress.

ᥟ Keep Your Options Open during Labour and Delivery

An important consideration in planning for your labour and delivery is the method(s) you may use to get through the process. Will you have epidural anaesthesia? Are you going to attempt a drug-free delivery? Will you need an episiotomy?

Every woman is different, and every labour is different. It's difficult to anticipate what will happen and what you will need during labour and delivery for pain relief. It's impossible to know how long labour will last—3 hours or 20 hours. It's best to adopt a flexible birth plan. Understand what's available and what options you can choose during labour.

During the last 2 months of your pregnancy, discuss these concerns with your doctor/midwife. Know what can be provided for you at the hospital at which you will give birth. Some medications may not be available in some areas.

ᥟ Pain Relief without Medication

Some women do not want medication during labour to relieve pain. They prefer to use different labouring positions, massage, breathing patterns, relaxation techniques or hypnotherapy to relieve their pain. Breathing patterns and relaxation techniques are usually learned in a childbirth-education class.

In some places, hypnosis to relieve pain during childbirth is used by some women. *HypnoBirthing* is a labour-pain management technique developed over 20 years ago and requires a period of practice sessions. It is not something you should try on a whim. Ask your midwife about it at one of your antenatal visits if you are interested in trying it or contact www.betterbirth.co.uk. Classes may be available in your area.

Aromatherapy, which consists of massage with certain aromatic oils, can be helpful for relaxation. *Birth pools* are available in most hospitals. Some women experience a reduction in pain and increased relaxation in the water. The water also softens the perineal area, so it may stretch more easily. In some places, you have to get out of the pool to give birth. Discuss it with your doctor if you are interested.

Acupressure uses pressure on specific parts of the body to help relieve pain and to relax you. It may give you a sense of well-being. However, for acupressure to work most effectively, it must usually be started at the beginning of labour.

ᴖ *Labouring Positions*

Different labouring positions may enable a woman and her partner to work together during labour to find relief. This interaction can help you feel closer, and it lets you share the experience. Some women say that using these methods brought them closer to their partner and made the birth experience a more joyful one.

Most women in Europe and North America give birth in bed, on their backs. However, some women are trying different positions to find relief from pain and to make the birth of their baby easier.

In the past, women often laboured and gave birth in an upright position that kept the pelvis vertical, such as kneeling, squatting, sitting or standing up. Labouring in this position enables the abdominal wall to relax and the baby to descend more rapidly. Because contractions are stronger and more regular, labour is often shorter.

Today, many women are asking to choose the birth position that is most comfortable for them. Freedom to choose the birth position can make a woman feel more confident about managing birth and labour. Women who choose their own methods may feel more satisfied with the entire experience.

If this is important to you, discuss the matter with your midwife. Ask about the facilities at the hospital you will use; some have special equipment, such as birthing chairs, squatting bars or birthing beds, to help you feel more comfortable. Positions you might consider for your labour are described below.

Walking and *standing* are good positions to use during early labour. Walking may help you breathe more easily and relax more. Standing in a warm shower may provide relief. When walking, be sure someone is with you to offer support (both physical and emotional).

Sitting can decrease the strength and frequency of contractions and can slow labour. Sitting to rest after walking or standing is acceptable; however, sitting can be uncomfortable during a contraction.

Kneeling on hands and knees is a good way to relieve the pain of back labour. *Kneeling against a support,* such as a chair or your partner, stretches your back muscles. The effects of kneeling are similar to those of walking and standing.

When you can't stand, walk or kneel, *lie on your side.* If you receive pain medication, you will need to lie down. Lie on your left side, then turn onto your right side.

Although *lying on your back* is the most common position used for labour, it can decrease the strength and frequency of contractions, which can slow the process. It can also make your blood pressure drop and cause your baby's heart rate to drop. If you lie on your back, elevate the head of the bed and put a pillow under one hip so you are not flat on your back.

Some women want to know if walking during labour makes labour easier and reduces the chance of a C-section. There has been some controversy about walking during labour. Some believe that walking helps move the baby into position more quickly, dilates the cervix faster and makes labour more pain free. Others note that walking puts the woman at risk of falling, and it doesn't allow for foetal monitoring, which can put the foetus at risk. A recent study of more than 1000 pregnant women demonstrated that walking had no effects, either way. We believe the bottom line is that it is a personal decision on your part, and you should be allowed to make the decision as to what feels best for you.

✑ *Massage for Relief*

Massage is a wonderful, gentle way to help you feel better during labour. The touching and caressing of massage helps you relax. One study showed that women who were massaged for 20 minutes every hour during active labour felt less anxiety and less pain.

Many parts of the body of a labouring woman can be massaged. Massaging the head, neck, back and feet can offer a great deal of comfort and relaxation. The person doing the massage should pay close attention to the woman's responses to determine correct pressure.

Different types of massage affect a woman in various ways. You and your partner may want to practise the two types of massage described below before labour for use during labour.

Effleurage is light, gentle fingertip massage over the abdomen and upper thighs; it is used during early labour. Stroking is light, but doesn't tickle, and fingertips never leave the skin.

Start with hands on either side of the navel. Move the hands upwards and outwards, and come back down to the pubic area. Then move the hands back up to the navel. Massage may extend down the thighs. It can also be done as a crossways motion, around foetal-monitor belts. Move fingers across the abdomen from one side to the other, between the belts.

Counterpressure massage is excellent for relieving the pain of back labour. Place the heel of the hand or the flat part of the fist (you can also use a tennis ball) against the tailbone. Apply firm pressure in a small, circular motion.

Your Nutrition

A woman often gets nauseated when she's in labour, which may cause vomiting.

Eating probably won't be of interest to you, but you may be thirsty. You will be allowed water or ice chips to suck on. You may even be offered a wet flannel to suck on. If your labour is long, your body may be hydrated with fluids intraveneously.

You Should Also Know

෨ Your Partner

In most instances, your partner is with you during labour. However, this isn't an absolute requirement. A close friend or relative, such as your mother or sister, can accompany you instead. Ask someone ahead of time; don't wait until the last minute. Give the person time to prepare for the experience and to make sure he or she will be able to be there with you.

Not everyone feels comfortable watching the entire labour and delivery. This may include your partner. Don't force your partner or whoever is with you to watch the delivery if he or she doesn't want to. It's not unusual for a partner to get lightheaded, dizzy or pass out during labour and delivery. On more than one occasion, partners have fainted or become extremely lightheaded just from talking about plans for labour and delivery or a C-section.

Preparing ahead of time, as with antenatal classes, helps avoid some problems. In the past, you would have been alone with the midwives and doctor while your partner paced in the waiting room. Things have changed!

The most important thing to consider when choosing who you want with you in the delivery room is the support he or she will give you. Choose this person carefully.

Coaching Tips. Once you arrive at the hospital, both of you may be nervous. Your partner can do the following to help you both relax:

- talk to you while you're in labour to distract you and to help you relax
- encourage and reassure you during labour and when it comes time for you to push
- keep a watch on the door and protect your privacy
- help relieve tension during labour
- touch, hug and kiss (If you don't want to be touched during labour, tell your partner.)

- reassure you it's OK for you to deal vocally with your pain
- wipe your face or your mouth with a flannel
- rub your abdomen or back
- support your back while you're pushing
- help create a mood in the labour room, including music and lighting (Discuss it ahead of time; bring things with you that you would like to have available during labour.)
- take pictures (Many couples find still pictures taken of the baby after the delivery help them best remember these wonderful moments of joy.)

What Can a Partner Do? Your partner may be one of the most valuable assets you have during labour and delivery. He (or she, if you have your mother, sister or friend with you) can help you prepare for labour and delivery in many ways. He can be there to support you as you go through the experience of labour together. He can share with you the joy of the birth of your baby.

An important role is to make sure you get to the hospital! Work out a plan during the last 4 to 6 weeks of pregnancy so you know how to reach your partner. It's helpful to have an alternate driver, such as a neighbour or friend, who is available in case you are unable to reach your partner immediately and need to be taken to the hospital. Before going to the hospital, your partner can time your contractions so you are aware of the progress of your labour.

It's all right for your partner to rest or to take a break during labour. This is especially true if labour lasts a long time. It's better if your partner eats in the lounge or hospital cafeteria.

Many couples do different things to distract themselves and to help pass time during labour. These include picking names for the baby, playing games, watching TV or listening to music. A partner should not bring work into the labour room—it is inappropriate and shows little support for the labouring woman.

Talk to your doctor about your partner's participation in the delivery, such as cutting the umbilical cord or bathing the baby after birth.

Things like this vary from one place to another. Understand that the responsibility of your doctor is the well-being of you and your baby—don't make requests or demands that could cause complications.

Decide ahead of time about who needs to be called. Bring a list of names and phone numbers with you. There are some people you may want to call yourself. In most places, a telephone is available in the labour and delivery area.

Discuss showing the baby to those who are waiting with your partner. If you want to be with your partner when friends or relatives first see the baby, make it clear to him or her. Don't allow your baby to be taken out of the room unless that's what you want. In most instances, you need some cleaning up. Take some time for yourselves with your new baby. After that you can show baby to friends and relatives, and share the joy with them.

ᨀ *Vaginal Delivery of Your Baby*

We have already covered Caesarean delivery in Week 37. Luckily, most women don't have to have a Caesarean delivery—they have a vaginal birth.

There are three distinct stages of labour. In the first stage of labour, your uterus contracts with enough intensity, duration and frequency to cause thinning (effacement) and dilatation of the cervix. The first stage of labour ends when the cervix is fully dilated (usually 10 cm) and sufficiently open to allow the baby's head to come through it.

The second stage of labour begins when the cervix is completely dilated at 10 cm. Once full dilatation of the cervix is reached, pushing begins. Pushing can take 1 to 2 hours (first or second baby) to a few minutes (an experienced mum). This stage of labour ends with the delivery of the baby.

The third stage of labour begins after delivery of the baby. It ends with delivery of the placenta and the membranes that have surrounded the foetus. Delivery of the baby and placenta, and repair of the episiotomy (if you have one) usually takes 20 to 30 minutes.

Following delivery, you and the baby are evaluated. During this time, you finally get to see and to hold your baby; you may even be able to feed baby.

Depending on whether you deliver in a hospital or birthing centre, you may deliver in the same room you have been labouring in (often called *LDRP* for labour, delivery, recovery and postpartum). Or you may be moved to a delivery room nearby. After the birth, you will go to a post-natal ward until you're ready to go home.

You will probably stay in the hospital from 24 to 48 hours after delivery, if you have no complications. If you do have any complications, you and your doctor/midwife will decide what is best for you.

ᴪ What Happens to Your Baby after It's Born?

When your baby is delivered, the doctor/midwife clamps and cuts the umbilical cord. The baby is passed to a paediatrician for initial evaluation and attention. The Apgar scores (see page 416) are recorded at 1- and 5-minute intervals. An identification band is placed on the baby so there's no mix-up on the post-natal ward.

It's important to keep the baby warm immediately after birth. To do this, the midwife will dry the baby and wrap it in warm blankets. This is done whether the baby is on your chest or attended to by a midwife or doctor.

The baby's well-being and health are of primary concern. You'll be able to hold and to nurse the baby, but if your child is having trouble breathing or needs special attention, such as monitors, immediate evaluation is the most appropriate procedure at this time.

If this is the case, your baby will be taken to the special care unit (SCBU) by a midwife or paediatrician and your partner. There are

> *Dad Tip* Discuss your role in labour and delivery with your partner. Learn what you can do to assist your partner. You may be able to help maintain privacy. When people visit during or after labour, be sure they don't get too loud or it doesn't become too crowded. Let your partner rest and recuperate; be her knight in shining armour.

many different reasons for admitting babies to SCBU, such as premature birth, breathing difficulties, feeding problems, and infections. In the SCBU, your baby may be placed in an incubator to keep her at the desired temperature. With your consent, your baby will be given vitamin K to help with her blood-clotting factors.

Your Baby's Apgar Score. After a baby is born, it is examined and evaluated at 1 minute and 5 minutes after delivery. The system of evaluation is called the *Apgar score*. This scoring system is a method of evaluating the overall well-being of the newborn infant.

In general, the higher the score, the better the infant's condition. The baby is scored in five areas. Each area is scored 0, 1 or 2; 2 points is the highest score for each category. The top total score is 10. Areas scored include the following.

Heart rate of the baby. If the heart rate is absent, a score of 0 is given. If it is slow, less than 100 beats per minute (bpm), a score of 1 is given. If it's over 100 bpm, 2 points are scored.

Respiratory effort of the baby. Respiratory effort indicates the newborn's attempts at breathing. If the baby isn't breathing, the score is 0. If breathing is slow and irregular, the score is 1. If the baby is crying and breathing well, the score is 2.

Baby's muscle tone. Muscle tone evaluates how well the baby moves. If arms and legs are limp and flabby, the score is 0. If some movement is observed and the arms and legs bend a little, the score is 1. If the baby is active and moving, the score is 2.

Response to Stimulus. This is scored 0 if the baby doesn't respond to stimulus, such as rubbing his or her back or arms. If there is a small movement or a grimace when the baby is stimulated, the score is 1. A baby who responds vigorously is scored with 2 points.

Baby's colour. The baby's colour is rated 0 if the baby is blue or pale. A score of 1 is given if the baby's body is pink and arms and legs are blue. A completely pink baby is scored at 2.

A perfect score of 10 is unusual. Most babies receive scores of 7, 8 or 9 in a normal, healthy delivery. A baby with a low 1-minute Apgar may need to be resuscitated. This means a paediatrician or midwife must help stimulate the baby to breathe and to recover from the delivery. In most cases, the 5-minute Apgar is higher than the 1-minute score because the baby becomes more active and more accustomed to being outside the uterus.

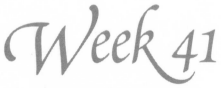

Week 41

When You're Overdue

*Y*our due date has come and gone. You haven't delivered yet, and you're getting tired of being pregnant. You are anxious to get labour and delivery over and finally meet your baby.

You keep seeing the doctor/midwife, and he or she tells you, 'I'm sure it'll be soon. Just sit tight.' You feel ready to scream. But hang in there. It *will* be over soon—the wait just seems never-ending right now.

What Happens When You're Overdue?

You've been anticipating the delivery of your baby. You counted the days to your due date—but that day has come and gone. And still no baby! As we've mentioned, not every woman delivers by her due date. Nearly 10 per cent of all babies are born more than 2 weeks late.

A pregnancy is considered to be overdue (*post-term*) only when it exceeds 42 weeks or 294 days from the first day of the last menstrual period. (A baby that is 41½ weeks is *not* post-term!)

Your doctor/midwife will examine you and determine if the baby is moving around in the womb and if the amount of amniotic fluid is healthy and normal. If the baby is healthy and active, you are usually monitored until labour begins on its own.

Tests may be done as reassurance that an overdue baby is fine and can remain in the womb. These tests include a *non-stress test,* a *contraction stress test* and a *biophysical profile.* They are all discussed below. If signs of foetal stress are found, labour is often induced.

✌ *Keep Taking Good Care of Yourself*

It's often hard to keep a positive attitude when you're overdue. But don't give up yet!

Maintain good nutrition, and keep up your fluid intake. If you can do so without any problems, get some mild exercise, like walking or swimming.

One of the best exercises you can do at this point in your pregnancy is to exercise in the water. You can swim or do water exercises without the fear of falling or losing your balance. You can even just walk back and forth in the pool!

Rest and relax now because you're baby will be here soon, and you'll be very busy. Use the time to get things ready for baby so you'll be all set when you both come home from the hospital.

✌ *Post-term Pregnancies*

The majority of babies born 2 weeks or more past their due date are delivered safely. However, carrying a baby longer than 42 weeks can cause some problems for the foetus and the mother, so tests are done on these babies and labour is induced, when necessary.

While the foetus is growing and developing inside your uterus, it depends on two important functions performed by the placenta—respiration and nutrition. The baby relies on these functions for continued growth and development.

When a pregnancy is post-term, the placenta may fail to provide the respiratory function and essential nutrients the baby needs to grow, and an infant may begin to suffer nutritional deprivation. The baby is called *post-mature.*

At birth, a post-mature baby has dry, cracked, peeling, wrinkled skin, long fingernails and abundant hair. It also has less vernix covering its body. The baby appears almost malnourished, with decreased amounts of subcutaneous fat.

Because the post-mature infant is in danger of losing nutritional support from the placenta, it's important to know the true dating of your pregnancy. This is one reason it's important to go to all of your antenatal visits.

Tests You May Have

As we mentioned above, various tests may be done to reassure you and your doctor/midwife that your overdue baby is doing OK and can remain in the womb. In evaluating the baby, the doctor/midwife looks at various pieces of data to see how your baby is doing. For example, if you are having contractions, it's important to know how your baby is affected.

The tests are done on you to determine the health of your baby. One of the first tests you'll receive is a vaginal exam.

You may also be asked to record kick counts. See the discussion in Week 27. In some high-risk pregnancies a weekly ultrasound may be performed to determine how big your baby is and how much amniotic fluid is present at any given time. It also helps to identify abnormalities in the placenta, which could cause problems for the baby.

Three other tests you may have will help determine foetal well-being inside the womb. These tests are often done when a baby is overdue. They are the non-stress test, the contraction stress test and the biophysical profile. They are discussed below.

ᗡ The Non-stress Test

A non-stress test (NST) is sometimes performed at your local midwifery-led unit, but more usually in the maternity department of a hospital. While you are lying down, a midwife attaches a foetal monitor to your abdomen. Every time you feel your baby move, you push a button to make a mark on a strip of monitor paper. At the same time, the monitor records the baby's heartbeat.

When the baby moves, its heart rate usually goes up. Doctors/midwives use the findings from the NST to help them evaluate how well a baby is tolerating life inside the uterus. Your doctor/midwife will decide if further action is necessary.

✑ *The Contraction Stress Test*

A contraction stress test (CST) gives an indication of how the baby is doing and how well the baby will tolerate contractions and labour. If the baby doesn't respond well to contractions, it can be a sign of foetal stress. Some believe this test is more accurate than the non-stress test in evaluating the baby's well-being.

To perform a CST, a monitor is placed on your abdomen to monitor the baby. You are attached to an IV that dispenses small amounts of the hormone oxytocin to make your uterus contract. The baby's heartbeat is monitored to see its response to the contractions.

This test gives an indication of how well the baby will tolerate contractions and labour. If the baby doesn't respond well to the contractions, it can be a sign of foetal distress. However, this is not routine in the U.K.

✑ *The Biophysical Profile*

A biophysical profile is a comprehensive test used to examine the foetus during pregnancy. It helps determine foetal health and is done when there is concern about foetal well-being. The test evaluates the well-being of your baby inside your uterus.

A biophysical profile uses a particular scoring system. The first four of the five tests listed below are made with ultrasound; the fifth is done with external foetal monitors. A score is given to each area. The five areas of evaluation are:

- foetal breathing movements
- foetal body movements
- foetal tone
- amount of amniotic fluid
- reactive foetal heart rate (non-stress test)

During the test, doctors evaluate foetal 'breathing'—the movement or expansion of the baby's chest inside the uterus. This score is based on the amount of foetal breathing that occurs.

Movement of the baby's body is noted. A normal score indicates normal body movements. An abnormal score is applied when there are few or no body movements during the allotted time period.

Foetal tone is evaluated similarly. Movement, or lack of movement, of the arms and legs of the baby is recorded.

Evaluation of the volume of amniotic fluid requires experience in ultrasound examination. A normal pregnancy has adequate fluid around the baby. An abnormal test indicates no amniotic fluid or decreased amniotic fluid around the baby.

Foetal heart-rate monitoring (non-stress test) is done with external monitors. It evaluates changes in the foetal heart rate associated with movement of the baby. The amount of change and number of changes in the foetal heart rate differ, depending on who is doing the test and their definition of normal.

A normal score is 2; an abnormal score is 0 for any of these tests. A score of 1 in any of the tests is a middle score. From these five scores, a total score is obtained by adding all the values together. Evaluation may vary depending on the sophistication of the equipment used and the expertise of the person doing the test. The higher the score, the better the baby's condition. A lower score may cause concern about the well-being of the foetus.

If the score is low, a recommendation may be made to deliver the baby. If the score is reassuring, the test may be repeated at a later date. If results fall between these two values, the test may be repeated the following day. It depends on the circumstances of your pregnancy and the findings of the biophysical profile. Your doctor will evaluate all the information before making any decision.

Inducing Labour

There may come a point in your pregnancy that your doctor decides to induce labour. If this happens, it might help you if you realize this is a fairly common practice. Each year, doctors induce labour for about 1 in 5 births. Labour is induced for overdue babies, but it is also used for a number of other reasons, including chronic high blood pressure in the mother, pre-eclampsia, gestational diabetes, intrauterine-growth restriction and Rh-isoimmunization.

The midwife may carry out a pelvic exam at approximately 41 weeks gestation to evaluate how ready you are for induction. The *Bishop score* is used to help make this determination. It is a method of cervical scoring, used to predict the success of inducing labour. Scoring includes dilatation, effacement, station, consistency and position of the cervix. A score is given for each point, then they are added together to give a total score. A stretch and sweep of your cervix may be carried out at the same time to encourage spontaneous labor.

✑ *Ripening the Cervix for Induction*
Depending on your past obstetric history, the cervix may be ripened before labour is induced. *Ripening the cervix* means medication is used to help the cervix soften, thin and dilate.

Various preparations are used for this purpose. The most common are prostaglandin tablets or gels, which are placed in the top of the vagina, behind the cervix. Medication is released directly onto the cervix, which helps it to ripen for induction of labour. This is carried out in the hospital, so the baby can be monitored.

✑ *Inducing Labour*
If your doctor induces labour, you may first have your cervix ripened, as described above, then you will receive oxytocin intravenously. This medication is gradually increased until contractions begin. The amount of oxytocin you receive is controlled by a pump, so you can't receive too much of it. While you receive oxytocin, you are monitored for the baby's reaction to your labour.

The oxytocin starts contractions to help you go into labour. The length of the entire process—ripening your cervix until the birth of your baby—varies from woman to woman.

It is important to realize that being induced or having an induction does not guarantee a vaginal delivery. In many instances, the induction doesn't work. In that case, a C-section is usually necessary.

What Happens after Your Pregnancy?

*A*fter your baby is born, there will be a lot of changes in your life. Take a look at this overview so you'll have an idea of what to anticipate as you begin your life as a new mother.

In the Hospital

- Muscles are sore from the effort of childbirth and labour.
- Your bottom is sore and swollen. If you had an episiotomy, it also hurts.
- Your incision may be uncomfortable, if you had a C-section or tubal ligation.
- Use the nurse-call button whenever necessary!
- Try different ways for you and your partner to bond with baby.
- Feeding (breast or bottle) the new miracle in your arms may be a little scary, but you'll soon be doing it like a pro!
- Heavy bleeding or passing blood clots larger than an egg can indicate a problem.
- High or low blood pressure may be a cause for further testing.
- Pain should be relieved by medication. If it isn't, tell the nurse.
- Fever over 25.25°C (101.5°F) may be a cause for concern.
- It's normal if you cry or feel emotional.
- The hospital will be able to give you the address of the nearest local registry office. By law, every birth must be notified within 6 weeks in England, Wales and Northern Ireland, and within 3 weeks in Scotland. Do register your baby as soon as possible because child benefit is only paid from the date of registration, not the date of birth.

- Try to rest. Ask to turn off your phone (if you have one) and to restrict visitors.
- Even though you just lost 4.5 to 6.8 kg (10 to 15 lb) with baby's birth, it'll take a while for the rest of your weight to come off.
- Eat nutritiously to keep up energy and for milk production, if you breastfeed.
- Write down thoughts and feelings about labour, delivery and the first hours with your new baby. Encourage your partner to do the same.

- Watch hospital videos (if they have them) about baby care. Ask staff for clarification or help.
- Ask questions, and get help from the nurses and staff in the hospital.
- Ask your partner to take you for a walk outside your hospital room.
- Take time for you, your partner and your baby to bond as a family.
- Experts recommend that you start using contraception within 4 weeks of delivery. You will be asked about your contraception plans and given a prescription of the pill if necessary.

- If you weren't immune to rubella (German Measles) during your pregnancy, you will be immunized.
- Before you leave the hospital, your baby may be thoroughly examined by a paediatrician to make sure that there are no problems. She will also be given a blood test, between days 5 and 7, usually by means of a tiny heel prick, to check for phenylketonuria (PKU), a rare metabolic disease, and for thyroid underactivity.

1st Week Home

- You will be visited at home by a midwife, who will continue to visit for the following 10 days, or as necessary. She will be able to answer many of the questions you have.
- You'll still have painful uterine contractions, especially during nursing.
- It's normal for your breasts to be full of milk, engorged and leaking.
- The area of your episiotomy or tear is probably still sore.
- Muscles may also be sore.

- Maternity clothes may be the most comfortable clothes to wear.
- Your legs may still be swollen.
- You may leak urine or stool and can't control it.
- If bleeding gets heavier, or you pass blood clots, call your doctor.
- It may indicate a problem if you get red streaks or hard spots in your breasts.
- Call your doctor if you develop a fever.

- Take it easy; don't worry about the housework.
- It's normal to cry, sigh or laugh for no reason.
- Be sure to ask for help from friends and family.
- You may still look pregnant from the side.
- You still carry some of the extra weight you gained during pregnancy.
- Give both yourself and your partner time and space to bond with your baby. Don't feel obliged to play hostess. Put a

note on the front door saying you are resting if you don't feel like seeing anyone just then—they can always come back another time.

- Make your 6-week postpartum checkup appointment with your doctor.
- Give your partner a job or assignment to help you and to make him feel useful.
- Contact La Leche League or the NCT, if you have any problems breastfeeding.

2nd Week Home

- Your breasts (whether or not you breastfeed) are full and uncomfortable.
- Haemorrhoids still hurt, but they should be getting better.
- With swelling and water retention diminishing, you can wear some of your clothes and shoes again.
- Feeding baby is starting to work better.
- When you cough, laugh, sneeze or lift something heavy, you may lose stool or urine and not be able to control it.
- You are probably fatigued. Taking care of baby requires a lot of time and energy.
- A foul odour or yellow-green vaginal discharge may indicate a problem; it should be decreasing at this point. If it isn't, contact your doctor.
- It's OK to let baby cry a little before checking on him or her.
- You can almost see your feet when you look down (your tummy is getting smaller).
- Keep your appointment with your doctor if you had a C-section or tubal ligation; you need your incision checked.
- Write down some of your thoughts and feelings in your diary.

3rd Week Home

- Swelling and soreness around your bottom are decreasing, but sitting for a long time still may not feel very comfortable.
- Swelling in hands decreases. If you took off your rings during pregnancy, try them on again.
- Baby doesn't know the difference between night and day, so your sleep patterns are also disturbed.
- Getting ready to go anywhere is like planning a major trip. It takes three times longer to get ready with baby.
- Call your doctor if you develop red streaks or tender, hard spots on your legs, particularly the back of the calves. It could be a blood clot.
- You may feel sad or depressed some of the time. You may even cry.
- You may have varicose veins, just like your mother! They'll get better as you recover from pregnancy and begin exercising again.
- Skin on your abdomen still looks stretched out when you stand up.

- If you live in Scotland, make sure you have registered the birth of your baby.
- Take lots of pictures and videos! You'll be amazed how quickly baby will change and grow.
- Keep your partner involved. Let him try his hand at caring for baby. Ask for his help with household chores.
- By this point, you've changed over 200 nappies—you're an expert.

4th Week Home

- Muscles feel better, and you can do more now. Be aware—it's easy to pull or to strain muscles you haven't used for a while.
- Control of urine and stool are improving. Doing your Kegel (pelvic floor) exercises is paying off.
- Baby is showing signs of adjusting to a regular schedule.
- Things that once were easy to do, such as bending over or lifting, may be harder now.

Take things slowly, and allow yourself plenty of time for even the easiest chores.

- Your first menstrual period after delivery could happen at any time. If you don't breastfeed, your first period is usually 4 to 9 weeks after delivery, but it can happen earlier.
- Blood in your urine, dark or cloudy urine, or severe cramping or pain with urination may be symptoms of a urinary-tract infection (UTI). Call your doctor.
- You've been walking and doing light exercise, and it feels OK. Keep it up!
- Check on your 6-week postpartum appointment. Write down any questions you have as they come to you.
- A night out with your partner is a good plan. Grandparents, other family members and friends can babysit, if you ask them.

5th Week Home

- As you get back to regular activities, sore muscles and a sore back may be expected.
- Bowel movements may still be uncomfortable in the area of your episiotomy or rectum from time to time.
- Bladder and bowel control have returned.
- Baby blues should be getting much better, if they haven't disappeared already.
- Clothes may still be snug, even if they were loose before pregnancy.
- Remind yourself that it took you 9 months of pregnancy to gain the weight you did. It will take awhile to return to your pre-pregnancy figure.

6th Week Home

- Having a pelvic exam at your 6-week checkup isn't usually as bad as you might expect.
- In the 6 weeks since baby's birth, your uterus has gone from the size of a watermelon to the size of your fist; it now weighs about 55 g (2 oz).
- At your 6-week postpartum appointment, plan to discuss several important subjects, such as contraception, your current activity level, limitations and future pregnancies.
- If you still have baby blues or feel depressed every day, tell your doctor.
- If you bleed vaginally or have a foul-smelling discharge, inform you doctor.
- If you have pain or swelling in your legs, or your breasts are red or tender, bring it up at your visit.
- Ask questions; make a list. Good questions include:

    What are my choices for contraception?

    Do I have any limitations as far as exercise or sex?

    Is there anything I should know from this pregnancy and delivery if I decide to get pregnant again?

- If you live in England, Wales or Northern Ireland, make sure you have registered the birth of your baby.
- If you take baby with you to your postpartum checkup, take plenty of supplies. You may have to wait.
- If you intend to return to work, begin making plans for daycare arrangements, if you haven't started yet.
- Continue to involve your partner as much as possible.
- Keep writing your thoughts and feelings in your diary. Encourage your partner to do the same.

3 Months

- Muscles may be sore from exercising—a little more than a month ago, you were given the OK to do any exercises you wanted.
- You may have your first period around this time. It could be heavier, longer and different from those before pregnancy.
- If you haven't done anything about contraception, do it now! (Unless you want to celebrate two birthdays in the same year.)
- It's OK to let baby cry when she's a little fussy and needs to soothe herself.
- Your excess weight may not be disappearing as quickly as you would like. Keep exercising and eating nutritiously. You'll get there!
- Write down baby's milestones as they

happen; write them in baby's book or keep a diary.
- Look for things your partner can do to be involved in baby's care. Let him help out when he can.
- If you've stopped breastfeeding, let baby's dad give him a bottle.

6 Months

- Getting on the scales may still be a daunting task. But hang in there, and keep working hard on eating well and exercising!
- Your first period may occur around this time, if you are breastfeeding. It could be heavier, longer and different from those before pregnancy.
- Don't try to do it all yourself. Let your partner and others help.
- Baby's feeding schedule should be well established by now.
- Take time for yourself.
- Arrange time for regular activities, such as exercising, baby play groups and meeting with other new mums.
- You're starting to fit into some of your clothing from before pregnancy.
- Share special baby moments with your partner.
- Record baby's noises, or take pictures. A tape recorder and videocamera are great for this!
- Find a friend with a baby, and trade child-care duties. It's a good way for each of you to find time for yourself.

1 Year

- All systems are go! It's taken time, energy and hard work, but your life is going smoothly now.
- Baby is on a schedule and sleeps through the night most of the time.
- Your body is returning to its pre-pregnancy shape. Your tummy is flat, you've lost most of the pregnancy weight and you feel great.
- Continue taking care of yourself. Eat nutritiously, get enough rest and exercise.
- Write down feelings about this time in your life. Encourage your partner to do the same.
- Sharing child care can be a good way to develop baby play groups. Interacting with other children is good for baby.
- Baby's 1st birthday is just around the corner. Celebrate!
- Enjoy baby's first words, first steps and every other first that will happen.
- Continue taking pictures of baby.
- You may be considering another pregnancy.

Resources

General Information for Parents

ARC (Antenatal Results and Choices)
73-75 Charlotte Street
London W1T 4PN
0207 631 0285 (Mon to Fri, 10 am to 5 pm)
www.arc-uk.org
A national charity providing non-directive
support and information to parents
throughout the antenatal testing process,
aimed at helping parents arrive at the most
appropriate decision for them in the
context of their family life.

Baby Centre
www.babycentre.co.uk
All aspects of fertility, pregnancy,
childbirth and babies.

Baby Doppler
www.babybeat.com
To buy a home-use doppler to hear baby's
heartbeat at home.

BBCi Parenting
www.bbc.co.uk/parenting/
Offers practical solutions to help with the
challenges of everyday parenting.

Boots On-line
www.boots.com
Information and advice covering
preconception to pre-school, with regular
features relating to pregnancy and parenting.

Consumer Health Information Centre
www.chic.org.uk

Family Planning Association
2-12 Pentonville Road
London N1 9FP
0207 837 5432

helpline: 0845 310 1334 (9 am to 7 pm,
Mon to Fri)
www.fpa.org.uk
Trained staff provide confidential
information.

Genetic Interest Group
Unit 4d Leroy House
436 Essex Road
London N1 3QP
0207 704 3141

Gingerbread Association for One-Parent
Families
1st Floor
7 Sovereign Close
Sovereign Court
London E1W 3HW
0207 488 9300
helpline: 0800 018 4318 (9 am to 5 pm,
Mon to Fri)
www.gingerbread.org.uk
Help, advice and contact with other lone
parents.

mom-e.com
www.mom-e.com
Aims to inform couples about pregnancy
in a medically accurate and easily
digestible way.

National Childbirth Trust
Alexandra House
Oldham Terrace
Acton
London W3 6NH
0208 992 8637
www.nct-online.org
Antenatal classes and postnatal help.

General Information for Parents *(continued)*

National Council for One Parent Families
255 Kentish Town Road
London NW5 2LX
0207 428 5400
www.oneparentfamilies.org.uk
Free advice and information for people
bringing up children on their own.

On-line Announcements
www.senda.com
www.growingfamily.com

Send on-line announcements and
invitations for almost every occasion.

SANDS (Stillbirth and Neonatal
Death Society)
28 Portland Place
London W1N 4DE
0207 436 5881
National support network for bereaved
parents.

At-Home Mums

Contact-a-Family
170 Tottenham Court Road
London W1P 0HA
0207 383 3555
www.cafamily.org.uk
Offers support to families of children with
special needs.

Home-Start
2 Salisbury Road
Leicester LE1 7QR
0116 233 9955
Trained volunteers give support if you've
just had a baby and are under stress.

MAMA (Meet-a-Mum Association)
Waterside Centre
25 Avenue Road
London SE25 4DX
0208 768 0123 (7 to 10 pm, Mon to Fri)
www.mama.org.uk
Help for new parents, especially mothers
who feel depressed and isolated when their
babies are born.

Mothers At Home
www.mah.org

National Childbirth Trust
(see above)
Runs local postnatal groups in all areas
where new parents can get to know each
other.

Parentline Plus
520 Highgate Studios
53-79 Highgate Road
Kentish Town
London NW5 1TL
0808 800 2222
www.parentlineplus.org.uk
Help and information for parents
concerning a range of topics.

Serene (formerly known as Cry-sis)
helpline: 0207 404 5011 (8 am to 11 pm, 7
days a week)
www.our-space.co.uk/serene.htm
Provides emotional support and practical
advice to parents dealing with excessive
crying, demanding behaviour and sleep
problems.

Websites for further information
www.momsonline.com
www.parentsplace.com
www.parentssoup.com
www.parenttime.com
www.ukparents.co.uk

Breastfeeding Information

Association of Breastfeeding Mothers
PO Box 207
Bridgewater TA6 7YT
0207 813 1481
24-hour helpline for breastfeeding mothers.

Breastfeeding Network
helpline: 0870 900 8787 (9.30 am to 9.30
pm, 7 days a week)
www.breastfeeding.co.uk
Independent support and information
about breastfeeding.

La Leche League
BM3424
London WC1N 3XX
0207 242 1278 (9 am to 6 pm Mon to Fri,
answering machine at weekends)
www.lalecheleague.org

National Childbirth Trust Breastfeeding Line
0870 444 8708 (8 am to 10 pm, 7 days a week)
Can put you in touch with a local NCT
breastfeeding counsellor. You do not need to
be an NCT member to get this help.

Websites for further information
www.moms4milk.org
www.breastfeed.com

Childbirth Information

Active Birth Centre
25 Bickerton Road
London N19 5JT
0207 482 5554 (9.30 am to 5.30 pm Mon
to Fri, 10 am to 4 pm Sat)
www.birthcentre.com
Information and classes on non-
mechanized childbirth.

AIMS (Association for Improvements in
Maternity Services)
2 Bacon Lane
Hayling Island
Hampshire P011 0DN
01753 652781
Voluntary pressure group giving support
and advice on choices in maternity care.

Birthworks
Unit 4E
Brent Mill Trading Estate
South Brent
Devon TQ10 9YT
01364 72802
www.birthworks.co.uk
Advice on water births, videos for sale and
birth pools for hire.

The British Homeopathic Association
27a Devonshire Street
London W1N 1RJ
0207935 2163
Will put you in touch with qualified
practitioners.

Hypnobirthing
www.betterbirth.co.uk

Independent Midwives Association
The Wessex Maternity Centre
Mansbridge Road
West End
Southampton SO18 3HW
www.independentmidwives.org.uk
Send SAE for register of midwives offering
private care. Free advice on home births.

The International Society of Professional
Aromatherapists
01455 637987

Sheila Kitzinger
www.sheilakitzinger.com
This website mainly offers a 'reflective
listening' service for women who have had
a bad birth experience - such as an
emergency caesarean - but it also has
information on home births, water births
and local classes.

The Register of Qualified Aromatherapists
01235 227957
Will put you in touch with qualified
practitioners.

Royal College of Midwives
15 Mansfield Street
London W1M 0BE
0207 312 3535
www.rcm.org.uk.

Childbirth Information *(continued)*

Royal College of Obstetricians and
Gynaecologists
27 Sussex Place
Regent's Park

London NW1 4G
www.rcg.org.uk
Will put you in touch with qualified
practitioners.

Child Care

Daycare Trust
Shoreditch Town Hall Annexe
380 Old Street
London EC1V 9LT
0207 739 2866
www.daycaretrust.org.uk
Charity campaigning to improve
conditions for working parents and
promoting high quality, affordable
childcare for all.

FRS (Federation of Recruitment and
Employment Services)
36-38 Mortimer Street

London W1N 7RB
0207 323 4300
Send SAE for a list of nanny and au pair
agencies.

International Nanny Association
www.nanny.org

Parents at Work
45 Beech Street
London EC2Y 8AD
0207 628 3565 (answer machine)
Advice and information on childcare and
employment issues relating to pregnancy
and working parents.

Dads

Fathers Direct
0207 920 9491 (10 am to 6 pm, Mon to Fri)
www.fathersdirect.com
The national information centre for
fatherhood.

Websites for further information
www.daddyshome.com
www.edads.com
www.fathersforum.com
www.fathersonline.com
www.fathersworld.com
www.newdads.com

Maternity and Paternity Rights and Benefits

Child Tax Credit and Working Tax Credit
www.taxcredits.inlandrevenue.gov.uk/
Home.aspx
Explains the tax credits and has a
calculator that will help you work out how
much you are entitled to. Also allows you
to apply online.

Department of Trade and Industry
www.dti.gov.uk

Maternity Alliance
3rd Floor West
2-6 Northburgh Street
London EC1V 0AY
0207 7490 7639
www.maternityalliance.org.uk

Advice and information about maternity
rights and benefits.

National Association of Citizens Advice
Bureaux
www.nacab.org.uk
email: adviceguide@nacab.org.uk

Parents at Work
45 Beech Street
London EC2Y 8AD
0207 628 3565 (answer machine)
Advice and information on childcare and
employment issues relating to pregnancy
and working parents.

Paternity Leave
ACAS helpline: 08457 47 47

Mother's Health

Active for Life
www.active.org.uk

APEC (Action on Pre-eclampsia)
84-88 Pinner Road
Harrow
Middlesex HA1 4HZ
0208 863 3271
helpline: 0208 427 4217 (weekday mornings)

Association for Postnatal Illness
25 Jerdan Place
London SW6 1BE
0207 386 0868
Advice for women with postnatal illness, including depression.

BBC Online Health and Fitness
www.bbc.co.uk/health/fightingfat

Breast Cancer Care
210 New Kings Road
London SW6 4NZ
020 7384 2984
www.breastcancercare.org.uk

Diabetes UK (formerly The British Diabetic Association)
0207 636 6112 (9 am to 4 pm, Mon to Fri)
www.diabetes.org.uk
Advice for pregnant diabetic women.

Epilepsy Action
Freephone helpline: 0808 800 5050
www.epilepsy.org.uk
Offers advice and information over the phone.

Miscarriage Association
Clayton Hospital
Northgate
Wakefield
West Yorkshire WF1 3JS
01924 200799
helpline: 01924 200795
www.the-ma.org.uk
Advice and information on a national network of miscarriage support groups.

Quitline
0800 0022 00
www.healthnet.org.uk/quit/guide
Counselling for those who are trying to give up smoking. Puts you in touch with local support groups.

Ovacome
St Bartholomew's Hospital
London EC1A 7BE
07071 781861
www.ovacome.org.uk
UK-wide support group for all those concerned with ovarian cancer.

SOS Morning Sickness
www.sosmorningsickness.com
For information on, and remedies for, nausea and vomiting.

Sickle Cell Society
54 Station Road
Harlesdon
London NW10 4UA
0208 961 4006/7795
www.sicklecellsociety.org

UK Thalassaemia Society
19 The Broadway
Southgate Circus
London N14 6PH
0208 882 0011
www.ukts.org

Toxoplasma Infection
0207 593 1150
Up-to-date information plus advice for women who may have had toxoplasma infection during pregnancy.

Women's Health
52 Featherstone Street
London EC1Y 8RT
0207 251 6580
email: womenshealth@pop3.poptel:org.uk
Telephone service, or send SAE for advice on reproductive health.

Multiples

Multiple Births Foundation
0208 383 3519
Telephone counselling.

TAMBA (Twins and Multiple Birth
Association)
2 The Willows
Gardner Road
Guildford
Surrey GU1 4PG
0870770 3305
helpline: 01732 868 000 (7 to 11 pm Mon
to Fri, 10 am to 11 pm weekends)
www.tamba.org.uk
Provides information and support network
for parents of multiple birth babies.

Twins Hope
www.twinshope.com
International centre for twin-related
diseases.

Twins World
www.twinsworld.com
Good resource for couples expecting
multiples.

Nutrition

British Nutrition Foundation
52-54 High Holborn
London WC1V 6RQ
0207 404 6504
www.nutrition.org.uk

Food Standards Agency
Aviation House
125 Kingsway
London WC2B 6NH
0207 276 8000
www.foodstandards.gov.uk

Health Supplement Information Service
www.hsis.org

Wellbeing
27 Sussex Place Regent's Park
London NW1 4SP
0207 772 6400
www.wellbeing.co.uk
Advice on what to eat during pregnancy
and while breastfeeding.

Premature Babies

Baby Life Support Systems (BLISS)
68 South Lambeth Road
London SW8 1RL
0870 770 0337
helpline: 0500 618 140 (10 am to 5 pm,
Mon to Fri)
www.bliss.org.uk
National charity offering support and
information for families of sick newborn
babies.

www.earlyarrivals.com
For information on, and products for,
premature infants.

Tommy's The Baby Charity
1 Kennington Road
London SE1 7RR
0207 620 0188
www.tommys.org
Charity that raises funds for research into
prematurity and provides advice on
pregnancy and premature birth.

Safety

Child Accident Prevention Trust
0207 608 382
Answers queries on specific matters to do with child safety.

ROSPA (Royal Society for the Prevention of Accidents)
353 Bristol Road
Edgbaston
Birmingham B5 7ST

0121 248 2000
www.rospa.co.uk
Registered charity actively involved in the promotion of safety in all areas of life. Provides information, advice, resources and training.

Websites for further information
www.dti.gov.uk/homesafetynetwork

Special Care and Special Needs

Association for Spina Bifida and Hydrocephalus
42 Park Road
Peterborough PE1 2UQ
01733 555988
www.asbah.demon.co.uk

Birth Defects Foundation
Martindale
Hawks Green
Cannock
Staffordshire WS11 2XN
01543 468888
www.birthdefects.co.uk

Cleft Lip and Palate Association (CLAPA)
235-37 Finchley Road

London NW3 6LS
0207 431 0033
www.cleft.com
Information and counselling for parents and contacts for local groups.

Down's Syndrome Association
155 Mitcham Road
London SW17 9PG
0208 682 4001
www.downs-syndrome.org.uk
Advice on the care of children with Down's syndrome.

AUSTRALIAN RESOURCES

Australian Breastfeeding Association
1818-1822 Malvern Road
East Malvern, VICT 3145
Ph: (03) 9885 0855
Breastfeeding Helplines:
NSW (02) 9639 8686
VICT (03) 9885 0653
QLD (07) 3844 8977
SA & NT (08) 8411 0050
WA (08) 9340 1200
ACT (02) 6258 8928
TAS (03) 6223 2609
Email: info@breastfeeding.asn.au

Internet: www.breastfeeding.asn.au
National organisation aimed at the promotion and protection of breastfeeding and offers education, counselling and support to breastfeeding women.

Australian Multiple Birth Association
PO Box 105
Coogee, NSW 2034
Email: secretary@amba.org.au
Internet: www.amba.org.au
Support for families with twins, triplets, quadruplets or more.

AUSTRALIAN RESOURCES *(continued)*

Centrelink
Ph: 131 305
For information on childcare benefits, maternity allowance, parenting payments, family assistance and maintenance enquiries.

Childbirth Education of Australia
PO Box 240
Sutherland, NSW 2232
Ph: (02) 8539 7188
Email: cea-nsw.com.au
Provides prenatal education courses and is affiliated with national and international childbirth education groups.

Early Childhood Australia
PO Box 105
Watson, ACT 2602
Ph: (02) 6242 1800
Freecall: 1800 356 900
Email: eca@earlychildhood.org.au
Internet: www.aeca.org.au
Works with government, early childhood professionals, parents and carers to secure the best range of options for children as they grow.

Family Planning Australia
Suite 4, Level 1
217 Northbourne Ave
Turner, ACT 2612
Ph: (02) 6230 5255
Email: fpa@fpa.net.au
Internet: www.fpa.net.au
A national organisation with clinics around Australia aimed at improving the reproductive and sexual health of Australians.

Foresight Association for the Promotion of Preconceptual Care
133 Rowntree Steet
Birchgrove, 2041 NSW
Ph: (02) 98188111
Internet: www.acnem.org/journal/14-2_november_1995/foresight_program.htm
Association aimed at preparing couples for pregnancy with preconceptual care and advice.

Homebirth Australia
Freecall 1800 222 180
Information on finding a midwife and on homebirths.

Immunise Australia
Freecall 1800 653 809
Internet: www.immunise.health.gov.au
Information on standard childhood immunisations.

Karitane
Cnr The Horsley Drive & Mitchell St
Carramar, NSW 2163
Ph: (02) 9794 1800
Internet: swsahs.nsw.gov.au/karitane

24-hour parent counselling
Ph: (02) 9794 1852
Freecall 1800 677 961
Supports, guides and informs families experiencing parenting difficulties.

Maternity Coalition
PO Box 1190
Blackburn North, VICT 3130
Email: inquiries@maternitycoalition.org.au
Internet: www.maternitycoalition.org.au
National organisation aimed at providing the best-practice maternity care for all Australian women and their families.

Medicare
Ph: 132 011

Nutrition Australia
University of Wollongong
Northfields, NSW 2522
Ph: (02) 4221 5346
Email: nsw@nutritionaustralia.org
Internet: www.nutritionaustralia.org
Provides scientifically based nutrition information to encourage all Australians, especially pregnant women, to achieve optimal health through food variety and exercise.

Playgroup Australia
Internet: www.playgroupaustralia.com.au
Freecall 1300 887 674

NSW (02) 9604 5513
Email: admin@playgroupnsw.com.au
Internet: www.playgroupnsw.com.au

NT (08) 8945 7775
Email: playgroupnt@octa4.net.au

QLD (07) 3368 2622
Email: info@playgroupqld.com.au

AUSTRALIAN RESOURCES *(continued)*

SA (08) 8344 2722
Email: info@playgroupsa.com.au

WA (08) 9228 8088
Email: admin@playgroupwa.com.au
Informal groups where parents, carers,
babies and children aged 0 to school age
get together in a relaxed and friendly
environment to learn through play.

Pre and Postnatal Depression
Karitane Parent and Baby Unit
130 Nelson St
Fairfield Heights, NSW 2165
Ph: (02) 9754 2655
Internet: www.swsahs.nsw.gov.au/karitane

Pre and Postnatal Depression Association
270 Church Street
Richmond, VICT 3121
Ph: (03) 9428 4600
Email: panda@vicnet.net.au
Internet: http://home.vicnet.net.au

Stillbirth and Neonatal Death Support
(SANDS)
ACT (02) 6287 1389
NSW (02) 9721 0124
QLD (07) 3252 2865
SA (08) 8277 0304
TAS (03) 6344 6811
VIC (03) 9899 0217
WA (08) 9474 3544
Support Line 1800 686 780
National organisation aimed at supporting
and counselling parents affected by
stillbirth or neonatal death.

Sudden Infant Death Syndrome
PO Box 431
Camperdown, NSW 1450
Ph: (02) 98188400
Freecall: 1300 308 307
Email: sydney@sidsandkids.org
Internet: www.sidsaustralia.org.au
National organisation aimed at educating,
supporting and counselling parents affected
by SIDS.

Tresillian
Tresillian Family Care Centre
McKenzie St
Belmore, NSW 2192
Ph (02) 9787 0800
Email: tresillian@tres.cant.cs.nsw.gov.au
Internet: www.cs.nsw.gov.au/tresillian

24-hour Parent's Helpline
Ph: (02) 9787 0855
Freecall 1800 637 357
Aimed at optimising the health and
wellbeing of families with babies and
young children.

Glossary

a

Abdominal measurement—Measurement taken of the growth of the baby in the uterus at antenatal visits. Measurement is from the pubic symphysis to the fundus. Too much growth or too little growth may indicate problems.

Abruptio placenta—See *placental abruption.*

Acquired immune deficiency syndrome (AIDS)—Debilitating, frequently fatal illness that affects the body's ability to respond to infection. Caused by the human immune deficiency virus (HIV).

Active labour—When a woman is dilated between 4 and 8 cm. Contractions are usually 3 to 5 minutes apart.

Aerobic exercise—Exercise that increases your heart rate and causes you to consume oxygen.

Afterbirth—Placenta and membranes expelled after baby is delivered. See *placenta.*

Alpha-foetoprotein (AFP)—Substance produced by the unborn baby as it grows inside the uterus. Large amounts of AFP are found in the amniotic fluid. Larger-than-normal amounts are found in the maternal bloodstream if neural-tube defects are present in the foetus.

Alveoli—Ends of the ducts of the lung.

Amino acids—Substances that act as building blocks in the developing embryo and foetus.

Amniocentesis—Process by which amniotic fluid is removed from the amniotic sac for testing; fluid is tested for some genetic defects and for foetal lung maturity.

Amniotic fluid—Fluid surrounding the baby inside the amniotic sac.

Amniotic sac—Membrane that surrounds baby inside the uterus. It contains baby, placenta and amniotic fluid.

Ampulla—Dilated opening of a tube or duct.

Anaemia—Any condition in which the number of red blood cells is less than normal. Term usually applies to the concentration of the oxygen-transporting material in the blood, which is the red blood cell.

Anencephaly—Defective development of the brain combined with the absence of the bones normally surrounding the brain.

Angioma—Tumour, usually benign, or swelling composed of lymph and blood vessels.

Anovulatory—Lack, or cessation, of ovulation.

Antenatal care—Programme of care for a pregnant woman before the birth of her baby.

Anti-D—Medication given during pregnancy and following delivery to prevent isoimmunization. Also see *isoimmunization*.

Anti-inflammatory medications—Drugs to relieve pain or inflammation.

Apgar scores—Measurement of a baby's response to birth and life on its own. Taken 1 minute and 5 minutes after birth.

Areola—Pigmented or coloured ring surrounding the nipple of the breast.

Arrhythmia—Irregular or missed heartbeat.

Aspiration—Swallowing or sucking a foreign body or fluid, such as vomit, into an airway.

Asthma—Disease marked by recurrent attacks of shortness of breath and difficulty breathing. Often caused by an allergic reaction.

Atonic uterus—Uterus that is flaccid; relaxed; lacking tone.

Augmented labour—When labour is 'stalled' or progress is not being made during labour, medication (oxytocin) is given.

Autoantibodies—Antibodies that attack parts of your body or your own tissues.

b

Baby blues—Mild depression in woman after delivery.

Back labour—Pain of labour felt in lower back.

Beta-adrenergics—Substances that interfere with transmission of stimuli. They affect the autonomic nervous system.

Bilirubin—Breakdown product of pigment formed in the liver from haemoglobin during the destruction of red blood cells.

Biophysical profile—Method of evaluating a foetus before birth.

Biopsy—Removal of a small piece of tissue for microscopic study.

Birthing centre—Facility specializing in the delivery of babies. Usually a woman labours, delivers and recovers in the same room. It may be part of a hospital or a freestanding unit. Sometimes called *LDRP*, for labour, delivery, recovery and postpartum.

Bishop score—Method of cervical scoring, used to predict the success of inducing labour. Includes dilatation, effacement, station, consistency and position of the cervix. A score is given for each point, then they are added together to give a total score to help doctor decide whether to induce labour.

Blastomere—One of the cells the egg divides into after it has been fertilized.

Blood pressure—Push of the blood against the walls of the arteries, which carry blood away from the heart. Changes in blood pressure may indicate problems.

Blood typing—Test to determine if a woman's blood type is A, B, AB or O.

Blood-pressure check—Check of a woman's blood pressure. High blood pressure can be significant during pregnancy, especially nearer the due date. Changes in blood pressure readings can alert the doctor to potential problems.

Blood-sugar tests—See *glucose-tolerance test.*

Bloody show—Small amount of vaginal bleeding late in pregnancy; often precedes labour.

Braxton-Hicks contractions—Irregular, painless tightening of uterus during pregnancy.

Breech presentation—Abnormal birth position of the foetus. Buttocks or legs come into the birth canal before the head.

C

Caesarean section or delivery—Delivery of a baby through an abdominal incision rather than through the vagina.

Canavan's disease screening—Blood test performed on people of Ashkenazi Jewish background to determine if a foetus is affected with Canavan's disease.

Cataract, congenital—Cloudiness of the eye lens present at birth.

Cell antibodies—See *autoantibodies.*

Cervical cultures—To test for STDs; when a Pap smear is done, a sample may also be taken to check for chlamydia, gonorrhoea or other STDs.

Cervix—Opening of the uterus.

Chadwick's sign—Dark-blue or purple discoloration of the mucosa of the vagina and cervix during pregnancy.

Chemotherapy—Treatment of disease by chemical substances or drugs.

Chlamydia—Sexually transmitted venereal infection.

Chloasma—Increased pigmentation or extensive brown patches of irregular shape and size on the face (commonly has the appearance of a butterfly) or other parts of the body. They may be extensive. Also called *mask of pregnancy.*

Chorion—Outermost foetal membrane found around the amnion.

Chorionic villus sampling (CVS)—Diagnostic test that can be done early in pregnancy to determine pregnancy abnormalities. A biopsy of tissue is taken from inside the uterus through the abdomen or the cervix.

Chromosomal abnormality—Abnormal number or abnormal makeup of chromosomes.

Chromosomes—Thread in a cell's nucleus that contains DNA, which transmits genetic information.

Cleft palate—Defect in the palate, a part of the upper jaw or mouth.

Colostrum—Thin yellow fluid, which is the first milk to come from the breast. Most often seen towards the end of pregnancy. It is different in content from milk produced later during nursing.

Complete blood count (CBC)—Blood test to check iron stores and to check for infections.

Condyloma acuminatum—Skin tags or warts that are sexually transmitted. Also called *venereal warts.*

Congenital deafness screening—If a couple has a family history of inherited deafness, this blood test may identify the problem before baby's birth.

Congenital problem—Problem present at birth.

Conization of the cervix—Surgical procedure performed on pre-malignant and malignant conditions of the cervix. A large biopsy of the cervix is taken in the shape of a cone.

Conjoined twins—Twins connected at the body; they may share vital organs. Previously called *Siamese twins.*

Constipation—Bowel movements are infrequent or incomplete.

Contraction stress test—Test of foetal response to uterine contractions to evaluate foetal well-being.

Contractions—Uterus squeezes or tightens to push the baby out of the uterus during birth.

Corpus luteum—Area in the ovary where the egg is released at ovulation. A cyst may form in this area after ovulation. Called a *corpus luteum cyst.*

Crown-to-rump length—Measurement from the top of the baby's head (crown) to baby's buttocks (rump).

Cystitis—Inflammation of the bladder.

Cytomegalovirus (CMV) infection—Group of viruses from the herpes virus family.

d

D&C (dilatation and curettage)—Surgical procedure in which the cervix is dilated and the lining of the uterus is scraped.

Developmental delay—Condition in which the development of the baby or child is slower than normal.

Diastasis recti—Separation of abdominal muscles.

Diethylstilbestrol (DES)—Non-steroidal synthetic oestrogen. Used in the past to try to prevent miscarriage.

Dilatation—Amount, in centimetres, the cervix has opened before birth. When a woman is fully dilated, she is at 10 cm.

Dizygotic twins—Twins derived from two different eggs. Often called *fraternal twins.*

Doppler—Device that enhances the foetal heartbeat so the doctor and others can hear it.

Down's syndrome—Chromosomal disorder in which baby has three copies of Chromosome 21 (instead of two); results in mental retardation, distinct physical traits and various other problems.

Due date—Date baby is expected to be born. Most babies are born near this date, but only 1 of 20 are born on the actual date.

Dysuria—Difficulty or pain urinating.

e

Early labour—When a woman experiences regular contractions (one every 20 minutes down to one every 5 minutes) for longer than 2 hours. The cervix usually dilates to 3 or 4 cm.

Eclampsia—Convulsions and coma in a woman with pre-eclampsia. Not related to epilepsy. See *pre-eclampsia.*

Ectodermal germ layer—Layer in the developing embryo that gives rise to developing structures in the foetus. These include skin, teeth and glands of the mouth, the nervous system and the pituitary gland.

Ectopic pregnancy—Pregnancy that occurs outside the uterine cavity, most often in the Fallopian tube. Also called *tubal pregnancy.*

ECV (External cephalic version)—Procedure done late in pregnancy, in which doctor manually attempts to move a baby in the breech presentation into the normal head-down birth position.

EDC (estimated date of confinement)—Anticipated due date for delivery of the baby. Calculated from the first day of the last period, counting forward 280 days.

Effacement—Thinning of cervix; occurs in the latter part of pregnancy and during labour.

Electroencephalogram—Recording of the electrical activity of the brain.

Embryo—Organism in the early stages of development; in a human pregnancy from conception to 10 weeks.

Embryonic period—First 10 weeks of gestation.

Endodermal germ layer—Area of tissue in early development of the embryo that gives rise to other structures. These include the digestive tract, respiratory organs, vagina, bladder and urethra. Also called *endoderm* or *entoderm.*

Endometrial cycle—Regular development of the mucous membrane that lines the inside of the uterus. It begins with the preparation for acceptance of a pregnancy and ends with the shedding of the lining during a menstrual period.

Endometrium—Mucous membrane that lines inside of the uterine wall.

Enema—Fluid injected into the rectum for the purpose of clearing out the bowel.

Engorgement—Filled with fluid; usually refers to breast engorgement in a breast-feeding mother.

Enzyme—Protein made by cells. It acts as a catalyst to improve or cause chemical changes in other substances.

Epidural block—Type of anaesthesia. Medication is injected around the spinal cord during labour or other types of surgery.

Episiotomy—Surgical incision of the perineum (area behind the vagina, above the rectum). Used during delivery to avoid tearing vaginal opening and rectum.

Estimated date of confinement—See *EDC.*

Exotoxin—Poison or toxin from a source outside the body.

Expressing breast milk—Manually forcing milk out of the breast.

f

Face presentation—Baby comes into the birth canal face first.

Fallopian tube—Tube that leads from the uterine cavity to the area of the ovary. Also called *uterine tube.*

False labour—Tightening of uterus without dilatation of the cervix.

Familial Mediterranean fever screening—Blood test performed on people of Armenian, Arabic, Turkish and Sephardic Jewish background to identify carriers of the recessive gene. Permits diagnosis in a newborn so treatment can be started.

Fasting blood sugar—Blood test to evaluate the amount of sugar in the blood following a time period of fasting.

Ferrous gluconate or sulfate—Iron supplement.

Fertilization—Joining of the sperm and egg.

Fertilization age—Dating a pregnancy from the time of fertilization; 2 weeks shorter than gestational age. Also see *gestational age.*

Fibrin—Elastic protein important in the coagulation of blood.

Foetal anomaly—Foetal malformation or abnormal development.

Foetal arrhythmia—See *arrhythmia.*

Foetal distress—Problems with the baby that occur before birth or during labour; often requires immediate delivery.

Foetal fibronectin (fFN)—Test done to evaluate premature labour. A sample of cervical-vaginal secretions is taken; if fFN is present after 22 weeks, it indicates increased risk for premature delivery.

Foetal goiter—Enlargement of the thyroid in the foetus.

Foetal monitor—Device used before or during labour to listen to and to record the foetal heartbeat. Monitoring baby inside the uterus can be external (through maternal abdomen) or internal (through maternal vagina).

Foetal period—Time period following the embryonic period (first 10 weeks of gestation) until birth.

Foetoscopy—Test that enables doctor to look through a foetoscope (a fibre-optics scope) to detect subtle abnormalities and problems in a foetus.

Foetus—Refers to the unborn baby after 10 weeks of gestation until birth.

Forceps—Instrument sometimes used to deliver baby. It is placed around baby's head, inside the birth canal, to help guide baby out of the birth canal during delivery.

Frank breech—Baby presenting buttocks first. Legs are straight and knees extended.

Fraternal twins—See *dizygotic twins.*

Fundus—Top part of the uterus; often measured during pregnancy.

g

Genes—Basic units of heredity. Each gene carries specific information and is passed from parent to child. A child receives half of its genes from its mother and half from its father. Every human has about 100,000 genes.

Genetic counselling—Consultation between a couple and specialists about genetic defects and the possibility of presence or recurrence of genetic problems in a pregnancy.

Genetic tests—Various screening and diagnostic tests done to determine whether a couple may have a child with a genetic defect. Usually part of genetic counselling.

Genital herpes simplex—Herpes simplex infection involving the genital area. It can be significant during pregnancy because of the danger to a newborn foetus becoming infected with herpes simplex.

Genitourinary problems—Defects or problems involving genital organs and the bladder or kidneys.

Germ layers—Layers or areas of tissue important in the development of the baby.

Gestational age—Dating a pregnancy from the first day of the last menstrual period; 2 weeks longer than fertilization age. Also see *fertilization age.*

Gestational diabetes—Occurrence or worsening of diabetes that occurs only during pregnancy (gestation).

Gestational trophoblastic disease (GTN)—Abnormal pregnancy with cystic growth of the placenta. Characterized by bleeding during early and middle pregnancy.

Globulin—Family of proteins from plasma or serum of the blood.

Glucose-tolerance test (GTT)—Blood test done to evaluate the body's response to sugar. Blood is drawn from the mother-to-be once or at intervals following ingestion of a sugary substance.

Glucosuria—Glucose (sugar) in the urine.

Gonorrhoea—Contagious venereal infection, transmitted primarily by intercourse.

Grand mal seizure—Loss of control of body functions. Seizure activity of a major form.

Group-B streptococcal (GBS) infection—Serious infection occurring in the mother's vagina, throat or rectum. Infection can be in any of these areas.

Group-B streptococcus (GBS) test—Near the end of the pregnancy, samples may be taken from the expectant woman's vagina, perineum and rectum to check for GBS. A urine test may also be done. If the test is positive, treatment may be started or given during labour.

h

Habitual miscarriage—Occurrence of three or more spontaneous miscarriages.

Haematocrit—Determines the proportion of blood cells to plasma. Important in diagnosing anaemia.

Haemoglobin—Pigment in red blood cells that carries oxygen to body tissues.

Haemolytic disease—Destruction of red blood cells. See *anaemia*.

Haemorrhoids—Dilated blood vessels, most often found in the rectum or rectal canal.

Heartburn—Discomfort or pain that occurs in the chest. Often occurs after eating.

Heparin—Medication used to thin the blood.

Hepatitis-B antibodies test—Test to determine if the pregnant woman has ever contracted hepatitis-B.

High-risk pregnancy—Pregnancy with complications that requires special medical attention, often from a specialist. Also see *perinatologist*.

HIV/AIDS test—Test to determine if a woman has HIV or AIDS (the test cannot be done without the woman's knowledge and permission).

Homan's sign—Pain caused by flexing the toes towards the knees when a person has a blood clot in the lower leg.

Home uterine monitoring—Contractions of a pregnant woman's uterus are recorded at home, then transmitted by telephone to the doctor (no special equipment is needed other than the monitor and a telephone). Used to identify women at risk of premature labour.

Human chorionic gonadatropin (HCG)—Hormone produced in early pregnancy; measured in a pregnancy test.

Human placental lactogen—Hormone of pregnancy produced by the placenta and found in the bloodstream.

Hyaline membrane disease—Respiratory disease of the newborn.

Hydatidiform mole—See *gestational trophoblastic disease*.

Hydramnios—Increased amount of amniotic fluid

Hydrocephalus—Excessive accumulation of fluid around the brain of the baby. Sometimes called *water on the brain*.

Hyperbilirubinaemia—Extremely high level of bilirubin in the blood.

Hyperemesis gravidarum—Severe nausea, dehydration and vomiting during pregnancy. Occurs most frequently during the first trimester.

Hyperglycaemia—Increased blood sugar.

Hypertension, pregnancy-induced—High blood pressure that occurs during pregnancy. Defined by an increase in the diastolic or systolic blood pressure.

Hyperthyroidism—Elevation of the thyroid hormone in the bloodstream.

Hypoplasia—Defective or incomplete development or formation of tissue.

Hypotension—Low blood pressure.

Hypothyroidism—Low or inadequate levels of thyroid hormone in the bloodstream.

i

Identical twins—See *monozygotic twins.*

Imaging tests—Tests that look inside the body, including X-rays, CT scans (or CAT scans) and magnetic resonance imaging (MRI).

Immune globulin preparation—Substance used to protect against infection with certain diseases, such as hepatitis or measles.

In utero—Within the uterus.

Incompetent cervix—Cervix that dilates painlessly, without contractions.

Incomplete miscarriage—Miscarriage in which part, but not all, of the uterine contents are expelled.

Induced labour—Labour started using a medication. See *oxytocin.*

Inevitable miscarriage—Pregnancy complicated with bleeding and cramping. Usually results in miscarriage.

Insulin—Peptide hormone made by the pancreas. It promotes the use of glucose.

Intrauterine-growth restriction (IUGR)—Inadequate growth of the foetus during the last stages of pregnancy.

Iodides—Medications made up of negative ions of iodine.

Iron-deficiency anaemia—Anaemia produced by lack of iron in the diet; often seen in pregnancy.

Isoimmunization—Development of specific antibody directed at the red blood cells of another individual, such as a baby in utero. Often occurs when an Rh-negative woman carries an Rh-positive baby or is given Rh-positive blood.

j–k

Jaundice—Yellow staining of the skin, sclera (eyes) and deeper tissues of the body. Caused by excessive amounts of bilirubin. Treated with phototherapy.

Ketones—Breakdown product of metabolism found in the blood, particularly from starvation or uncontrolled diabetes.

Kick count—Record of how often a pregnant woman feels her baby move; used to evaluate foetal well-being.

Kidney stones—Small mass or lesion found in the kidney or urinary tract. Can block the flow of urine.

l

Labour—Process of expelling a foetus from the uterus.

Laparoscopy—Minor surgical procedure performed for tubal ligation, diagnosis of pelvic pain or diagnosis of ectopic pregnancy.

Leucorrhoea—Vaginal discharge characterized by a white or yellowish colour. Primarily composed of mucus.

Lightening—Change in the shape of the pregnant uterus a few weeks before labour. Often described as the baby 'dropping.'

Linea nigra—Line of increased pigmentation that often develops during pregnancy; line runs down the abdomen from bellybutton to pubic area.

Lochia—Vaginal discharge that occurs after delivery of the baby and placenta.

m

Malignant GTN—Cancerous change of gestational trophoblastic disease. See *gestational trophoblastic disease.*

Mammogram—X-ray study of the breasts to identify normal and abnormal breast tissue.

Mask of pregnancy—Increased pigmentation over the area of the face under each eye. Commonly has the appearance of a butterfly.

McDonald cerclage—Surgical procedure performed on an incompetent cervix. A drawstring-type suture holds the cervical opening closed during pregnancy. Also see *incompetent cervix.*

Meconium—First intestinal discharge of the newborn; green or yellow in colour. It consists of epithelial or surface cells, mucus and bile. Discharge may occur before or during labour or soon after birth.

Melanoma—Pigmented mole or tumour. It may or may not be cancerous.

Meningomyelocele—Congenital defect of the central nervous system of the baby. Membranes and the spinal cord protrude through an opening or defect in the vertebral column.

Menstrual age—See *gestational age.*

Menstruation—Regular or periodic discharge of endometrial lining and blood from the uterus.

Mesodermal germ layer—Tissue of the embryo that forms connective tissue, muscles, kidneys, ureters and other organs.

Metaplasia—Change in the structure of a tissue into another type that is not normal for that tissue.

Microcephaly—Abnormally small development of the head in the developing foetus.

Microphthalmia—Abnormally small eyeballs.

Midwife—Nurse who has received extra training in the care of pregnant patients and the delivery of their babies.

Miscarriage—Termination or premature end of pregnancy; giving birth to an embryo or foetus before it can live outside the womb, usually defined as before 20 weeks of pregnancy.

Missed miscarriage—Failed pregnancy without bleeding or cramping. Often diagnosed by ultrasound weeks or months after a pregnancy fails.

Mittelschmerz—Pain that coincides with release of an egg from the ovary.

Molar pregnancy—See *gestational trophoblastic disease.*

Monilial vulvovaginitis—Infection caused by yeast or monilia. Usually affects the vagina and vulva.

Monozygotic twins—Twins conceived from one egg. Often called *identical twins.*

Morning sickness—Nausea and vomiting, with ill health, found primarily during the first trimester of pregnancy. Also see *hyperemesis gravidarum.*

Morula—Cells resulting from the early division of the fertilized egg at the beginning of pregnancy.

Mucus plug—Secretions in the cervix; often released just before labour.

Multiple-markers test—See *quad-screen test* and *triple-screen test.*

Mutations—Change in the character of a gene. Passed from one cell division to another.

n

Natural childbirth—Labour and delivery in which the mother has as few interventions as possible. This may include no medication or monitoring. The woman usually has taken classes to prepare her for labour and delivery.

Neural-tube defects—Abnormalities in the development of the spinal cord and brain in a foetus. Also see *anencephaly; hydrocephalus; spina bifida.*

Non-stress test—Test in which movements of the baby felt by the mother or observed by a healthcare provider are recorded, along with changes in the foetal heart rate. Used to evaluate foetal well-being.

Nuchal translucency screening—Detailed ultrasound that allows the doctor to measure the space behind baby's neck. When combined with blood test results, can measure a woman's probability of her baby having Down's syndrome.

O

Obstetrician—Doctor who specializes in the care of pregnant women and the delivery of their babies.

Oligohydramnios—Lack or deficiency of amniotic fluid.

Omphalocele—Presence of congenital outpouching of the umbilicus containing internal organs in the foetus or newborn infant.

Opioids—Synthetic compounds with effects similar to those of opium.

Organogenesis—Development of the organ systems in the embryo.

Ossification—Bone formation.

Ovarian cycle—Regular production of hormones from the ovary in response to hormonal messages from the brain. The ovarian cycle governs the endometrial cycle.

Ovulation—Cyclic release of an egg from the ovary.

Ovulatory age—See *fertilization age.*

Oxytocin—Medication that causes uterine contractions; used to induce or augment labour. Also the hormone produced by pituitary glands.

p

Paediatrician—Doctor who specializes in the care of babies and children.

Palmar erythema—Redness of palms of the hands.

Pap smear—Routine screening test that evaluates presence of pre-malignant or cancerous conditions of the cervix.

Paracervical block—Local anaesthetic to relieve pain of cervical dilatation.

Pelvic exam—Physical examination by the doctor who feels inside the pelvic area to evaluate the size of the uterus at the beginning of pregnancy and to help the doctor determine if the cervix is dilating and thinning towards the end of pregnancy.

Percutaneous umbilical-cord blood sampling (PUBS, cordocentesis)—Test done on the foetus to diagnose Rh-incompatibility, blood disorders and infections. Also called *cordocentesis.*

Perinatologist—Doctor who specializes in the care of high-risk pregnancies.

Perineum—Area between the rectum and vagina.

Petit mal seizure—Attack of a brief nature with possible short impairment of consciousness. Often associated with blinking or flickering of the eyelids and a mild twitching of the mouth.

Phosphatidyl glycerol (PG)—Lipoprotein present when foetal lungs are mature.

Phospholipids—Fat-containing phosphorous; the most important are lecithins and sphingomyelin, which are important in the maturation of foetal lungs before birth.

Phototherapy—Treatment for jaundice in a newborn infant. Also see *jaundice.*

Physiologic anaemia of pregnancy—Anaemia during pregnancy caused by an increase in the amount of plasma (fluid) in the blood compared to the number of cells in the blood. Also see *anaemia.*

Placenta previa—Low attachment of the placenta, very close to, or covering, the cervix.

Placenta—Organ inside the uterus that is attached to the baby by the umbilical cord. Essential during pregnancy for growth and development of the embryo and foetus. Also called *afterbirth.*

Placental abruption—Premature separation of the placenta from the uterus.

Pneumonitis—Inflammation of the lungs.

Polyhydramnios—See *hydramnios.*

Postmature baby—Baby born 2 weeks or more past its due date.

Postpartum—The 6-week period following a baby's birth. Refers to the mother, not the baby.

Postpartum blues—Mild depression after delivery.

Postpartum distress syndrome (PPDS)—A range of symptoms including baby blues, postpartum depression and postpartum psychosis.

Postpartum haemorrhage—Bleeding greater than 450 ml (17 fl oz) at time of delivery.

Post-term birth—Pregnancy of 42+ weeks gestation.

Pre-eclampsia—Combination of significant symptoms unique to pregnancy, including high blood pressure, oedema, swelling and changes in reflexes.

Pregnancy diabetes—See *gestational diabetes*.

Premature delivery—Delivery before 38 weeks gestation.

Preterm premature rupture of membranes (PPROM)—Rupture of foetal membranes before 37 weeks of pregnancy.

Prepared childbirth—Woman has taken classes so she knows what to expect during labour and delivery. She may request pain medication if she needs it.

Presentation—Describes which part of the baby comes into the birth canal first.

Propylthiouracil—Medication used to treat thyroid disease.

Proteinuria—Protein in urine.

Pruritis gravidarum—Itching during pregnancy.

Pubic symphysis—Bony prominence in the pelvic bone found in the middle of a woman's lower abdomen. Landmark from which the doctor often measures the growing uterus during pregnancy.

Pudendal block—Local anaesthesia during labour.

Pulmonary embolism—Blood clot from another part of the body that travels to the lungs. Can close passages in the lungs and decrease oxygen exchange.

Pyelonephritis—Serious kidney infection.

q–r

Quad-screen test—Measurement of four blood components to help identify problems. The four tests include alpha-foetoprotein, human chorionic gonadotropin, unconjugated oestriol and inhibin-A.

Quickening—Feeling the baby move inside the uterus.

Radiation therapy—Method of treating various cancers.

Radioactive scan—Diagnostic test in which radioactive material is injected into a particular part of the body and scanned to find a problem within that part of the body.

Rh-factor—Blood test to determine if a woman is Rh-negative.

Rh-negative—Absence of rhesus antibody in the blood.

Rh-sensitivity—See *isoimmunization.*

Round-ligament pain—Pain caused by stretching the ligaments on the sides of the uterus during pregnancy.

Rubella titers—Blood test to check for immunity against rubella (German measles).

Rupture of membranes—Loss of fluid from the amniotic sac. Also called *breaking of waters* or *water breaking.*

S

Seizure—Sudden onset of a convulsion.

Sexually transmitted disease (STD)—Infection transmitted through sexual contact or sexual intercourse.

Sickle-cell anaemia—Anaemia caused by abnormal red blood cells shaped like a sickle or a cylinder.

Sickle-cell trait—Presence of the trait for sickle-cell anaemia. Not sickle-cell disease itself.

Sickle crisis—Painful episode caused by sickle-cell disease.

Silent labour—Painless dilatation of the cervix.

Skin tag—Flap or extra buildup of skin.

Sodium—Element found in many foods, particularly salt. Ingestion of too much sodium may cause fluid retention.

Sonogram or sonography—See *ultrasound.*

Spina bifida—Birth defect in which membranes of the spinal cord and the spinal cord itself protrude outside the protective bony canal of the spine. Can cause paralysis or malfunctioning of lower extremities.

Spinal anaesthesia—Anaesthesia given in the spinal canal.

Spontaneous miscarriage—Loss of pregnancy during the first 20 weeks of gestation.

Stasis—Decreased flow.

Station—Estimation of the baby's descent into the birth canal in preparation for birth.

Stillbirth—Death of a foetus before birth, usually defined as after 20 weeks gestation.

Stress test—Test in which mild contractions of the mother's uterus are induced; foetal heart rate in response to the contractions is noted.

Stretch marks—Areas of the skin that are torn or stretched. Often found on the abdomen, breasts, buttocks and legs.

Syphilis test—To test for syphilis; if a woman has syphilis, treatment will be started.

t

Teratology—Study of abnormal foetal development.

Term—Baby is considered 'term' when it is born after 38 weeks. Also called *full term*.

Transition—Phase after active labour during which the cervix fully dilates. Contractions are strongest during this stage.

Trimester—Method of dividing pregnancy into three equal periods of about 13 weeks each.

Triple-screen test—Measurement of three blood components to help identify problems. The three tests include alpha-foetoprotein, human chorionic gonadotropin and unconjugated oestriol.

u

Ultrasound—Non-invasive test that shows a picture of the foetus inside womb. Sound waves bounce off foetus to create a picture.

Umbilical cord—Cord that connects the placenta to the developing baby. It removes waste products and carbon dioxide from baby and brings oxygenated blood and nutrients from mother through the placenta to baby.

Urinalysis and urine cultures—To test for any infections and to determine the levels of sugar and protein in the urine.

Uterus—Organ an embryo/foetus grows in. Also called a *womb*.

v

Vacuum extractor—Device sometimes used to provide traction on fetal head during delivery; used to help deliver a baby. Also called a *ventouse*.

Vagina—Birth canal.

Varicose veins—Blood vessels (veins) that are dilated or enlarged.

Vena cava—Major vein in the body that empties into the right atrium of the heart. It returns unoxygenated blood to the heart for transport to the lungs.

Venereal warts—See *condyloma acuminatum*.

Vernix—Fatty substance made up of epithelial cells that covers foetal skin inside the uterus.

Vertex—Head first.

Villi—Projection from a mucous membrane. Most important within the placenta in the exchange of nutrients from maternal blood to the placenta and foetus.

W

Weight check—Weight is checked at every antenatal visit; gaining too much weight or not gaining enough weight can indicate problems.

Womb—See *uterus.*

Y–Z

Yeast infection—See *monilial vulvovaginitis; thrush.*

Zygote—Cell that results from the union of a sperm and egg at fertilization.

Index

Page numbers in italics indicate boxed information.

Abdominal muscles, stretching, 209
Abdominal pain, severe, 198
Abnormal foetal development, 57–60
    and amniocentesis, 171–172
    congenital malformations, 115–116
    and embryonic period, 77
    and miscarriage, 102
    and premature birth, 293
    and roaccutane, 101
    See also Birth defects
Accident. *See* Injuries
ACE inhibitors, 137
Acne, 101, *106*
Acupressure and acupuncture
    and labour, 409
    and nausea, 66, *67*
Adipose tissue, 179
Afrazine, 200
Age of foetus and calculating due date,
    29–31, *30*
Age of parents, risks associated with
    father, 16, 18–19, 62, 173–174
    mother, 15, 16–18, 172–173
    See also Older mothers
AIDS. *See* HIV/AIDS
Air embolus, 182
Air travel during pregnancy, 127–128
Alcohol, 3, 38–39, 312
    and breastfeeding, 391–392
    in cooking, *39*
    and drugs, 38–39
    and foetal alcohol syndrome (FAS) or
        exposure (FAE), 24, 38
    and folic acid, 51
    and placental abruption, 334
    response differs depending on foetus, 58
    risk with any use, 24, 38
    See also Substance abuse
Allergies, *53*, 200–201
Alpha-foetoprotein testing (AFP), 162, 164
    and triple-screen test, 169
Alpha-hydroxy acid, 144
Aluminum, 91
Amniocentesis, 122–123, 171–172
    and Anti-D, 177
    and cystic fibrosis, 140
    and foetal-lung maturity, 355
    and sex of baby, 253
    and sickle-cell anaemia, 226
    and terminating pregnancy, 171
    and triple-screen test, 169
Amniotic fluid, 243–245, 356
    and amniocentesis, 171
    and breaking of waters, 336

    and breech presentation, 380
    and polyhydramnios, 239
    and post-term pregnancy, 422
    swallowing of by baby and digestive
        system, 213–214, 243
    volume of, 136, 243
    weight of, *108*, 194
Amniotic sac, 243–245, 282, 368
Anaemia, 7–8, 110, 224–227
    in baby from Rh-sensitivity of mother,
        176
    and dizziness and fatigue, 197
    and folic acid, 51
    and intrauterine-growth restriction, 312
    iron-deficiency, 225–226
    sickle-cell, 226–227
    and thalassaemia, 227
Anaesthesia
    and broken bones, 256
    and Caesarian delivery, 368
    for dental treatment, 158
    and labour, 396–399
    problems and complications, 399
    spinal, 398
Analgesics, 38, 50–51, *51*, 91, *92*, 397
    See also Paracetamol
Anencephaly, 51, 171
    and alpha-foetoprotein, 162, 164
Angiomas, 136–137
Antacids, 79, 91, 225
Antenatal care and clinics, 33–35
Antenatal classes, 275–277
Antibiotics, *59*, 105–106
    and appendicitis, 232
    and dental treatment, 158
    and Lyme disease, 152
    and urinary-tract infection, 192
Anti-D, 84, 104
    and amniocentesis, 172
    and chorionic villus sampling, 122
    and foetoscopy, 123
    given after birth, 177
    injection of at twenty-eight weeks, 288
    and percutaneous umbilical-cord blood
        sampling (PUBS), 208
    use of, 177
Antidepressants, 38, 246
    Paxil, 62–63
Antihistamines, 200
Antioxidants, 144
Apgar scores, 397, 399, 415, 416
Appendicitis, 157, 230–232
Areola of breast, 145
Armed forces, *25*, 159

Aromatherapy, 409
Artificial sweeteners, 210–211
Aspartame, 210–211
Aspirin, 50–51, *51*, 91
Asthma, 8, *53*, *106*, 285–287
Arteriosclerosis, 237
Atonic uterus, 400

"Baby blues," 377, 378, 427
    See also Postnatal (postpartum)
        depression (PND)
Baby's development in womb
    and adipose tissue, 179
    amniotic sac and fluid, 136, 243, 245
    and differentiation into male or female,
        125, 134, 154
    ears, 108, 154, 162
    eyes and eyelids, 109, 154, 270
    and foetal digestive system and
        swallowing, 213
    and head size, 143
    heart and circulatory system, 185–186
    and lanugo hair, 162, 168, 169, 235
    and liver function, 223
    and lungs and respiratory system, 355
    nervous system, 195
    organ development in first 13 weeks, 13
    and ossification of bones, 134, 162
    and pancreatic function, 235
    and skin, 206
Backache, 186, 188
Back labour, 373
Bag of waters
    rupture of, 301, 303
    See also Waters, breaking of
Balance, *186*, 188, 255
Bathing, 110–111, 156, 303
Bed rest, *290*, 294, *295*
    and intrauterine-growth restriction, 311
    and multiple births, 327
    and pre-eclampsia, 320
Bellybutton, *340*
Benefits of pregnancy, 53
Beta-adrenergic agents, 294
Bicycling, 47, 189
Bilirubin, 223, 403
Biophysical profile, 421–422
Bipolar disorder, *106*
Birth control
    after childbirth, 425
    discontinuing of, 3, 6–7
    getting pregnant while using, 69
    and molar pregnancy, 115
    and sexually transmitted diseases, 26–27
Birth control pills, 6
Birth defects, 57–60
    and AIDS/HIV medications, 84
    charts of drug and chemical agents of, 59,
        60
    and chorionic villus sampling (CVS), 122
    and cocaine use, 24
    correcting in utero, 122, 197
    and Debendox, 66
    and diabetes, 9

and genetic counselling, 15–16, 173–174
    and lupus, 12
    and maternal epilepsy, 10
    and premature birth, 293
    and rubella, 57–58
    and seizure medications, 268
    and smoking, 36
    and teratogens, 57
    and ultrasound, 131
    and use of folic acid, 3
    See also Abnormal foetal development
Birth pools, 409
Bladder and ultrasound examination,
    131–132
Bladder infections (urinary-tract infection or
    UTI), 8–9, 191–193, 427
Blastocyst, 45, 46
Bleeding, 52
    after childbirth, 424, 425
    and age of mother, 17
    and anaemia, 225
    and "bloody show," 346
    and exercise, 50, 52
    from foetus to mother and different RH
        factors, 172
    at implantation of fertilized egg into
        uterine cavity, 46, 52
    and miscarriage, 102–104
    and molar pregnancy, 115
    and placenta previa, 353
    and placental abruption, 335
    postpartum, and haemorrhage, 331
    prior to delivery of placenta, 400
    with uterine contractions, 99
    from uterus and multiple births, 328–329
    from vagina and contractions of uterus,
        99
    from vagina and round ligament pain,
        181
    from vagina as warning sign of difficulty,
        198
Blood
    and anaemia, 224–227
    composition of, 110
    decreased flow of or stasis, 215
    and diabetes, 237
    foetal, 110
    increase in volume of, 39, 110
    knowing type, 5
    sampling baby's, 208, 376
    See also Red blood cells
Blood clots in legs, 215–217
Blood. *See* Rh-sensitivity
Blood-sugar level, 197–198
    checking and diabetes, 237
    See also Diabetes
"Bloody show," 346
Blurring of vision, 199
Bones, broken, 256
Bone tumours, 309
Boredom relievers for bed-resting, *295*
Bottlefeeding, 394–395, 396
Bowel control after childbirth, 425, 427
Brain, baby's, 121, 195, 265

Bras, *353*, 393
Braxton-Hicks contractions, 344
Breaking of waters. *See* Waters, breaking of
Breast cancer, 274, 308
    inflammatory breast cancer (IBC), 308
    and weight gain during pregnancy, 61
Breastfeeding, 389–396
    benefits of, 389–391
    and breast pump, 392
    and caffeine effects on baby, 150–151, 391
    and engorgement, 392, 425, 426
    learning to, 391–392
    nipples and, 393
    nutritional requirements during, *352*, 425
    and pasteurising, 84
    reasons may not be able to, 394
    with silicone implants, 394
    vs. bottlefeeding, 394–395
Breasts
    after childbirth, 426
    cancer of, 61, 274, 303
    changes in, 68, 145, 147
    enlargement of, 46, *108*, 145
    enlargement of alveoli, 391
    lumps discovered in, 273–274, 308
    preparatory examination of, 4, 5
    and production of colostrum, 147
    sagging and older mothers, 174
    tingling and soreness in, *121*, 145, 147
    weight of, 194
Breathing and sleeping on back, 165
Breathing problems in newborn
    and anaesthesia use, 399
    and caffeine use, 150
Breech presentation, 64, 359, 361, 364, 366,
    379–382
    attempts to turn baby (external cephalic
      version), 382
    delivery of, 380–382
    reasons for and types of, 380
    See also Presentation of foetus

Caesarean delivery, 2, 6, 365–372
    and abnormal presentations, 382–383
    and active herpes infection, 80
    advantages and disadvantages of, 369
    and age of mother, 17, 175
    and breech presentation, 380, 382
    and cephalo-pelvic disproportion (CPD),
      366
    determining necessity of, 348, 369
    and diabetes, 237
    and general anaesthesia, 397
    and HIV/AIDS, 84
    and intrauterine-growth restriction, 312
    and multiple babies, 329
    and ON-Q drug-pump for pain, 369
    and placenta previa, 353
    and post-term pregnancy, 423
    reasons for, 365, 366
    recovery from, 369–370, 426
    rising rate of, 366, 368
    types of, 368
    and venereal warts, 81

    vs. natural childbirth, 317
    See also Vaginal birth after Caesarean
      (VBAC)
Caffeine, *60*, 91, *142*, 150–151, *150*
    amounts from sources, 151
    and breastfeeding, 391, 396
    and sleep, 166
Calcium, 92–94, *105*, 200
    adding by cooking with skim milk, *212*
    and breastfeeding, 396
    and caffeine, 150
    foods interring with absorption of, 94
    and heparin use, 216
Caloric intake, increased, 39
Canavan's disease, 16
Cancer, 9, 306–309
    before pregnancy, 306
    breast, 61, 274, 308
    cervical, 164–165
    cervical and pelvic, 308
    and cord blood, 400
    and hormone levels and blood flow, 307
    pregnancy protects against breast and
      ovarian, *53*
    special types of, 309
    treatment of while pregnant, 274
Car
    infant-restraint seats, 277, *310*, 362
    safety during pregnancy, 128–129, *129*,
      228
Carbohydrates, 129–130
Carpal tunnel syndrome, *314*
Cat and precautions against infections,
    106–107
Cataracts, congenital, 270
Cephalo-pelvic disproportion (CPD), 366
Cervical cancer, 164–165, 308
Cervical smear, 4, 5
    during pregnancy, 164–165
Cervix
    dilatation and effacement of, 356–358,
      364, 414
    incompetent, 50, 102, 249–250, 293
    and pelvic exam late in pregnancy, 364
    ripening of, 423
    See also Labour
Chadwick's sign, 181
Chemicals, toxic
    avoiding of prior to pregnancy, 3, 26
    and ejaculate, 249
    and genetic defects, 15
    and military services, *25*, 159
    pollutants to avoid, *63*
Chicken pox, 3, 119–120
Childbirth education classes, *247*, *269*,
    275–277
Childbirth facility and care choices, 33–35
Childbirth methods, 315–318
Child-care decisions, 304–306
Children Act 1989, 305
Chills, 199
Chlamydia, 72, 81–83
Chloasma, 136
Chlophenamine, 245

Cholesterol
    and breastfeeding, 390
    checking, 345
    minimizing prior to pregnancy, 3
Choline, 121
Chorionic villus sampling (CVS), 122, 131,
    177
    and sickle-cell anaemia, 226
Chromosome analysis, 104
Chromosomal abnormalities, 18–19, 171
Chromosomes and fertilization, 44–46
Cigarettes. See Smoking
Cimetidine, 91
Citric acid, 144
Cleft lip and palate, 132
Clomiphene, 325
Cocaine, 24, 60
Coffee, 70, 229
Colostrum, 147, 391
Colposcopy, 164, 165
Computer use during pregnancy, 253
Conception
    and diabetes, 9, 236
    herbs interfering with, 3
Cone biopsy, 165
Congenital cataracts, 270
Congenital malformations, 115–116
Congestive heart failure, 227
Conjoined twins, 323
Constipation, 79, 91, 200
    and iron, 95, 226
Consultant Obstetrician, 199
Contraception. See Birth control
Contractions
    premature, and muscle relaxants, 294,
        296
    timing of, 346
    See also Labour
Contraction stress test (CST), 421
Convulsions. See Seizures
Cord-blood banking and storage, 400–401
    See also Umbilical cord
Cordocentesis, 208
Corpus luteum, 56–57
Corticosteroids and lupus, 279
Coughs, 106
Cramps
    and ectopic pregnancy, 72
    leg, 181
    and miscarriage, 101–104
    stomach, and vitamin C, 113
    uterine, 229
Cranberry juice, 192
Crohn's disease, 51
Crown-to-rump length, 76
C-section. See Caesarean delivery
CT scans, 5, 157
Cyst
    in abdomen, ultrasound picture of,
        217–218
    in ovaries, 115
Cystic fibrosis, 5, 5, 16, 140–141
Cystitis. See Bladder infections
Cytomegalovirus (CMV), 120, 272

Dairy products, 92, 93
Deafness, inherited, 16
Death rate for newborn babies, 292
Debendox, 66
Decongestants, 92, 200, 245
Deep-vein thrombosis, 215–217
Defects. See Abnormal foetal development;
    Birth defects
Dehydration, 67
Delivery
    and blood loss, 225
    and episiotomy, 317, 338–339, 424
    forceps, 339, 374
    keeping options open, 408
    and lupus, 279
    and multiple babies, 328–329
    post-delivery procedures, 259,
        414–416
    preparing for successful, 263
    vacuum extractor (ventouse), 339, 374
    See also Caesarean delivery; Labour
Dental care, 4, 147, 157–158, 158
Depo provera, 7
Depression, 106, 245–246
    See also Emotional changes; Postnatal
        (postpartum) depression
DES (diethylstilbestrol), 72
DHA (Docosahexaenoic acid), 121
Diabetes, 9–10, 236–239, 400
    and age of mother, 17
    and birth defects, 9
    gestational, 2, 10, 174, 238–239, 288
    and insulin levels in foetus, 235
    and miscarriage, 104
    and sugar in the urine, 241
    symptoms of and diagnosing, 238
    testing for, 5, 105, 240–241
    Type 1 and 2, 237
    See also Gestational diabetes
Diarrhoea, 113, 137, 227–228
Diastasis recti, 209
Dick-Read, Grantley, 316
Dieting, 71, 121, 158, 337
    before pregnancy, 20, 22
Digestive system, foetal, 213–214
Dilatation and curettage (D&C)
    and incompetent cervix, 250
    for miscarriage, 104
    and molar pregnancy, 115
    and placental abruption, 334
Dilatation of cervix. See Cervix, dilatation
Dioxin, 266
Diptheria, 118
Dizziness, 72, 191, 197–198, 224
Docosahexaenoic acid (DHA), 121
Doctors and doctor visits, 1, 315
    and emotional changes, 118
    father's attendance at, 113
    first antenatal visit to, 85–86
    lab tests ordered at first or second visit,
        105
    number of visits to, 86, 329
    pre-pregnancy visit with, 4–6
    taking others including children to, 160

visiting when pregnancy first suspected, 69
visit when pregnancy confirmed, 33
See also Paediatrician; Consultant Obstetrician
Donor (artificial) insemination, 201, 203
Doppler device, 134, *154*
Douching, 182
Down's syndrome, 5, 15, 131
 and age of parents, 16, 18, 62, 174
 and alpha-foetoprotein, 162, 164
 and amniocentesis, 171, 174
 and chorionic villus sampling, 122, 174
 and quad-screen test, 183
 and triple-screen test, 169
 and ultrasound, 186
DPT (diphtheria, pertussis [whooping cough], tetanus) vaccine, 118, 119
Dropping of foetus (lightening), 341–342
Drugs, prescription. *See* Medications
Drugs, recreational, 22–25, *60*, 62, 312
 and alcohol use, 38–39
 and birth defects, 58–60
Duchenne muscular dystrophy, 5, 71, 171
Due date, 162
 calculating and birth control methods, 6, 7
 determining with ultrasound, 205, 208
 how to calculate, 29–31, *30*
Due week, 30–31

Eating out, 247–248
Echinacea, 3
Eclampsia, 320, 321
 See also Pre-eclampsia
Ecstasy (drug), *60*
Ectopic pregnancy, 6, 71–75
 and chlamydia, 82
 and pelvic inflammatory disease, 26–27
 and Rh-sensitivity, 177
 symptoms of, 72
 treatment for, 74–75
Effacement, 364
 See also Labour
Egg (ovum)
 fertilization of, 44
 number of, 32
Electric blankets, 111
Electroencephalogram (EEG), 268
Electromagnetic fields, 111
Embryonic period, 77, 117
Emotional changes, 424, 425, 426, 428
 and baby blues, 377, 378, 427
 and depression, 245–246
 during pregnancy, 116, 118, 236
 in late pregnancy, 350–351
 and postnatal (postpartum) depression (PND), 245, 376–379
 and sharing feelings, *177*
 and upset and miscarriage, 102
Encephalocele, 51
Endometrial cycle, 32
Endometriosis, *53*
Enemas, 372–373, 407
Engorgement, 392, 425, 426

Epidural and other pain blocks, 317, 389, 397–398, 408
 and C-section, 368
 and low blood pressure, 398
Epilepsy and seizures, 10
Episiotomy, 317, 338–339, 424, 427
Equipment, baby, *310*
Erythromycin, 83, 106
Evaluation of baby after delivery, 415–416
Exercise, 46–50, *186*
 aerobic, 47, 48–49
 and balance, *186*, 188
 before pregnancy, 2, 22, 49
 and constipation, 79
 focus on lower back and abdominal muscles, 22
 general advantages of, 46–47
 guidelines for, 49, *50*
 and older mothers, 174
 with partner, *145*
 post-term, in the water, 419
 in second and third trimester, 188–190
 and sleep, 166
 sports activities, 47, 188, 190
 and stress, 230
 and target heart rates, *47*
External cephalic version (ECV), 382
External foetal monitoring, 376
Eyes
 and congenital cataracts, 270
 development of, 270
 infection and chlamydia, 82
 infection from gonorrhoea, 81
 and microphthalmia, 272

Falls, injuries from, 255–256
False-labour, 343–344, *344*
Famotidine, 91
Father
 age of and associated risks, 16, 18–19, 62, 173–174
 and alcohol and drug use, *24*, 25, 38–39, 60, 62
 and attendance at doctor's office, 113
 baby equipment, *310*
 during delivery, *347*, 412–414, *415*
 and exercise with mother, 145
 and movement of baby, 286
 not legally married to mother, 202–203
 and paternity leave, 148–149, *237*
 and pregnancy symptoms (couvade), *291*
 and ultrasound, *206*
Fatigue, 68, 191
 after childbirth, 426
 and anaemia, 197
 and depression, 246
 and older mothers, 174
Fats and sweets, 139, 144
Feet, swelling in, 214–215, 314
Ferning test, 336
Fertility
 checking cycle of, 3
 monitors of, 14–15
 preserving and ectopic pregnancy, 74

Fertility drugs, 325–326
    and postnatal depression, 378
Fertilization, 44, 46
Fever, high, 199
Fifth disease (parvo virus B19 or 'slapped
    cheek'), 139–140
First Response Fertility Monitor, 14
Fish, eating, 63, 144, *201*, 264–267, 338
    cautions regarding, 265–267
    good choices, *266*
    methyl-mercury poisoning, 265–266
    and omega–3 fatty acids, 264, 265
Floating, 342
Flouride supplementation, 96–97
Fluconazole (Difulucan), 80
Fluid loss, major or continuous, 198, 235–236
    See also Waters, breaking of
Fluids
    and constipation, 79
    drinking lots of, 67, 70, 150, *221*, 228–229
    and haemorrhoids, 156
    intake during breastfeeding, 395
    not drinking before sleep, 166
    and stretch marks, 144
    and ultrasound, 131
    and urinary-tract infections, 192
Flu vaccine, 14, 119
Foetal alcohol exposure (FAE) and syndrome
    (FAS), 24, 38
Foetal distress
    and Caesarean delivery, 366
    and delivering multiple babies, 328
    and intrauterine-growth restriction
        (IUGR), 312
    and meconium, 214
    monitoring during labour, 376
    and placental abruption, 335
    testing for in overdue pregnancy, 420–422
Foetal fibronectin (fFN), 224, 293
Foetal monitoring, 341, 375–376
Foetal period, 115
Foetoscopy, 122–123
Foetus, regarding as a person, 116
Folic acid, 51–52, *105*
    and armed forces, *25*, 159
    and depression, 246
    foods containing, 20–21, 51
    and fruits and vegetables, 112
    and placental abruption, 334
    preparatory to pregnancy, 3, 20
    and smoking, 30
Food additives, 210, 337
Food aversion, 291
Food cravings, 219, *219*
Food Pyramid (USDA), 85
Foods and nutrition
    alcohol in, *39*
    and artificial sweeteners, 210–211
    before pregnancy, 19–22
    and bottlefeeding, 396
    and breastfeeding, 391–392, 395
    and choline and DHA, 121
    and cutting down saturated fat, *21*
    dairy products, 92

    and eating out, 247–248
    and fibre and haemorrhoid, 156
    and food cravings, 219, *219*
    and frequent, small meals, *198*
    and gestational diabetes, 239
    increasing food intake, 39, 40
    and intrauterine-growth restriction, 312
    junk, 122, 138
    and mineral deficiency, 95
    and multiple babies, 330–331, *330*
    and nausea and morning sickness, *22*, 67,
        70
    need for balance in, 40
    and omega–3 fatty acids, 264, 265
    and parties, 372
    and snacks, 139, 175, 298, 345, 383–384
    and sodium intake and content of foods,
        239–240, *240*
    and USDA Food Pyramid, *85*
    variety in, 299
    and vegetarian diet, 182–183
    and weight gain during first trimester, 61
    what to avoid, 337–338
    See also Folic acid; Iron; Vitamins
Foods and nutrition, choices and servings
    for adding 300 calories, 165–166
    and alternative food choice suggestions,
        257
    caffeine, 151
    of calcium sources, 93–94, *105*
    carbohydrates, 129–130
    fats and sweets servings, 139
    fish and shellfish, *266*
    fruits and vegetables, 111–112, 144
    low-fat protein sources, 120–121
    and servings and food groups, 85, *85*
    sources of nutrients, *105*, 112
    sources of Vitamin C, 112, *112*, 359
    for third trimester, *287*
Foramen ovale, 185, 186
Forceps delivery, 339, 374
Forty-week timetable, 31–32
Fraternal twins, 323
Fruits, 111–112, 144
Full-term baby, 291

Genetic counselling, 15–16, 173–174
Genetics and abnormalities, 18–19, 104, 171
Genital herpes simplex infection, 79–80
Genital warts, 80–81
German measles. *See* Rubella
Germ layers, 56
Gestational age, 30, *30*, 162
Gestational diabetes, 2, 10, 174, 238–239
    and home birth, *288*
    See also Diabetes
Gestational trophoblastic neoplasia (GTN),
    115
Ginger, 70
Glucose-tolerance test (GTT), 240–241, 288
Glucosuria, 240
Gonorrhoea, 72, 81
Government benefits during pregnancy, 147
GP/community midwife care, 34

Grave's disease, 12
Group-B streptococcus infection, 299

Haematocrit reading, 224–225
Haemoglobin level, 225
Haemophilia, 5, 71, 171
Haemorrhage, postpartum, 331, 400
Haemorrhoids, 79, 154, 156, 426
  relief for, 156
Hair, baby's
  growth of, 206, 282
  lanugo, 162
Hair, mother's
  curling of, *111*
  increase or loss of, 125, 127
  pubic, 384–385
Head, feeling of foetal, 359
Headaches, 12, *106*, 191, 199, 229
Head size
  diminished and use of caffeine, 150
  and hydrocephalus, 195
  and medicine for seizures, 268
Health insurance, 4
Hearing, baby's, and exposure to noise, 247
Heart and circulatory system, development of
  baby's, 185–186
Heart arrhythmia (foetal), 261
Heart attack and diabetes, 237
Heartbeat, foetal, 116, 211
  distinguishing from mother's, 211
  and distress in labour, 366
  and doppler device, 134, *154*
  hearing, 134, *134*, *154*, 160, 211
  monitoring in post-term pregnancy, 422
  monitoring of during labour, 375–376
  and multiple births, 326
  speed of and gender, 253
  and ultrasound, 130, 185
Heartburn, 77, 79, 139, *198*, *243*, 359
  and sleep, 166, *243*
Heart disease, 10–11
Heparin therapy, 216
Hepatitis, 5, 40–41
Herbal teas, 175, 303–304, *304*
Herbs
  interfering with conception, 3
  for nausea and caution, 67
  as remedies and consultation with doctor,
    20, 199–200
Hernia of abdominal muscles, 209
Herpes simplex virus, 79–80, 171
High blood pressure, 2, 11, 18
  after childbirth, 424
  and age of mother, 17, 173, 174
  and aspirin use, *51*
  and calcium, 92
  entering pregnancy with, 137
  and foetal growth, 312
  and home birth, *288*
  and maternal overweight, 2
  and omega–3 fatty acids, 264
  and pre-eclampsia, 319
  pregnancy-induced, 318–319
  and premature delivery, 264

  risks from, 137
  safe medications for, *106*
  and third trimester, 31
HIV/AIDS, 4, 5, 83–84, 400
Hodgkin's disease, 309
Homan's sign, 216
Home birth, *288*
Home uterine monitoring, 264
Hormones
  and beginning of labour, 356
  and food aversion, 219
  increases of and backache, 186
  and postnatal depression, 377, 378
  used to induce labor and uterine rupture,
    371
Hospital
  admission questions, 406–407
  and antenatal clinic, 35
  choosing, 33
  and deep-vein thrombosis, 216–217
  going to, 405–406, 412–413
  packing for, 361–362, *383*
  questions regarding, 33–34
  with specialized facilities, 199
  touring ahead of time, *281*, 351
  what happens after pregnancy, 424–425
Hot baths, 110–111
Hugging and cuddling, *39*
Human chorionic gonadotropin (HCG), 65, 69
  and ectopic pregnancy, 74
  and molar pregnancy, 115
  production of in placenta, 284
  and triple-screen test, 169
Human papillomavirus, HPV (Condyloma
    acuminata), 80–81
Humidifier, 245
Hyaline membrane disease, 355
Hydatidiform mole, 115
Hydramnios, 327
Hydrocephalus, 195, 197, 380
Hydrocortisone, 91, 144, 287
Hydroxyurea, 8, 227
Hyperactivity and smoking, 36–37
Hyperemesis gravidarum, 66
Hyperglycaemia, 197
Hypertension. *See* High blood pressure
Hyperthyroidism. *See* Thyroid problems
Hypnosis, 409
Hypoglycaemia, 197, 237
Hypotension, 197, 398, 424
Hypothyroidism. *See* Thyroid problems

Ibuprofen, 91
Identical twins, 323
Immune globulin, 41
Immunizations. *See* Vaccinations and
    immunizations
Incompetent cervix, 50, 102, 249–250, 293
Indigestion, 191, *198*
Inducing labour, 422–423
Infant-restraint seats, 277, 362
Infections
  and amniocentesis, 172
  avoiding of prior to pregnancy, 3

Infections *(continued)*
  bacterial, *106*
  bladder or urinary-tract (UTI), 8–9
  breast, 393
  dental, 158
  E.sakazakii, 390
  eye (gonorrhoeal ophthalmia), 81
  fifth disease, 139–140
  and gestational diabetes, 39
  group-B streptococcus infection (GBS), 299
  and increased vaginal discharge, 181–182
  Lyme disease, 151–152
  maternal, effects on foetus, 120, *120*
  and microphthalmia, 272
  and miscarriage, 102, 104
  and premature delivery, 264
  protection against in breast milk, 390
  pyelonephritis, 8–9, 188, 192–193
  and sickle-cell anaemia, 227
  toxoplasmosis, 102, 105–106, *120*, 272
  viral with diarrhoea, 228
  and washing hands, *98*
  See also Sexually transmitted diseases;
    Urinary-tract infections
Infertility, 12, 172
Inflammatory breast cancer (IBC), 308
Inhibin-A level, 183
Injuries, physical, 102, 137–138, 199
  and falling, 255–256
  and incompetent cervix, 250
Insulin, 10, 235, 236, 237, 238
Insurance coverage, 26
Intelligence, baby's
  and breastfeeding, 390
  enhanced by fish oils, 265
  and substance use, 23, 24, 36–37
Internal foetal monitor, 376
Intestines, baby's, 143
Intrauterine device (IUD), 7, 69, 72, 131, 293
Intrauterine-growth restriction (IUGR),
    311–312
  causes of, 312
  concerns relative to, 311, 312
  and C-section delivery, 312
  and exercise, 50
  and father's use of alcohol, 38–39
  and high blood pressure, 12, 137
  and lupus, 12
  and small placenta, 285
  and smoking, 23, 312
Intrauterine therapy, for hydrocephalus, 195,
    197
In-vitro fertilization, 5, 326
Iron, 3, 95, *105*, 191
  and anaemia, 8
  and fruits and vegetables, 112
  getting enough, 95
  and iron-deficiency anaemia, 225–226
  and military services, *25*, 159
  and nausea and vomiting, 95, 226
  use of previous to pregnancy, 3
Iron-deficiency anaemia, 225–226
Isoimmunization, 172, 176
  See also Anti-D

Isotonic, isometric, and isokinetic exercise, 48
Itching, 254
IUD (intrauterine device), 7, 69, 72, 131, 293

Jaundice, baby's, 223, 237, 403
Jogging, 190
Joint mobility, 186
Junk food, 122, 138

Kernicterus, 403
Ketoprofen, 91
Kick count of baby's movement, 273, 428
Kidney problems, 192–193, 312
  and diabetes, 237
  and lupus, 279
  stones, 9, 188, 193
Kitzinger, Sheila, 317
Knot in umbilical chord, 301, 302, 387

Labour, 356–358
  back labour, 373
  and determining if baby will fit through
    birth canal, 348, 350
  as dilatation of cervix, 356–358, 364
  eating and drinking during, 411–412
  effacement, 364
  and enemas, 372–373, 407
  false, 342, 344, *344*
  and foetal heart arrhythmia, 261
  foetal monitoring during, 375–376
  and gestational diabetes, 239
  inducing, 422–423
  and *labour check*, 406
  length of, 357
  and older women, 175
  and pain relief, 396–399
  and partner, 412–414
  positions in, 409–411
  preparing for, 263, 351
  and single mother, 202
  three stages of, 357, 414
  and timing of contractions, 346
  who should attend, *401*, 406, 412
  See also Delivery; Hospital; Pain relief
    during labour; Premature labour
Lactic acid, 144
Lactose intolerance, 94–95
Lamaze, 316
Lanugo hair, 162, 168, 169, 235
Laparoscopy
  and appendicitis, 232
  and ectopic pregnancy, 74
Laser treatment for stretch marks, 145
Lead, *63*, 94
Leaking from vagina, 198, 235–236, 301, 303,
    336–337, 364
Leboyer, Frederick, 316
Legal questions, and single mothers, 202–203
Legs
  blood clots in, 215–217
  cramps, *181*
  swelling in, 214–215, 314, 320, 425
  and varicose veins, 219–220, 426
Length of pregnancy, 30

Leucorrhoea, 181
Leukaemia, 309
Lightening, 341
Light therapy, 246
Linea nigra, 136
Listeriosis, 95, 102
Liver function, baby's, 223, 403
Loss of fluid
  major or continuous, 198, 236
  See also Leaking from vagina; waters,
    breaking of
Low birthweight, risks for
  asthma, 286
  and bladder infections, 192
  and caffeine use, 150
  and hyperthyroidism, 12
  and infections, 79
  and multiple babies, 326, 330
  and periodontal disease, 4
  and smoking, 23, 36, 37
  and standing at work, 149
  underweight mother, 2, 36
Low blood pressure, 197, 398, 424
L/S ratio test, 355
Lumps, breast, 273–274, 308
Lunar months, *30*, 31
Lungs, 186, 355
Lupus or systemic lupus erythematosus
  (SLE), 11–12, 104, 261, 278–279
Lying on side while resting, *260*
  See also Sleeping and resting positions
Lyme disease, 151–152

Magnesium, 91, *105*
Magnesium sulphate, 296, 321
Mammary glands in embryo, 147
Mammogram, 5, 19, 274
Marijuana, 24–25, *60*
Mask of pregnancy, 136
Massage, 66, 145, *182*, 408, 411
Maternity clothes, 153
Maternity leave, 26, 148
McDonald cerclage, 250
Measles, 14, 118
Measuring uterus, 203–204
Meconium, 214
Medical history, 4, 6, 16, 86
Medications
  ACE inhibitors, 137
  alcohol in, 36, 91
  analgesics, 38, 50–51, *51*, 91, *92*, 397
  antacids, 79, 91, 225
  antibiotics, 13, 105–106, 152, 158
  antidepressants, 246
  antidepressants, analgesics, and
    anticonvulsants, 38
  antihistamines, 200
  aspirin, 50–51, *51*, 91
  AZT, 84
  Bendectin, 66
  beta-adrenergic, 294
  and birth defects, 15
  and broken bones, 256
  Caesarean, pain following, 368

caffeine in, *142*
clomiphene (Clomid), 325
considering before pregnancy, 2
coumadin derivatives, *59*
Debendox, 66
decongestants, 92, 200, 245
effects on foetal development, *59*
epidural block, 397–398
erythromycin, 83, 106
fluconazole, 80
guidelines for using, *13*
heparin, 216–217
herbal, 3, 20, 67, 199–200, *304*
hydrocortisone, 144
insulin, 237
magnesium sulphate, 296, 321
methotrexate, 75
metronidazole, 80
milk of magnesia, *137*
over-the-counter, 39, 66, 89, 91–92, *91*, *92*
oxymetazoline, 200
oxytocin, 329, 371, 423
paracetamol, 50–51, *92*, *106*, 188, 215,
  339, 392
Paxil, 62–63
penicillin, 81
phenobarbital, 10, 268
prior to pregnancy, 13–14
progesterone, 104
propylthiouracil, 259
prostaglandin tablets, 423
pyrimethamine, 105
Retin-A or Retinova, 144, 267
RhoGAM, 84, 104, 122, 123, 177, 288
ritodrine, 294, 296, 327
roaccutane, 101
"safe" to use during pregnancy, *106*
safety dangers during pregnancy, 13
steroid creams, 144
steroids, 279
StriVectin-SD, 144
sulfadiazine, 105
suppositories and stool softeners, 156
surfacant, 355
teracycline, 83
terbutaline, 296
thyroid replacement (thyroxin), 259
VZIG, 120
warfarin, *59*, 217
  See also Antibiotics
Medications, conditions treated by, *106*
  allergies, 200–201
  asthma, 8, 286, 287
  bladder infections, 191–192
  bleeding, 329
  chicken pox, 120
  chlamydia, 83
  deep-vein thrombosis, 216–217
  dental treatment, 158
  depression, 62–63, 246
  diabetes, 237
  diarrhoea, *137*
  ectopic pregnancy, 75
  epilepsy, 10

Medications, conditions treated by *(continued)*
  gonorrhoea, 81
  haemorrhoids, 156
  high blood pressure, 11, *51*, 137
  HIV/AIDS, 84
  hypertension (high blood pressure), 11
  inducing labor, 423
  infertility, 325
  kidney stones, 193
  labour and delivery pain, 396–399
  lupus, 278–279
  Lyme disease, 152
  miscarriage, 104
  morning sickliness, 66
  nasal problems, 91, 245
  nausea and vomiting, 66
  pain in delivery, 396–399
  pre-eclampsia, 296, 321
  premature baby lung immaturity, 355
  premature labour, 294, 296, *296*, 327
  pyelonephritis, 193
  Rh-sensitivity, 84, 104, 122, 123, 177, 288
  ripening cervix, 423
  seizures, 268
  and sickle-cell anaemia, 8
  stretch marks, 144
  thyroid problems, 12, 258–259
  trichomonal vaginitis, 80
  yeast infections, 80
Melanoma, 309
Membranes, rupture of, 299, 301, 303,
    336–337
Meningomyelocele, 195
Menstrual cycle and period, 32–33
  and cramps, *53*
  return of after childbirth, 427, 429
  two or three before pregnancy, 6, 7
Mercury poisoning, *63*, 265–266
Metformin, 238
Methotrexate, 75
Microphthalmia, 272
Microwave ovens, 111
Midwifery, 34, 35
Migraine headaches, 12, *53*, *106*
Military, pregnancy in, *25*, 159
Milkaid, 95
Milk of magnesia, *137*
Minimal-brain-dysfunction syndrome
    (hyperactivity), 3–37
Miscarriages, 101–104
  and alcohol use, 38, 102
  and amniocentesis, 172
  and caffeine, 150
  causes and types of, 102–103
  and chorionic villus sampling (CVS), 122
  and cocaine use, 24
  and diabetes, 9
  and exercise, 50
  and foetoscopy, 123
  and intrauterine device (IUD), 69
  and lupus, 12, 279
  most occur in first trimester, 31
  and percutaneous umbilical-cord blood
    sampling, 208

  recurrent, 16, 104
  and Rh-sensitivity, 177
  and roaccutane, 101
  and senna, 200
  and sexual activity, 249
  and sickle-cell anaemia, 227
  and smoking, 102
  and stress, 254
  and thyroid problems, 12, 258
Mitral-valve prolapse, 11
Mittelschmerz, 32–33
MMR. *See* Rubella
Molar pregnancy, 115
Moles, 154
Moods. *See* Emotional changes
Morning sickness, 65–66, 89, 142, *167*
  and cutting down saturated fats prior to
    pregnancy, *21*
  emergency bag for, *67*
  and first trimester, 66, 69–70
  improvement of around week 12, 136
  nutritional and practical help for, 67, 70
Movement, foetal, 116, 124, 272–273
  change in or lack of, 199
  and kick count, 273, 420
  in last four to five weeks, 356
  mother's feeling of, 169, 179
  and pain under ribs, 273
  and post-term pregnancy, 421
  and stretching and separation of
    abdominal muscles, 208–209
  and ultrasound, 131, 169
MRIs (magnetic resonance imaging), 5, 157
Multiple foetuses, 322–329
  and age of mother, 17
  and breech presentation, 380
  and Caesarian delivery, 371
  delivery of, 328–329
  frequency of, 323, 325
  and gender, 326
  and length of pregnancy, 327
  and premature labour and birth, 293
  problems of, 326–327
  and twins, 174, 205, 322–323
  See also Twins
Multiple pregnancy
  and breech presentation, 380
  and multiple placentas, 285
Mumps, 14
Muscular dystrophy, *5*

Nails, 125, 127
Names for baby, *213*
Naproxen, 91
Nasal problems, maternal, 91, 245
Natural childbirth, 315–316, 317–318
Nausea, 65–68, *67*, 70, *106*, 139, *173*
  and appendicitis, 230
  dietary measures for, 67, 70, *198*
  and ectopic pregnancy, 72
  and iron, 95, 226
  and molar pregnancy, 115
  See also Morning sickness; Vomiting
NdLYAG laser treatments, 145

Nervous system, foetal, 121, 195, 265
Neural-tube defects, 183, 195
  and alpha-foetoprotein level, 169, 171
  folic acid to prevent, 3, 20–21, 51
  and smoking, 36
Nicotine substitutes, *36*
Nipples
  and breastfeeding, 393
  stimulation of and uterine contractions, 249, 345
Nitrazine test, 336
Noise, baby's exposure to, 247
Non-stress test (NST), 420
Norplant, 7
Numbers of births daily and each year, 28
Nursing. *See* Breastfeeding
Nutrition. *See* Foods and nutrition

Oestrogen
  and placenta, 284
  and postnatal depression, 378
  and skin changes, 137
Older mothers, 16–19, 172–175
  differences in pregnancy, 174–175
  and exercise, 174
  and fatigue, 174
  and genetic counselling, 15, 173–174
  growing trend of, 172
  and increased testing, 174
  and pre-eclampsia and high blood pressure, 320
  risks associated with, 15, 16–18, 172–173
  and twins, 174
Omega–3 fatty acids, 246, 264, 265
Omphalocele, 143, 195
ON-Q drug pump, 369
Oral contraceptives and chlamydia, 82
Ovarian cycle, 32
Ovarian cysts and molar pregnancy, 115
Overdue pregnancy. *See* Post-term pregnancy
Over-the-counter medications, 39, 66, 89, 91–92, *91*, *92*
Overweight. *See* Weight
Ovulation, 32–33
  and corpus luteum, 56
  noticing of, 46
Ovulation-predictor kit, 3
Ovulatory age, 30, *30*
Oxygen
  consumption of, 287
  foetus gets from mother, 185–186
Oxymetazoline, 200, 245
Oxytocin, 329, 371, 423

Paediatrician
  and examination of newborn, 425
  present at delivery when foetal heart arrhythmia during labour, 261
  present at delivery with use of general anaesthesia, 397
Pain relief during labour, 396–399
  and epidural block, 317, 368, 397–398
  and intrathecal anaesthesia, 399
  and pudendal block, 397, 398

  and waiting to go to hospital, 405
  without medication, 408
Palmar erythaema, 137
Palms, moist, 258
Pancreatic function, foetal, 235
Paracetamol, 50–51, *92*, *106*
  for back pain, 188
  and breastfeeding, 392
  and episiotomy, 339
  and thrombosis, 215
Parental leave, 148–149
Paternity leave, 148–149, *237*
Paxil, 62–63
Pelvic cancer, 308
Pelvic exam, 86
  in late pregnancy, 364–365
  upon admission to hospital for delivery, 407
Pelvic inflammatory disease (PID), 26–27
  and chlamydia, 82
  and Ectopic pregnancy, 72
Penicillin, 81
Peptic ulcer disease, *106*
Percutaneous umbilical-cord blood sampling (PUBS), 131, 208
Periods, menstrual. *See* Menstrual cycle and period
PERSONA fertility monitor, 14
Pesticides, 15, *63*, 337–338
Pets, *102*
Phenobarbital, 10, 268
Phenylketonuria (PKU), 210
Philosophers of childbirth, 316–317
Phosphatidyl glycerol (PG) test, 355
Phototherapy, 223, 403
"Pins-and-needles" sensation in pelvis region, 342
Pituitary gland, foetal, 134
Placenta, 282–285
  and chorionic villus sampling (CVS), 122
  delivery of, 357, 400
  formation of, 282, 284
  functions of, 185–186, 284
  initial formation of, 56
  and progesterone, 57
  retained, 331, 384
  weight of, *108*, 194, 284
Placental abruption, 332–336
  and age of mother, 17
  and Caesarian delivery, 366
  causes of, 334
  and cocaine use, 24
  and falls, 256
  and multiple foetuses, 326
  and premature labour and birth, 293
  and smoking, 37
  symptoms and treatment of, 335
Placenta previa, 349, 352–353, 407
  and breech presentation, 380
  and Caesarian delivery, 366
  and sexual activity, 249
  and smoking, 37
Pneumonia
  baby's, and meconium, 214
  and chicken pox, 120

Pneumonia *(continued)*
  from chlamydia, 82
  and X-rays, 157
Police force, pregnancy, 159
Polio vaccination, 119
Pollutants, 62, *63*
Polychlorinated biphenyls (PCBs), 63, 266
Polyhydramnios, 239
Position of baby. *See* Presentation of foetus
Positions in labour, 409–411
Postdate baby, 291
Post-delivery procedures, 259, 414
Post-mature babies, 419–420
Postnatal (postpartum) depression (PND),
    245, 376–379
  and "baby blues," 377, 378, 427
  degrees of, 377–378
  handling, 378–379
Post-pregnancy care, maternal, 144–145
Post-term pregnancy, 418–423
  biophysical profile, 421–422
  and post-mature babies, 419–420
  tests to insure baby is fine, 419, 420–422
Postural hypotension, 197
Posture, *303*
Potassium, *181*
Pre-eclampsia, 319–321
  and age of pregnancy, 17
  and calcium, 92
  and diabetes, 37
  and foetal growth, 312
  and high blood pressure, 137
  and intrauterine-growth restriction
    (IUGR), 312
  and multiple babies, 326, 330
  and omega–3 fatty acids, 264
  and stress, 254
  and third trimester, 31
  treating of, 320–321
  and use of magnesium sulphate, 296
Pregnancy over 35. *See* Age of parents; Older
    mothers
Pregnancy risk and age vs. health status,
    172–173
Pregnancy tests, 65
  over the counter, earliest results from, *32*
  positive before period, 65
Pre-implementation genetic diagnosis, *5*
Premature baby, 292–293
  and breastfeeding vs. formula, 390–391
  definition of term, 291–292
  and respiratory-distress syndrome, 355
  survival of from week 25 on, 253, 292
Premature labour and delivery
  and age of mother, 17
  and amniocentesis, 172
  and aspirin use, *51*
  and asthma, 286
  benefits of stopping, 298
  and bilirubin levels, 223, 403
  and bladder infections, 192
  and breech presentation, 380
  and caffeine, 150
  and exercise, 50

factors associated with, 264
and gestational diabetes, 239
and home uterine monitoring, 264
and infections, 79
and lupus, 12, 279
medications to help stop, 294, 296, *296*
and multiple foetuses, 327
prevented by omega–3 fatty acids, 264
and standing at work, 149
and stress, 254
and thyroid problems, 258
treatment of, 294, 296
and urinary tract infections and
    pyelonephritis, 8
Prenatal vitamins, 2, *25*, 51, 93, *96*, 256, 330
  individuals needing special help,
    256–257
  and iron, 191, 225
  missing when sick, 228
  and nursing, 391
  taking under doctor's supervision, 258
Preparation for pregnancy, 1–27
  actions to take before pregnancy, 2–4
  and armed forces, *25*
  current medical problems, 7–13
  current medications, 13–14
  discontinuing contraception, 6–7
  exercise and nutrition, 19–22
  genetic counselling, 15–16
  good health before, 1–2
  and medical history, 4, 6, 16
  substance use, 22–25
  and treating your body as if you were
    pregnant, *23*
  vaccinations, 14, *25*
  work-related concerns, 25–26
Prescription drugs. *See* Medications
Presentation of foetus
  abnormal types of, 382–383
  and baby looking up (back labour),
    373
  breech, 64, 359, 361, 364, 366, 379–382
  and Caesarian delivery, 366
  determining, 288–289, 359–361, 365
  and multiple foetuses, 327, 328
  station determination, 365
Preterm baby or premature baby, 291–292
  See also Premature baby
Preterm delivery, 224
  See also Premature labour
Progesterone, 56, 57
  as hormone to reduce incidence of
    premature labour, *296*
  and placenta, 284
  and postnatal depression, 378
  and prevention of miscarriage, 104
Protein, 120–121, 144
Pubic hair, shaving of, 384–385
Pubic symphysis, 205
Pudendal block, 397, 398
Puerperal psychosis, 377
Pulmonary embolism, 216
Pulsed dye laser treatments, 145
Pyelonephritis, 8–9, 188, 192–193

Quad-screen test, 183
Quickening. *See* Movement, foetal

Radiation
    and CT scans, 157
    and deep-vein thrombosis, 216
    and dental X-rays, 158
    harm from, *59*, 102, 116, 156–157
    and mammogram, 274
    and microwave ovens, 111
    schedule needed X-rays before pregnancy,
        3, 5
    and X-rays during pregnancy, 157
Red blood cells
    and anaemia, 224
    and fifth disease, 140
    and sickle-cell anaemia, 226
Registration of baby, 424, 427
ReliefBand, *67*
Respiratory-distress syndrome, 355
Respiratory system, baby's, 355, 421
Restaurants, 247–248
Retin-A or Retinova, 144, 267
Rh-sensitivity, 176–177
    and bleeding from foetus to mother, 172
    and enlarged placenta, 285
    test prior to pregnancy, 5, 176
Rings, *319*
Rising slowly, 197
Ritodrine, 294, 296, 327
Roaccutane, 101, 267
Round-ligament pain, 179, 181
Rubella (MMR) or German measles, 3, 4, 5,
        14, 105, 425
    and amniocentesis, 171
    and anatomical defects, 57–58
    and congenital cataracts, 270
    during pregnancy, 119
    effects on foetus, *120*, 312
    vaccination, 118, 119

Saccharin, 210–211
SalEst, 293
Saliva-testing kit, 3
Salmonella poisoning, 318
Saunas, 110–111
Sciatic-nerve pain, 99, 101
Seat belt, *129*
Sedative or narcotics, to stop premature
    labour, 296
Seizures, 10, 268
    and eclampsia, 320, 321
Senna, 200
Sex of baby, *44*, 71
    and amniocentesis, 171, 253
    determining, 253–254
    and sperm separation, 71
    ultrasound determination of, 132, *205*,
        253
Sexual intimacy during pregnancy, 97,
        209–210
    and breaking of waters, 337
    and emptying bladder afterwards, 192
    and inception of labour, 345

practices to avoid, 249
    and stimulation of nipples and uterine
        contractions, 249, 345
    varies by trimester, 248
    when to avoid, 249
Sexually transmitted diseases (STDs), 26–27,
        79–84
    and chlamydia, 81–83
    and ectopic pregnancy, 72
    genital herpes simplex infection, 79–80
    gonorrhoea, 81
    and hepatitis B, 40
    HIV and AIDS, 83–84
    HPV-human papillomavirus, 80
    and preparation for pregnancy, 6
    syphilis, 81
    See also HIV/AIDS
Siamese twins, 323
Sickle-cell anaemia, 8, 11, 226–227, 400
Sickness while pregnant, 227–228
SIDS. *See* Sudden infant death syndrome
Signs and symptoms of pregnancy, 29
Silicone breast implants, nursing with, 394
Single mothers, 201–203
Sitz baths, 156
Size of baby
    and high blood pressure, 11
    large, and diabetes, 237
    smaller, and asthma, 286
    and standing, 26
Skiing, 190
Skin, baby's, 206
Skin, maternal
    after childbirth, 426
    changes in, 136–137, 426
    conditions, 267
    and melanoma, 309
    and stretch marks, 143–145
Skin tags, 154
Slapped cheek, 139–140
Sleep
    and foetal movements at night, 272
    patterns of foetus, 261
    and stress, 230
    tips for sleeping soundly, 166
Sleeping and resting positions, 165, *165*, 166
    for haemorrhoids, 156
    and lying on side, 188, *260*, 315
    and not sleeping on back, 165, 176, 197
    and shortness of breath, 170
    and waterbeds, 165
Smoking, 35–38
    and caffeine, 151
    and miscarriage, 102
    and placental abruption, 334
    quitting, 3, *37*, 38
    risks associated with, 23, 35–37, *60*
    secondary smoke, 38, *58*
    and size of baby, 312
    and vitamins and minerals, 256
Snacking, 70, 139, 175, 298, 345, 383–384
Sodium bicarbonate, 91
Sodium intake, 91, 239–240, *240*
    and eating out, 248

Sonography or sonogram. *See* Ultrasound
Spas, 110–111
Sperm, 44, 71
Spina bifida, 16, 20, 51
　　and alpha-foetoprotein, 162, 164, 171
　　and hydrocephalus, 195
Splenda, 211
Standing, hazards of, 26, 149
Stasis (decreased blood flow), 215
Station, 365
　　See also Presentation of foetus
Stationary bicycles, 47, 189
Statutory Maternity Pay, 148
Stem cells, 400–401
Sterilization, 387, 389
Steroid and steroid creams, 144, 267, 279, 287
Stillbirth
　　and caffeine, 150
　　and cocaine use, 24
　　definition of, 101
　　and diabetes, 9
　　and lupus, 12
　　and sickle-cell anaemia, 227
Stress, 3, 116, 229–230, 254
　　and working, 320
Stretching the vagina, 339
Stretch marks (straie distensae), 143–145
　　and older mothers, 174
　　treatment after pregnancy, 144–145
StriVectin-SD, 144
Substance abuse, 35–39, *60*, 62, 312
　　in first trimester, 23
　　in preparation for pregnancy, 22–25
　　See also Alcohol; Drugs, recreational;
　　　　Smoking
Sucralose, 211
Sudden infant death syndrome (SIDS), 24,
　　25, 60
　　and breastfeeding, 390
　　and caffeine, *150*
Sugar in the urine, 240–241
Sunlight, avoiding, 144
Superficial thrombosis, 215
Supine hypotension, 197
Swallowing, foetal, 213, 214, 243
Swelling
　　in bottom, 424, 425
　　of face or fingers, 198, *319*, 426
　　in legs and feet, 214–215, 314, 320, 425
　　and pre-eclampsia, 319
Swimming during pregnancy, 47, *145*, 189
Syphilis, 81, 102, 105, *120*, 285
Systemic lupus erythematosus (SLE), 11–12,
　　104, 261, 278–279

Tay-Sachs disease, *5*, 16
Temperature of body, maintaining, 48,
　　110–111
Teratogens, 57, 102
　　and pollutants, 62, *63*
　　prescription drugs and chemicals, *59*
　　and substance abuse, *60*
　　See also Substance abuse
Terbutaline, 296

Term baby, 291
Terminating the pregnancy, 171, 174
　　See also Miscarriage
Tests
　　alpha-foetoprotein (AFP), 162, 164
　　amniocentesis, 122–123, 140, 169,
　　　　171–172
　　antinuclear antibody, 279
　　before conception, 4–5, *5*, 19
　　biophysical profile, 421–422
　　blood-sugar level, 198
　　blood test for Lyme disease, 151
　　chorionic villus sampling, 122, 131, 177,
　　　　226
　　colposcopy, 164, 165
　　cone biopsy, 165
　　contraction stress test (CST), 341, 421
　　Cystic Fibrosis (CF) Complete Test,
　　　　140–141
　　ELISA, 84
　　fasting blood-sugar, 240–241
　　FBC (full blood count), 8, 105
　　ferning, 335
　　and first antenatal visit to doctor, 86
　　foetal blood sampling (pH), 376
　　foetal fibronectin test (fFN), 224, 293
　　foetoscopy, 122–123
　　GBS culture, 299
　　glucose-tolerance test (GTT), 240–241
　　haematocrit reading, 224–225
　　imaging, avoiding radiation from, 5
　　for kidney function prior to pregnancy, 9
　　lab, at first or second visit, 105
　　L/S ratio test, 355
　　lupus antibody, 279
　　mammogram, 5, 19, 274
　　non-stress test (NST), 341, 420
　　cervical smear, 4, 5, 80, 164–165
　　percutaneous umbilical blood sampling
　　　　(PUBS), 131, 208
　　phosphatidyl glycerol (PG) test, 355
　　pregnancy, measuring HCG, 65, 69
　　pre-implementation genetic diagnosis, 5
　　quad-screen test, 183
　　quantitative HCG, 65, 69, 74, 103, 115
　　Rh-factor, 5, 105, 176
　　SalEst, 293
　　screening vs. diagnostic, 171
　　thyroid panel, 258
　　triple screen test, 169
　　urinalysis, 192
　　Western Blot, 84
　　See also Amniocentesis; Ultrasound;
　　　　X-rays
Tests, conditions monitored by, 258
　　anaemia, 224–225
　　anencephaly, 162, 164
　　bladder infections, 192
　　bleeding, 52
　　breast lumps, 275, 308
　　cervical cancer, 164–165
　　chlamydia, 82–83
　　cystic fibrosis, 140–141
　　deep-vein thrombosis, 216

to determine cause of miscarriage, 104
diabetes, 238, 288
Down's syndrome, 162, 164, 169, 183
ectopic pregnancy, 74
fertility, 14
fifth disease, 140
foetal distress, 376
foetal-lung maturity, 355
genetic abnormality, 5, 122–123
group-B Streptococcus infection, 299
hepatitis B, 41
HIV/AIDS, 5, 84
lupus, 278–279
miscarriage, 103
molar pregnancy, 115
overdue pregnancy, 420–422
phenylketonuria (PKU), 425
post-term babies, 420–422
premature labour, 293
preterm delivery, 224
sickle-cell anaemia, 226
thyroid disease, 258
waters, breaking of, 336
See also Down's syndrome
Tetanus, 118
Tetracycline, 83
Thalassaemia, 227
Threatened miscarriages, 102–103
Thrombosis. *See* Deep-vein thrombosis
Thyroid problems, 12, *106*, 258–259
Tiredness. *See* Fatigue
Tobacco. *See* Smoking
Tocolytic agent, 327
Toxoplasmosis, 102, 105–106, *120*, 272
Transvaginal ultrasound, 132
Trauma, 102, 137–138
Travel during pregnancy, 127–129
Trichomonal vaginitis, 80
Trimester, definition of, *30*, 31
Triple-screen test, 169, 183
Triplets, 325
Trouble signs in pregnancy, symptoms of, 198–199
Tubal ligation, 387, 389, 426
Tubal pregnancy. *See* Ectopic pregnancy
Turner syndrome, *5*
Twins, 205
and age, 174
frequency of, 323, 325
See also Multiple foetuses

Ultrasound, 130–132, *130, 206*, 341
and amniocentesis, 171
and baby's movements in womb, 131, 169
and bleeding, 52
and breast lumps, 274
and cyst, picture of, 217–218
and deep-vein thrombosis, 216
and determining foetal weight, 348
and determining due date, 205, 208
and diagnosing ectopic pregnancy, 74
and falls, 255
and foetal swallowing, 213
and heart abnormalities, 186

and high blood pressure, 137
and hydrocephalus, 195
illustration of 20 weeks gestation exam, 206–208
and intrauterine-growth restriction, 311
and measurements of size of uterus, 205
and miscarriages, 103
and molar pregnancy, 115
and multiple foetuses, 324, 325, 326
and percutaneous umbilical-cord sampling (PUBS), 208
and placental abruption, 335
and placenta previa, 353
and position of baby, *380*
safety of, 217
and sex of baby, 132, *205*, 253
and size of baby, 366, 420
and triple-screen test, 169
Umbilical cord
and blood flow, 185
compressed and Caesarian, 366
and cord-blood banking and storage, 400–401
description of, 285
knots in, 301, 302, 387
tangling and multiple foetuses, 327
Unconjugated oestriol, 169
Underweight. *See* Low birthweight; Weight
Urinalysis, 192
Urinary-tract infections (UTIs), 8–9, 191–193, 427
Urine and urination
and bladder infection, 192–193
checking, 229
control of after childbirth, 427
foetus', 243
frequency of, 68
painful, 199
sugar in, 240–241
USDA Food Pyramid, *85*
Uterine rupture, 371
Uterus
and beginning of labour, 356
contractions of after childbirth, 400, 425
contractions of throughout pregnancy, 99
growth and size of, 39, 99, *108*, 124, 133–134, 179, 428
measuring of, 204–205
and multiple babies, 328–329
relaxation of during premature labour, 294
and round-ligament pain, 179, 181
shape of and breech presentation, 380
weight of, 133–134, 158, 194, 428

Vaccinations and immunizations, 3, 118–119, 159
complete before pregnancy, 14, *25*
risk of exposure, 118
Vacuum extractor (ventouse), 339, 374
Vaginal birth after Caesarean (VBAC), 366, 370–372
types of Caesarian incisions, 368
and uterine rupture, 371

Vaginal bleeding, 99, 181, 198
Vaginal discharge
    increased, 181–182
    major or continual, 198, 236
Varicellazoster immune globulin (VZIG), 120
Varicose veins, 219–220, 426
Vascular spiders (telangiectasias or
        angiomas), 136–137
Vegetables, 111–112
Vegetarian diet, 182–183
Vein stripping, 220
Venereal warts, 80–81
Vernix, 206
Viruses. *See* Infections
Vitamins
    absorption of and smoking, 36
    not overdoing, 20
    nutritional requirements during
        pregnancy and breastfeeding, *352*
    and sources of food nutrients chart, *105*
    those needing special help with, 256–257
    vitamin A, 20, *59*, 277–278, 359
    vitamin B, 246, 278
    vitamin B6, *105*
    vitamin C, 112–113, 359
    vitamin E, *105*, 278
    See also Prenatal vitamins
Vomiting, 65–68, *106*, 139
    and appendicitis, 230
    and iron, 226
    and molar pregnancy, 115
    severe, 199
    See also Morning sickness; Nausea

Walking
    during labor, 410–411
    for exercise, 47, *145*, 189–190
Warning signs of problem pregnancy, 198–199
Washing hands, *98*
Water, drinking. *See* Fluids
Waterbed, 165
Waters, breaking of, 301, 303, 336–337
    determining, 336
Ways to have great pregnancy, *87*
Weight, maternal
    achieving ideal weight prior to pregnancy,
        2, 19–20, *25*
    after childbirth, 425, 429
    and armed services, 159
    average gain, 70–71, *71*, 121

chart for pregnancy weight gain, 42
and dieting, 20, 71, 121, 158, 337
distribution of pregnancy weight, *108*,
    300–301
in first trimester and weight of baby, 61
and gestational diabetes, 238–239
and growth-restricted baby, 312
and increasing caloric intake, 39
loss of weight from nausea, 76
and multiple foetuses, 326, 327, 330
need to gain, 61, 121–122
and older mothers, 174
overweight when pregnancy begins,
    problems, 2, 158–159
and watching weight, 61, 71, 139, 184
and zinc for underweight, 96
Weight of baby, *108*, 142, 337, 348
    average, 291
    determining and ultrasound, 348
    of developing baby, 114, 194, 282
    gender differences, 291
    increases with more maternal births, 291
    of premature babies, 291, 292
    and weight gain of mother during first
        trimester, 61
    See also Low birthweight, risks for
Wellbutrin, *36*
Work
    and job stress, 320
    and pregnancy, 147–150
    and preparation for pregnancy, 25–26
    taking care of yourself at, 149–150

X-rays
    and broken bones, 256
    dangers of, 157
    dental, 158
    and diagnosing multiple foetuses, 326
    and mammogram, 274
    scheduling before pregnancy, 3, 5
    and study of thyroid, 254
    See also Radiation

Yeast infections (monilial vulvovaginitis), 80
Your Baby's First Year Week by Week (Curtis
        and Schuler), 223

Zinc, 96, *105*
Zyban, *36*
Zygote, 46